DERMATOLOGIC SURGERY AND PROCEDURES

Edited by **Pierre Vereecken**

Dermatologic Surgery and Procedures
http://dx.doi.org/10.5772/66008
Edited by Pierre Vereecken

Contributors

Eleni Papakonstantinou, Ulrike Raap, Florian Löhr, Diana Kitala, Agnieszka Klama-Baryła, Wojciech Łabuś, Marcelina Misiuga, Mariusz Nowak, Marek Kawecki, Suruchi Garg, Shweta Manchanda, Chandi Garg, Sevgi Akarsu, Işıl Kamberoğlu, Tatyana Kotova, Sergei Nikolaevich Tsybusov, Vladimir Ivanovich Kochenov, Hector Leal Silva, Merdan Serin, Caio Camargo, Paola Savoia, Paolo Boggio, Benedetta Miglino, Rossana Tiberio, Federica Veronese, Yohei Tanaka, Premjit Juntongjin, Chavanatda Chanyasak

Published by InTech

Janeza Trdine 9, 51000 Rijeka, Croatia

Publishing Process Manager Romina Skomersic
Technical Editor SPi Global
Cover InTech Design team

First published February, 2018
Printed in Croatia
Legal deposit, Croatia: National and University Library in Zagreb

Additional hard copies can be obtained from orders@intechopen.com

Dermatologic Surgery and Procedures, Edited by Pierre Vereecken
p. cm.
Print ISBN 978-953-51-3851-8
Online ISBN 978-953-51-3852-5

For EU product safety concerns:
IN TECH d.o.o., Prolaz Marije Krucifikse Kozulić 3, 51000 Rijeka, Croatia,
info@intechopen.com or visit our website at intechopen.com.

Meet the editor

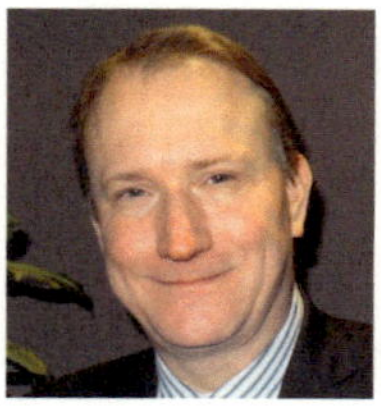

Dr. Pierre Vereecken, MD, PhD, is a Doctor of Medicine graduate and is certified and specialized in dermatology (general, aesthetic, and corrective) and skin oncology. He studied medicine in Brussels, Belgium (1991, ULB), and obtained his PhD degree from the same university in 2008, with a research work on the topic of cutaneous malignant melanoma biology and progression. After working for the Belgian Army (Belgium, Germany) and the United Nations Protection Force (Central Bosnia), he was the head of the Department of Dermatology in academic hospitals (Brugmann University Public Hospital, Belgium, and Saint-Luc University U.C.L. Hospital, Belgium). He is convinced that knowledge has to be shared with not only colleagues, specialists, or GPs but also nurses for the best care of our patients. He also emphasizes the need for a better communication of medical information with patients. In 2010, he decided to dedicate his own practice to patients and research and to build an international dermatologic network, Cliderm. He also founded the European Institute for Dermatological Practice and Research, a multifaceted organization that aims to promote clinical dermatology and dermatological research in the European Union. He has published more than 100 scientific papers in international medical literature and also edited and authored chapters for more than 20 books.

Contents

Preface

As dermatology grows as a speciality, numerous major procedures have been developed in order to better satisfy our patients. A better insight into the biology of the skin leads to new technological breakthroughs including techniques and medications. The advance of minimally invasive procedural dermatology allows, for instance, aging patients to ask their dermatologist for new options for improving the appearance of their skin.

The demand for skin procedures and surgery has increased considerably. A part of the skin surgery is now offered by not only dermatologists but also skin surgeons and general practitioners who therefore also need to gather high-quality knowledge and information. This book is dedicated to all of them.

This book is neither an extensive review of cosmetic and surgical dermatology nor a theoretical description of new techniques awaiting validation. This book is a practical guide, which focuses on different aspects of surgical dermatology. The basic information about local anesthesia is extensively described in the chapter by Dr. Caio Lamunier de Abreu Camargo, and the common dermosurgical procedures such as cryogenic methods and cryotherapy are discussed in the chapter by Prof. Tatyana Gennadyevna Kotova et al. Advanced surgical procedures, namely excision techniques (basic surgery, Mohs surgery, and skin reconstruction), are also treated in depth in the chapters by Dr. Merdan Serin and Dr. Paolo Boggio et al.

Moreover, a special emphasis has been placed on new dermatological procedures, photodynamic therapy, and platelet-rich plasma (PRP) in the chapters by Dr. Hector Leal Silva, Prof. Diana Kitala et al., Dr. Eleni Papakonstantinou et al., Dr. Yohei Tanaka, and Dr. Suruchi Garg et al.

Finally, a new approach using UV skin protection after skin surgery is described and will close this book.

What is most exciting nowadays is the active communication between researchers and clinicians who share a major interest in applying new procedures for the treatments of patients. This book brings a new proof that it is possible!

A remarkable lesson of dermatological research is that we can nowadays extend the strategies we offer to our patients. Besides the technology and the expertise, the daily challenges in surgical or corrective dermatology are to listen to patients' expectations, to discuss the procedures together with the patients, to answer their questions, and to remind them that follow-up visits are just as important as initial consultations.

Advice on various issues is proposed to the readers who will perform a new cutaneous procedure. The "pre-act" consultation can be complemented with printed handouts or other materials such as video presentations on the Internet. This first consultation should include the details of the procedure, the results of the patient, the possible complications based on the characteristics of the patient, and the alternative procedures available. This is the basis of what we can consider as a perfectly informed consent.

After the procedure, the patients may expect you to be available for any assistance or clarification. The first night and the next day are not only physically but also mentally critical for the patients. Patients will appreciate phone numbers if they can use it in case of a problem. If a patient needs more time, then the extra time should be provided.

In this book, the readers will discover major contributions from expert authors all over the world about all aspects of dermatological surgery and procedures. These authors have been selected for their expertise and reputations as educators. From the basic to the most advanced technologies, the readers will find topics that will enable them to extend their knowledge and skills.

Dr. Pierre Vereecken, MD, PhD
Cliderm Medical Offices
Brussels, Belgium

Section 1

Basic Techniques in Dermatology

Chapter 1

Local Anesthesia

Caio Lamunier de Abreu Camargo

Additional information is available at the end of the chapter

http://dx.doi.org/10.5772/intechopen.72930

Abstract

Local anesthesia is a routine procedure in dermatological practice. This chapter deals with the basic principles of pharmacology and pharmacodynamics related to the most commonly used anesthetics in dermatology as well as its side effects, the most common anesthetic solutions, anesthesia techniques, and topical anesthesia.

Keywords: anesthesia, dermatologic surgery, pharmacology, dermatology

1. Introduction

Anesthesia is a common procedure in all fields of dermatology. Knowing its pharmacological and clinical elements is essential to a good dermatological practice. Efficiency, safety, and comfort are the main concern. There are several anesthetics, and the choice of the correct one as the best application technique provides more safety, comfort, and efficiency.

It is not known exactly when the anesthesia began. Nitrous oxide is believed to have been used since 1772 by Joseph Priestley. The use of ether became famous after a public demonstration by William Thomas Green Morton in 1846, but its use is older and several other scientists have claimed the discovery of the ether as an anesthetic. The use of local anesthetics gained ground in medical science in 1884, and cocaine was widely used as a local anesthetic, although there is evidence of its use in ancient civilizations.

We can classify dermatological anesthesia in two different groups: general anesthesia and local anesthesia. General anesthesia is associated with increased risks of morbidity and mortality than local anesthesia. For this reason, local anesthesia is widely used in dermatological practice. Moreover, local anesthesia is cheaper, with less surgical time and faster recovery. Nevertheless, there are some limitations depending on the procedure's extension and patient discomfort and collaboration. Local anesthesia can be achieved by topical products, by infiltrative nerve blocks, and by infiltrative tumescent anesthesia [1].

2. Local anesthesia

Nerve impulse transmission occurs when voltage-gated sodium channels on the neuronal membrane open, allowing massive influx of sodium into peripheral nerve cells. In resting state, the intracellular electric potential is negative relative to the extracellular space thanks to the cellular membrane and by Na^+/K^+ ATPase. The influx of sodium causes membrane depolarization and propagation of the impulse. Local anesthetics prevent nerve impulse transmission by blocking sodium channels without causing central nervous system depression or altered mental status [2, 3].

The block generally occurs in a stepwise sequence with autonomic impulses blocked first, then sensory impulses, and finally motor impulses. Unmyelinated and smaller myelinated nerve fibers are easier to block than larger myelinated fibers. Therefore, C-type fibers are the first to be blocked in a local anesthesia. Pain is first controlled followed by heat and cold sensation. Then, B-type fibers are blocked, which are the preganglionic sympathetic fibers. Finally, A-type fibers are block. Proprioception, touch and pressure, and motor fibers are the last to suffer anesthetics effects [4].

The most used anesthetic agents have three structural components: an aromatic portion, an intermediate connecting chain, and an amine portion. The aromatic portion provides hydrophobic and lipophilic properties and facilitates the diffusion of the anesthetics through nerve cell membranes. Therefore, its efficiency is improved. However, the amine portion provides lipophobic and hydrophilic properties and can become soluble for injection. The intermediate connecting chain provides the main anesthetic properties and classifies the local anesthetics into two groups: the amino amides and the amino esters [5].

Amide anesthetics—these anesthetics all have an amide linkage (i.e., bupivacaine, ropivacaine, lidocaine, prilocaine, mepivacaine). They are metabolized by microsomal enzymes in the liver and excreted by the kidneys. Decreased liver function may lead to amide anesthetics toxic effects [2, 6].

Ester anesthetics—they have an ester linkage (i.e., procaine, chloroprocaine, tetracaine, benzocaine, cocaine). The ester anesthetics use to have a shorter duration. They are hydrolyzed by plasma pseudocholinesterases and excreted by the kidneys. Decreased levels of plasma pseudocholinesterases may lead to toxic effects. The metabolite para-aminobenzoic acid (PABA) is a major metabolic product and is associated with higher incidence of allergies [2, 6].

The main properties of anesthetics are potency, toxicity, onset of action, and duration of action (**Table 1**). Lipid solubility use to be directly associated with potency as the compound penetrates the nerve cells more easily. The protein type and its capacity of maintain the sodium

http://dx.doi.org/10.5772/intechopen.72930

channels receptor binding is association with duration of action. The dissociation constant (pKa) determines the proportion of the anesthetics base and its cation at a given pH and is associated with shorter onset of action and less toxicity. However, if the pH is raised too much, the anesthetic may precipitate out of solution [7].

Lidocaine is labeled pregnancy category B. However, it is recommended that lidocaine and all other anesthetic agents be used warily during first trimester of pregnancy. The anesthetic agents commonly cross the placenta barrier and achieve the fetus. For use in children, the maximum recommended dosage should be adjusted to child's weight. In infants, prilocaine is associated with major risk of methemoglobinemia [8] (**Tables 2** and **3**).

Anesthetic	pKa	Onset (min)	Duration (min) without epinephrine	Duration (min) with epinephrine	Max dose (mg/kg) without epinephrine	Max dose (mg/kg) with epinephrine
Chloroprocaine	9	5–6	30–60	N/A	11	14
Procaine	8.9	5	30–90	30–180	10	14
Tetracaine	8.6	7	120–240	240–480	2	2
Bupivacaine	8.1	2–10	120–240	240–480	2.5	3
Etidocaine	7.7	3–5	200	240–360	4.5	6.5
Lidocaine	7.7	<1	30–120	60–400	5	7
Mepivacaine	7.6	3–20	30–120	60–400	6	7
Prilocaine	7.7	5–6	30–120	60–400	7	10
Ropivacaine	8.2	1–15	120–360	Not yet defined	3.5	Not yet defined

Kouba et al. [9].

Table 1. Properties of local anesthetics.

		Duration (min)		Maximal recommended dose for adults	
Anesthetic	Onset (min)	Without epinephrine	With epinephrine	Without epinephrine	With epinephrine
Amides					
Articaine	2-4	30-120	60-240	5.0 mg/kg or 350 mg	7.0 mg/kg or 500 mg
Bupivacaine	2-10	120-240	240-480	2.5 mg/kg or 175 mg	3.0 mg/kg or 225 mg
Etidocaine	3-5	200	240-360	4.5 mg/kg or 300 mg	6.5 mg/kg or 400 mg
Lidocaine	<1	30-120	60-400	4.5 mg/kg or 300 mg	7.0 mg/kg or 500 mg
Mepivacaine	3-20	30-120	60-400	6.0 mg/kg or 400 mg	7.0 mg/kg or 550 mg
Prilocaine	5-6	30-120	60-400	7.0 mg/kg or 400 mg	10.0 mg/kg or 600 mg
Esters					
Chloroprocaine	5-6	30-60	N/A	11.0 mg/kg or 800 mg	14.0 mg/kg or 1000 mg
Procaine	5	15-90	30-180	10.0 mg/kg	14.0 mg/kg
Tetracaine	7	120-240	240-480	2.0 mg/kg	2.0 mg/kg

Table 2. Anesthetics used for local infiltration.

Anesthetic	Onset (min)	Duration (min)	Special considerations
Benzocaine	<5	15-45	Methemoglobinemia possible
Cocaine	1-5	30-60	
Dibucaine	<5	15-45	For mucous membranes
Dyclonine	2-10	<60	For mucous membranes but not conjunctiva
Lidocaine	<2	30-45	
Lidocaine/prilocaine eutectic mixture	<60	60-120 after removal of occlusive dressing	Only for use on intact skin, methemoglobinemia possible

Kouba et al. [9].

Table 3. Anesthetics for topical use.

3. Additions to local anesthetics

Many additives to local anesthetics have been studied. The aim of making complex anesthetic's solutions is to achieve better efficacy and safety during dermatologic surgery.

3.1. Other anesthetics

We can mix different local anesthetics in an attempt to take advantage of useful properties of each drug. For example, short-duration anesthetics like lidocaine can be mixed with a long-duration one like ropivacaine in an attempt to gain in durability. As well as, longer onset anesthetics can be mixed with shorter ones. However, this kind of association is not as logical as it seems, the nerve blockades obtained by mixing commercially available solutions of local anesthetics are unpredictable and may depend on a number of factors, which include not only the types of drugs but also the pH of the mixture. It is possible also to inject a rapid-onset anesthetic first to a longer-onset anesthetic, without mixing them [10].

3.2. Vasoconstrictors

Most local anesthetics promote vasodilatation by relaxation of vascular smooth muscle. Cocaine is the only example of local anesthetics that promotes vasoconstriction, and ropivacaine seems to be a local anesthetic that causes neither vasodilatation nor vasoconstriction. Cocaine is a norepinephrine reuptake inhibitor, thus potentiating sympathetic stimulation and causing hypertension and ventricular irritability.

Vasoconstriction at the operative site is commonly intended because it promotes less bleeding and facilitates the ease of surgery. Moreover, vasodilatation increases systemic absorption of anesthetics solution decreasing duration and efficacy of the anesthesia and increasing also systemic toxicity. Therefore, epinephrine can be useful decreasing bleeding and anesthetics systemic toxicity, and increasing their efficacy and duration [11].

Epinephrine is widely used in dermatologic surgery to promote vasoconstriction. It typically requires 5–15 min to reach full vasoconstriction effect. There are premixed solutions with epinephrine at a concentration of 1:100,000 and 1:200,000. However, effective vasoconstriction is achieved with a 1:100,000 concentration and risks of side effects are greater in 1:200,000 concentration. The maximum dose is 1 mg over approximately 8–10 h; however, this dosage should be much lower (or even absent) depending on patient age and concomitant health issues [12, 13]. Physicians using local anesthetic with epinephrine should be aware of this interaction. Epinephrine is a strong β- and α-agonist and can cause severe hypertension in patients using β-blocker medications [14]. Patients with severe cardiovascular disease may have their underlying diseases exacerbated with epinephrine use, as well as patients with narrow angle glaucoma. Patients taking monoamine oxidase inhibitors, tricyclic antidepressant, and phenothiazines are more sensitive to epinephrine. However, absolute contraindications to their use are hyperthyroidism and pheochromocytoma.

Systemic side effects of epinephrine can be self-limited or leaves to death. Therefore, it is important to avoid unintentional intravascular injection of epinephrine. Self-limited side effects include palpitations, anxiety, sweating, tremor, tachycardia, and elevated blood pressure. These signs and symptoms usually resolve within a few minutes, but the patient must be under continuous monitorization to identify a serious side effect. Serious side effects of epinephrine include cardiovascular and cerebral suffering. Arrhythmias, tachycardias, and ventricular fibrillation are between the most common severe side effects.

Epinephrine is labeled pregnancy category C. The effect of pregnancy on arterial sensitivity to vasoconstrictors is controversial. Pregnancy was demonstrated to be associated with a significant reduction in both uterine artery response and sensitivity to norepinephrine, epinephrine, and phenylephrine. However, there was no consistent pregnancy-associated effect on carotid artery response and sensitivity [15]. This reduction in artery response can be related to a fetal suffering, particularly in the first semester, and a premature labor in the third semester. Thereby, it is prudent to postpone nonurgent procedures requiring the use of epinephrine until after pregnancy.

Epinephrine found commercially available with lidocaine in premixed solutions contains acidic preservatives, such as sodium metabisulfite and citric acid [16]. As lower pH solutions use to cause more pain on injection, fresh lidocaine and epinephrine solutions are preferred than commercially lidocaine and epinephrine solutions [17].

The use of epinephrine on digits may prolong the duration of anesthesia and reduce the risk of bleeding during surgery, but it has been associated once with digital necrosis caused by vasoconstriction. Recent big studies recurrently demonstrate that evidence is insufficient to recommend use or avoidance of adrenaline in digital nerve blocks. However, there are case reports describing digital necrosis after injection of lidocaine with epinephrine. These digital necrosis cases can be as associated with vessel compression, constricting circumferential dressings, tourniquets, infection, hematoma, or patient's vascular disease. In absence of these conditions, the use of epinephrine on digits seems to be safe. However, if a tourniquet is used during the surgery, there is no benefit of using also epinephrine to control bleeding [18–20].

3.3. Sodium bicarbonate

Lower pH solutions use to cause more pain on injection [17]. That is why the pain of infiltrating lidocaine with epinephrine into skin is reduced by the addition of sodium bicarbonate.

Adding sodium bicarbonate to anesthetic solution of lidocaine plus epinephrine in a proportion of 1–10 can raise the solution's pH from approximately 5.0 to approximately 7.5. As epinephrine concentration declined approximately 25% per week in anesthetic solution containing sodium bicarbonate, it is recommended to use fresh solutions [21, 22].

In addition, alkalinization of local anesthetics solutions leads to a faster onset of action and a better anesthetic efficacy. However, it declines the duration of both anesthesia and vasoconstriction.

3.4. Hyaluronidase

Hyaluronidase is an enzyme that depolymerizes hyaluronic acid. Despite it is famous in correcting acid hyaluronic fillers defect, it can be used in dermatologic surgery as an addition to local anesthetics by facilitating diffusion of solutions through tissue planes further away from the injection point. Although the duration of anesthesia is slightly decreased, the addition of hyaluronidase to local anesthesia offers the benefits of minimizing loss of surface contour and enhanced ease in undermining and dissection through subcutaneous tissue planes [23, 24].

The decrease of anesthesia's duration and the major toxicity are explained due to increased absorption of the solution. That is why the tumescent technique must be avoided in hyaluronidase solution. The dosage usually recommended is one ampule to 30 ml anesthetic solution.

4. Side effects

Local anesthetics side injection frequently causes pain and local edema. Transient bruise and motor nerve paralysis can also occur. These are common local side effects. More rarely is nerve injuries. Intraneural injection can cause nerve damage and prolonged sensory nerve paresthesia may develop.

Despite local anesthetic systemic toxicity (LAST) is relatively rare, it must be considered whenever local anesthetic is administered. Difficulties in the clearance of these drugs can also be an important cause of LAST.

Central nervous system toxicity is due to intracellular voltage-gated fast sodium channels blockage in neuronal tissue. It all begins with blockade of cerebral cortical inhibitory pathways, leading to excitation, sensory and visual disturbance, muscle twitching, and convulsions. Perioral paresthesia is a classic early manifestation of LAST. CNS depression comes later with dizziness, confusion, unconsciousness, coma, and respiratory arrest [25].

Cardiovascular toxicity can be expressed by different kinds of arrhythmias. Local anesthetics block sodium channels in cardiovascular conducting cells and reduce the rate of depolarization and propagation of action potentials. Thereby, PR, QRS, and ST intervals become larger increasing the risk of bradyarrhythmia and re-entrant tachyarrhythmias. Myocardial depression and changes in systemic vascular resistance is also described. Among the commonly used local anesthetics, bupivacaine is the most cardiotoxic one [26].

Usually, central nervous systemic toxicity signs precede cardiovascular toxicity signs whereas it is not a rule. The majority of LAST events occurs within several minutes of local anesthetics injection, but onset of symptoms can be delayed up to 60 min. Intra-arterial injection of anesthetics deflagrates almost immediately the LAST symptoms, as in intravenous injection or in systemic abortion, and there is a delay in the onset of signs [27].

Risk factors for LAST include drug pharmacological properties, administration dynamics, and patient factors. Local anesthetics should be reduced by 15% in babies less than 4 months old due to immaturity of hepatic enzymes [28]. Elderly people can have clearance of anesthetics reduced. Renal dysfunction is not related to more LAST and routine dose reduction is usually unnecessary. Hepatic dysfunction is offset by an increased volume of distribution of anesthetic agents and injections doses should be limited accordingly to the severity of hepatic dysfunction. Severe cardiac dysfunction can cause reduced hepatic and renal perfusion taking to clearance deficiency. Pregnant patients also can have increased cardiac output in second and third semester pregnancy [29].

There are maximum doses permissible for each anesthetic agent, and it is usually bigger when vasoconstrictors are associated. However, LAST may occur despite adherence to these limits. Therefore, practitioners should always use the lowest dose necessary to achieve the desired result due to the significant risk of systemic toxicity [30].

Besides respect the maximum anesthetics dosage, it is important to avoid intravascular injection. Ultrasound-guided peripheral nerve blockade reduces risk of LAST [31].

The management of LAST is mainly clinical support. Intravenous access, oxygen, and standard monitoring should be a routine for all patients with suspect of LAST. However, there are other clinical evidences that must be distinct of LAST, as vasovagal or allergic reactions [32].

Vasovagal reactions are by far the most common situation that must be distinct of LAST. Patient anxiety can result in an increase in parasympathetic tone. Dizziness, nausea, distal paresthesia, and hypotension are the main symptoms [33].

Although allergic reactions to anesthetics are commonly reported, true allergic reactions are actually rare. Local anesthetics are too small to be antigenic by themselves but are sufficiently alien to bind as haptens to tissues with antigenic properties. Up to 14 days are required to develop sensitization (antibody production). Once sensitization occurs, exposure to fractional quantities of the offending agent invokes an antigen-antibody reaction. Responses are classified into four categories depending upon the response. Type I reactions are IgE-mediated and are characterized by a massive release of histamine, serotonin, leukotrienes, and other humoral substances from mast cells resulting in a sudden onset of bronchospasm, cardiovascular depression and airway compromise, otherwise known as anaphylaxis. This is a true medical emergency and requires immediate and aggressive treatment. Type IV reactions represent the other end of the spectrum. Characteristically, they have a slower onset, associated with a non-IgE mediated release of bioamines, including histamine. The severity of the reaction depends on the quantity of the mediator released and can vary from mild contact dermatitis to anaphylactoid shock [34, 35].

Allergies have been reported for each class of local anesthetics, but cross-over sensitivity does not occur. Ester local anesthetics are metabolized to a PABA-like compound, and anaphylaxis has been reported. Amide local anesthetics sometimes contain the preservative methylparaben, which has also been reported to cause severe allergic reactions. It is important to know which class of local anesthetic caused the reaction and avoid that class in the future [2].

Taking a thorough history in these cases and reviewing all relevant medical and dental records are the best way of doing it. Allergists usually carry out skin testing whereas they are equivocal in a large percentage of cases [34].

5. Topical anesthetics

Topical anesthetics act on the peripheral nerve endings in the dermis or mucosa, reduce the sensation of pain at the site of application, and avoid local pain caused by needling. They are useful aids during dermatologic treatment, especially in children, by mitigating discomfort and pain. Topical anesthetics also avoid tissue edema and surgical site distortions [36].

Their delivery and effectiveness can be enhanced by using free bases, by increasing the drug concentration, lowering the melting point, by using physical and chemical permeation enhancers and lipid delivery vesicles. Topical anesthetics are also able to penetrate mucosal surfaces, such as the mouth, genitals, and conjunctiva more easily than through a keratinized surface because of the absence of a stratum corneum [37].

Topical anesthetics seem to be safe, whereas systemic absorption occurs and systemic toxic events must be prevented. Extra caution is needed in damaged skin barrier, in infants, in mucosa, and in the extension of the applied corporal area [38].

The discovery of various amide and ester local anesthetics, their topical preparations and delivery systems in due course of time opened the gate of immense possible uses of topical anesthetics. The main topical anesthetics for mucous membrane and intact skin are benzocaine, dibucaine, lidocaine, prilocaine, proparacaine, and tetracaine. They exist in isolated form or in mixed different formulas.

Cryoanesthesia is the reduction of pain by applying cold agents to the skin. Various topical freezing agents are available: applying ice to the skin, the use of cooled gel or a cold glass, vapocoolant equipments, and cryogen sprays. The efficacy of cryoanesthesia is variable, and it has risk of causing scars and hyper or hypopigmentation [39].

6. Anesthetic injection techniques

Local anesthetic injection is often cited in literature as the most painful part of minor procedures. It is also very possible for all doctors to get better at giving local anesthesia with less pain for patients [40].

The pain of needle insertion can be reduced by verbal distraction, massage at neighborhood of the local of injection, pinching, quick and right need injection, the use of previously topic anesthetics, and accessory vibratory and cooler equipments. Small needles are related to less pain also. Additional sticks should be through an already numb area, and the injection should start on the side that the sensory innervations are coming from.

Sometimes, the injection of the anesthetic solution is more painful than the needle insertion itself due to tissue distension and solutions' pH. To minimize tissue distension, the slowly injection of the anesthetic fluid is recommended. This is better obtained by the use of smaller needles and syringes. Subcutaneous injections promote less pain because of better tissue distension than intradermal injection. Acid solutions are usually associated with major pain. That is one reason why doctors associate sodium bicarbonate with anesthetic solutions. Intracutaneous instillation of lidocaine at body temperature is no less painful than injection at lower temperature [41].

Nerve block anesthesia also can minimize multiple anesthetics injection, besides decreasing the amount of solution need and its side effects. It is good to anesthetize large areas with little surface distortion. In general, nerve blocks cause less discomfort to the patient, especially during a mucosal approach. The correct technique involves injection of the anesthetic solution around the nerve, never into the nerve, to avoid nerve injuries. It is important to remember the presence of accompanying vein and artery to the nerve. Caution is needed to prevent intravascular injection. Intraforaminal injection is not recommended due to nerve compression. It is recommended to wait for about 5–10 min for full effectiveness of nerve blocks [4].

Field block anesthesia is a technique used mainly in cyst and skin cancer surgery. Field block anesthesia involves injecting anesthetic solution around the proposed surgical site, thereby blocking surrounding innervations. It is useful to avoid tumor transection. There are case reports of neoplasm surgical skin implantation. That is why field block anesthesia is recommended. Puncturing the cyst during surgery should also be avoided to decrease cyst recurrent [42].

Tumescent anesthesia is technique, which consists in infiltrating a large volume of dilute anesthetic and epinephrine solution to produce swelling and firmness of the target areas. It was first described by Kein and Lillis for liposuction surgery. The tumescent technique for local anesthesia has made it possible to do liposuction, dermabrasion, facelifts, carbon dioxide laser full-face resurfacing, hair transplants, and large cutaneous excisions and repairs totally by local anesthesia without intravenous sedation or narcotic analgesia. These benefits are optimizing biochemical compartments, maximizing drug concentration locally, delaying systemic drug absorption, decreasing systemic toxicity, prolonging local anesthetic effects, and benefiting from augmented local hydrostatic pressure to reduce bleeding and facilitate tissue dissection [43, 44]. Lidocaine is the most used anesthetic agent, whereas prilocaine also seems to be safe and effective [45]. There is no data examining other anesthetics for use in tumescent local anesthesia.

Author details

Caio Lamunier de Abreu Camargo

Address all correspondence to: caiolamunier@yahoo.com.br

Universidade de São Paulo (USP), São Paulo, Brazil

References

[1] Koay J, Orengo I. Application of local anesthetics in dermatologic surgery. Dermatologic Surgery. 2002 Feb;**28**(2):143-148

[2] Garmon EH, Dulebohn SC. Topical, Local, and Regional Anesthesia and Anesthetics. StatPearls Publishing; 2017 June

[3] Ragsdale DS, McPhee JC, Scheuer T, Catterall WA. Molecular determinants of state-dependent block of Na+ channels by local anesthetics. Science. 1994 Sep 16;**265**(5179):1724-1728

[4] Grekin RC, Auletta MJ. Local anesthesia in dermatologic surgery. Journal of the American Academy of Dermatology. 1988 Oct;**19**(4):599-614

[5] Covino BG. Local anesthesia. 1. The New England Journal of Medicine. 1972 May 4;**286**(18):975-983

[6] Covino BG. Local anesthesia. 2. The New England Journal of Medicine. 1972 May 11;**286**(19):1035-1042

[7] Covino BG. Pharmacology of local anesthetic agents. Rational Drug Therapy. 1987 Aug;**21**(8):1-9

[8] Richards KA, Stasko T. Dermatologic surgery and the pregnant patient. Dermatologic Surgery. 2002 Mar;**28**(3):248-256

[9] Kouba DJ, LoPiccolo MC, Alam M, Bordeaux JS, Cohen B, Hanke CW, Jellinek N, Maibach HI, Tanner JW, Vashi N, Gross KG, Adamson T, Begolka WS, Moyano JV. Guidelines for the use of local anesthesia in office-based dermatologic surgery. Journal of the American Academy of Dermatology. 2016 Jun;**74**(6):1201-1219

[10] Galindo A, Witcher T. Mixtures of local anesthetics: Bupivacaine-chloroprocaine. Anesthesia and Analgesia. 1980 Sep;**59**(9):683-685

[11] Covino BG. Pharmacology of local anaesthetic agents. British Journal of Anaesthesia. 1986 Jul;**58**(7):701-716

[12] Siegel RJ, Vistnes LM, Iverson RE. Effective hemostasis with less epinephrine. An experimental and clinical study. Plastic and Reconstructive Surgery. 1973 Feb;**51**(2):129-133

[13] Fante RG, Elner VM. The use of epinephrine in infiltrative local anesthesia for eyelid reconstruction. Plastic and Reconstructive Surgery. 1998 Sep;**102**(3):917

[14] Foster CA, Aston SJ. Propranolol-epinephrine interaction: A potential disaster. Plastic and Reconstructive Surgery. 1983 Jul;**72**(1):74-78

[15] Weiner CP, Martinez E, Chestnut DH, Ghodsi A. Effect of pregnancy on uterine and carotid artery response to norepinephrine, epinephrine, and phenylephrine in vessels with documented functional endothelium. American Journal of Obstetrics and Gynecology. 1989 Dec;**161**(6 Pt 1):1605-1610

http://dx.doi.org/10.5772/intechopen.72930

[16] Moore DC. The pH of local anesthetic solutions. Anesthesia and Analgesia. 1981 Nov;**60**(11):833-834

[17] Howe NR, Williams JM. Pain of injection and duration of anesthesia for intradermal infiltration of lidocaine, bupivacaine, and etidocaine. The Journal of Dermatologic Surgery and Oncology. 1994 Jul;**20**(7):459-464

[18] Prabhakar H, Rath S, Kalaivani M, Bhanderi N. Adrenaline with lidocaine for digital nerve blocks. Cochrane Database of Systematic Reviews. 2015 Mar 19;**3**

[19] Denkler KA. Epinephrine in the digits. Plastic and Reconstructive Surgery. 2011 Aug;**128**(2):598-599

[20] Denkler K. Myth of not using lidocaine with epinephrine in the digits. American Family Physician. 2010 May 15;**81**(10):1188

[21] McKay W, Morris R, Mushlin P. Sodium bicarbonate attenuates pain on skin infiltration with lidocaine, with or without epinephrine. Anesthesia and Analgesia. 1987 Jun;**66**(6):572-574

[22] Stewart JH, Cole GW, Klein JA. Neutralized lidocaine with epinephrine for local anesthesia. The Journal of Dermatologic Surgery and Oncology. 1989 Oct;**15**(10):1081-1083

[23] Lewis-Smith PA. Adjunctive use of hyaluronidase in local anaesthesia. British Journal of Plastic Surgery. 1986 Oct;**39**(4):554-558

[24] Clark LE, Mellette JR Jr. The use of hyaluronidase as an adjunct to surgical procedures. The Journal of Dermatologic Surgery and Oncology. 1994 Dec;**20**(12):842-844

[25] Di Gregorio G, Neal JM, Rosenquist RW, Weinberg GL. Clinical presentation of local anesthetic systemic toxicity: A review of published cases, 1979 to 2009. Regional Anesthesia and Pain Medicine. 2010 Mar-Apr;**35**(2):181-187

[26] Groban L. Central nervous system and cardiac effects from long-acting amide local anesthetic toxicity in the intact animal model. Regional Anesthesia and Pain Medicine. 2003 Jan-Feb;**28**(1):3-11

[27] Mulroy MF. Systemic toxicity and cardiotoxicity from local anesthetics: Incidence and preventive measures. Regional Anesthesia and Pain Medicine. 2002 Nov-Dec;**27**(6):556-561

[28] Meunier JF, Goujard E, Dubousset AM, Samii K, Mazoit JX. Pharmacokinetics of bupivacaine after continuous epidural infusion in infants with and without biliary atresia. Anesthesiology. 2001 Jul;**95**(1):87-95

[29] Rosenberg PH, Veering BT, Urmey WF. Maximum recommended doses of local anesthetics: A multifactorial concept. Regional Anesthesia and Pain Medicine. 2004 Nov-Dec;**29**(6):564-575 discussion 524

[30] Neal JM, Bernards CM, Butterworth JF 4th, Di Gregorio G, Drasner K, Hejtmanek MR, Mulroy MF, Rosenquist RW, Weinberg GL. ASRA practice advisory on local anesthetic systemic toxicity. Regional Anesthesia and Pain Medicine. 2010 Mar-Apr;**35**(2):152-161

[31] Barrington MJ, Kluger R. Ultrasound guidance reduces the risk of local anesthetic systemic toxicity following peripheral nerve blockade. Regional Anesthesia and Pain Medicine. 2013 Jul-Aug;**38**(4):289-299

[32] El-Boghdadly K, Chin KJ. Local anesthetic systemic toxicity: Continuing professional development. Canadian Journal of Anaesthesia. 2016 Mar;**63**(3):330-349

[33] Baluga JC. Allergy to local anesthetics in dentistry. Myth or reality? Revista Alergia México. 2003 Sep-Oct;**50**(5):176-181

[34] Bhole MV, Manson AL, Seneviratne SL, Misbah SA. IgE-mediated allergy to local anaesthetics: Separating fact from perception: A UK perspective. British Journal of Anaesthesia. 2012 Jun;**108**(6):903-911

[35] Finucane BT. Allergies to local anesthetics—The real truth. Canadian Journal of Anaesthesia. 2003 Nov;**50**(9):869-874

[36] Lee HS. Recent advances in topical anesthesia. Journal of Dental Anesthesia and Pain Medicine. 2016 Dec;**16**(4):237-244

[37] Kumar M, Chawla R, Goyal M. Topical anesthesia. Journal of Anaesthesiology Clinical Pharmacology. 2015 Oct-Dec;**31**(4):450-456

[38] Sobanko JF, Miller CJ, Alster TS. Topical anesthetics for dermatologic procedures: A review. Dermatologic Surgery. 2012 May;**38**(5):709-721

[39] Plotkin S. Clinical comparison of preinjection anesthetics. Journal of the American Podiatric Medical Association. 1998 Feb;**88**(2):73-79

[40] Strazar AR, Leynes PG, Lalonde DH. Minimizing the pain of local anesthesia injection. Plastic and Reconstructive Surgery. 2013 Sep;**132**(3):675-684

[41] Arndt KA, Burton C, Noe JM. Minimizing the pain of local anesthesia. Plastic and Reconstructive Surgery. 1983 Nov;**72**(5):676-679

[42] Auletta MJ. Local anesthesia for dermatologic surgery. Seminars in Dermatology. 1994 Mar;**13**(1):35-42

[43] Klein JA. Tumescent technique chronicles. Local anesthesia, liposuction, and beyond. Dermatologic Surgery. 1995 May;**21**(5):449-457

[44] Behroozan DS, Goldberg LH. Dermal tumescent local anesthesia in cutaneous surgery. Journal of the American Academy of Dermatology. 2005 Nov;**53**(5):828-830

[45] Augustin M, Maier K, Sommer B, Sattler G, Herberger K. Double-blind, randomized, intraindividual comparison study of the efficacy of prilocaine and lidocaine in tumescent local anesthesia. Dermatology. 2010;**221**(3):248-252

Chapter 2

Cryotherapy for Common Premalignant and Malignant Skin Disorders

Sevgi Akarsu and Isil Kamberoglu

Additional information is available at the end of the chapter

http://dx.doi.org/10.5772/intechopen.70286

Abstract

Cryotherapy, also known as cryosurgery or cryoablation, is a common dermatological treatment that is an expanded area from benign to malignant lesions. The system has been designed as a localized freezing cold that causes the destruction of cell integrity. The treatment has been also used for all ages, which is not required to have a condition of wellness. It is convenient, fast, and easy to apply in clinics, and there is no need for anesthesia. Additionally, multiple lesions are also cured in the same sessions. After the treatment, recovery period has not taken much longer and also has simple adverse effects, which are tolerable. Lastly, cryotherapy has gained excellent cosmetic results. It is highly effective for actinic keratosis and is the treatment of choice for most old patients who show poor cooperation and recurrent multiple lesions. Additionally, due to increasing premalignant lesions all over the world associated with increasing age, it is a considerable choice for lentigo maligna and Bowen's disease. In non-melanoma skin cancers, it is also the most important option in patients who do not undergo surgery and when other options are not appropriate. In this chapter, the use of cryotherapy for premalignant and malignant cutaneous disorders has been mainly focused.

Keywords: cryotherapy, cryosurgery, treatment, cutaneous, premalignant, malignant, actinic keratosis, non-melanoma skin cancers

1. History

Cryotherapy (also called cryosurgery or cryoablation) method was produced by James Arnott in England in 1945 to reduce the size of cancerous cells based on the theory that cold blood cells destroy the cells. Campbell White of New York City used cryotherapy as the first dermatological indication in early-stage epithelioma patients in 1890. Later in 1907, Whitehouse described the use of this method in different diseases such as pigmented nevus and lupus. In addition, he has published a case series of skin cancers in different face regions. Beyond these series, he described that the spray method is superior to cotton swab. Lortat Jacobs and Solente first described the name "La Cryotherapie," which compounds with carbon dioxide in 1930s. Earlier in 1960s, Cooper and Lee introduced the cryosurgery technique as cooper apparatus cooled using liquid nitrogen. In the course of time, this technique has improved and has transformed in the present day [1, 2].

2. Mechanisms of action in cutaneous cryotherapy

If we consider the mechanism, mainly −196°C was required to transmit the cold over tissues. When freezing shock has just reached tissues due to intracellular hyperosmotic conditions, damage of cells begin. Rapid electrolyte transfer has started, thereby increasing the intracellular component, which has been incriminated for the damage of cell proteins and enzyme systems. Thrombosis has been observed in microcirculation system as a factor of irreversible tissue loss even in mild freeze. Furthermore, inflammation converts necrosis finally [3, 4].

The size of ice crystals is important, and larger crystals cause greater damage. Rapid freezing speeds are required in the treatment of malignant lesions where cryosurgery is required. Speed is also required, and repetitions of sequence increase cell deaths. This issue is also useful for malignant ones [3, 4].

The mechanism of extinction has referred melanocyte between −4 and −7°C, whereas keratinocyte and connective tissue cell destruction occur only at −20°C. Regarding basic mechanism, this technique has been applied in lower temperature, which is also available for such dermatological conditions having high success rates [3].

3. Techniques of cutaneous cryotherapy

Technical modalities have been divided into three main groups which include contact, spray, and intralesional types. The frequency of these methods, which are written in an order, extends to benign and malignant lesions. Contact method is applied using a cotton applicator that is usually used for common warts. The most widely used technique in dermatology clinic is the spray form directed from a 90° angle at a distance of 1–2 cm. The newly developed one is the intralesional technique mainly used in malignant lesions and keloid scars. Intralesional cryotherapy is the preferred choice than other methods due to preserving epidermis and absence of hypopigmentation and scarring. Local anesthesia is usually not necessary but may be recommended if large areas are being treated [5].

Cryotherapy and cryosurgery are the modalities used interchangeably. If we enlighten the terminology, cryotherapy accurately freezes the lesion, but when combined with curettage, it gets its name as cryosurgery. Nevertheless, most clinicians unintentionally confuse each other.

4. Indications of cutaneous cryotherapy

The most common indications change from country to country due to the mean age of population, education levels, and capability of the physicians. In a comprehensive study conducted between 1993 and 2010 in the USA, the cryotherapy method is the most frequently used in actinic keratosis (AK), common warts, and seborrheic keratosis [6]. An article investigated in our country suggested that the most common indications are common warts, anogenital warts, callosity, and AK. An interesting point of this article is the use of cryotherapy on leishmania cases, and it achieved good results [7]. Generally, authors receive attention regarding physicians who have to determine how many cycles and how long duration are required for each lesion. Especially, some of the skin areas having a thin dermis should take lesser freezing time even if malignant lesions should be repeated for more than one cycle. Additionally, cryotherapy is also reliable in pregnant women with anogenital warts. As expected, a combination with various therapeutical methods increases the success rate. Different dermatological indications of cryotherapy are summarized in **Table 1**. Our clinical experiences in cryotherapy of seborrheic keratosis and verruca plantaris (which are commonly seen as benign lesions) are also demonstrated in **Figures 1** and **2**, respectively.

Cryotherapy is also being discussed as an alternative to surgery in patients with premalignant or malignant lesions. The interesting point involved in our review is that the frequency of using cryotherapy has doubled compared to the first 10 years (1988–2000) than the second

Benign lesions	Premalignant lesions	Malignant lesions
Acne scars	Actinic keratosis	Basal cell carcinoma
Angioma	Bowen's disease	Squamous cell carcinoma
Dermatofibroma	Lentigomaligna	Keratoacanthoma
Fibroma molle		Kaposi sarcoma
Myxoid cyst		Inoperable melanoma metastases
Molluscum contagiosum		
Hidradenitis suppurativa [72]		
Idiopathic guttate hypomelanosis [73]		
Keloid, hypertrophic scar		
Lentigo solaris		
Pyogenic granuloma		
Sebaceous hyperplasia		
Seborrheic keratosis		
Warts		
Xanthelasma palpebrarum [74]		

Table 1. Different indications of cutaneous cryotherapy [6, 7, 10, 28, 36, 43, 54, 65, 69, 70, 71, 75].

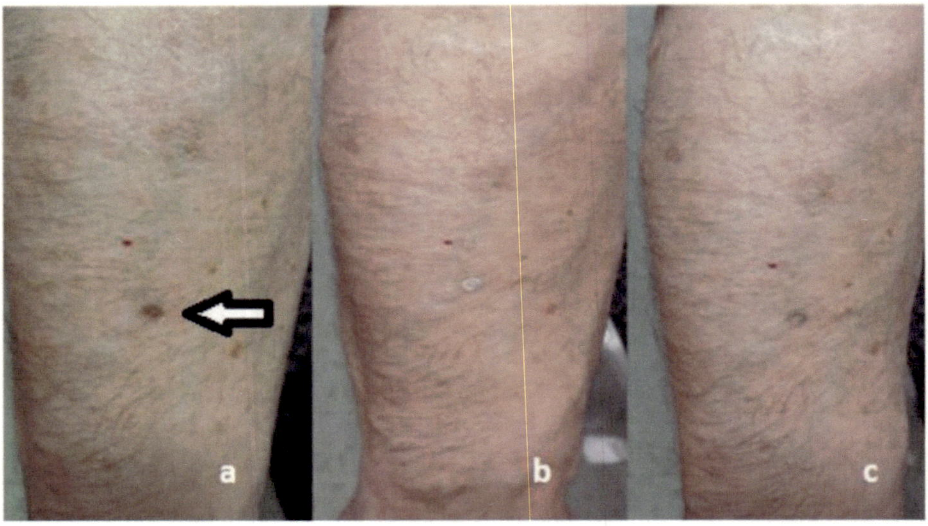

Figure 1. (a) Seborrheic keratosis in the right arm, (b) one cycle for 5–10-s freezing time via spray method, (c) before the second session of the treatment, reducing in size and fading in pigmentation of lesion.

decade (2008–2016). Additionally, it has been shown that the cryotherapy has lower cost than radiotherapy in patients who cannot undergo surgery in non-melanoma skin cancers. The average age increase in the second decade is also directly proportional to the increase in non-melanoma skin cancers [6]. For these reasons, the frequency of cryotherapy application in premalignant and malignant disorders may have been increased step by step over the years. In this chapter, premalignant and malignant cutaneous disorders have been mainly focused.

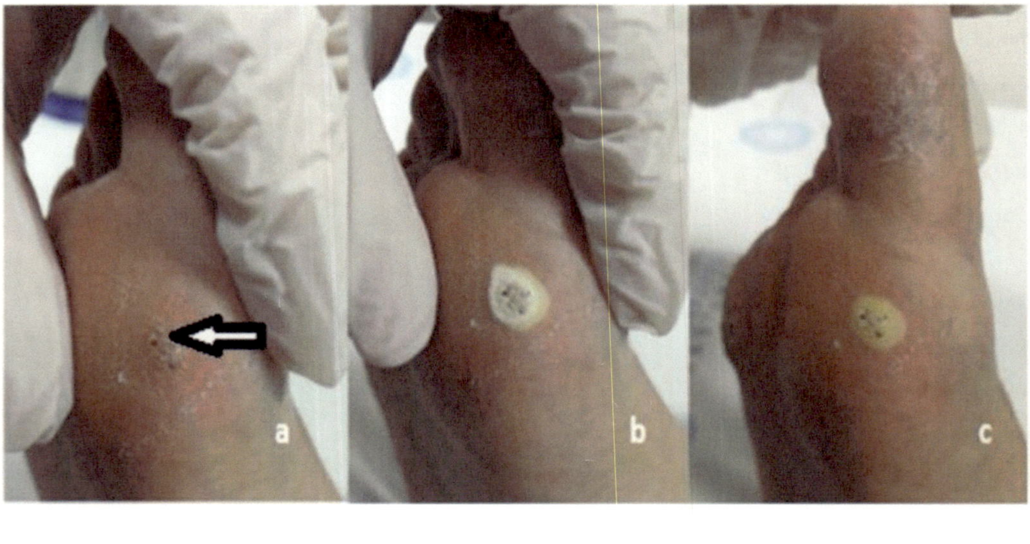

Figure 2. (a) Verruca plantaris in the sole of right foot, (b) two cycles for 15–20-s freezing time via spray method, (c) after 2 weeks, reduction in width and induration of lesion.

4.1. The use of cryotherapy in premalignant skin lesions

4.1.1. Actinic keratosis

AKs are common lesions consisting of epidermal keratinocytic dysplasia that are caused by chronic sun exposure. They are the most common premalignant skin lesions and clinically characterized by slow-growing, <1 cm, scaly, or hyperkeratotic papules in the areas exposed to the sun such as bald scalp, face, forearms, and hands. AKs are of public health importance because their presence is associated with the ability to progress to squamous cell carcinoma (SCC), especially when they are numerous and have coalesced into an area with severe photodamage. Nevertheless, lesions occasionally have spontaneous remission. Utility of the cured AKs reduces the metastases, death ratio, and health economic expenditure [8–10].

Dermatologists have been treating patients with AKs for many years with cryotherapy. Treatment of these lesions with a simple and inexpensive method prevents converting non-melanoma skin cancers (especially SCC), which may be more complicated in the future. According to an Italian consensus, it is the first treatment option for AK patients with a high degree (Olsen 3) of clinical severity [11]. On behalf of the British Association of Dermatologists Therapy Guidelines, cryotherapy is a recommendation strength belonging to A group, which means there is good evidence to support the use of the procedure [10].

There was no clear consensus on the cryotherapy method of AK treatment all over the world. Numerous variables can influence the success of cryotherapy: the skill and experience of the physician, freezing time, freezing depth, the pressure of the liquid nitrogen set, the size of the orifice on the device, the distance between the lesion, the number of sessions, size, and the presence of hyperkeratotic lesions [12–14]. To get a point of view, Zouboulis published the meta-analysis via 26 studies which compared the regional regimens; they declared that the response rate depends on the clinicians' technique, freezing time, and extended area [13].

In this chapter, we focus on the most suitable method. As we wish to enlighten, we have evaluated a large number of group samples. Up to 98.8% cure rate has been reported, but more recent data indicate smaller cure rates [15]. Ianhez et al. had cryotherapy for 5–10 s in the form of two sessions between 5 and 50 tumors on the arm and face area of 92 patients at baseline and after 120 days. The same examiner counted the lesions before the treatment, at 120th and 300th days. After all, they found 57% reduction of lesion numbers. An interesting point of view was that higher education level of AK patients and lower number of lesions showed more successful results [12]. If we increase the sample size, Goldberg et al. performed a single session for 180 AK lesions for the same time as 5–10 s. At the end of 6 weeks, complete recovery was observed for all lesions. Though they occasionally focused on non-hyperkeratotic lesions, more success rates have been expected also due to freezing depth reaching the underlying lesions [14]. **Figure 3** shows the result of one-cycle cryotherapy of a patient with bowenoid AK on the third week.

By the way, authors also investigated the freeze time for line of best fit. An article was investigated in Australia where 90 adult patients who had 421 eligible AK lesions were cured by cryotherapy. They found that higher freezing time is correlated with the higher complete

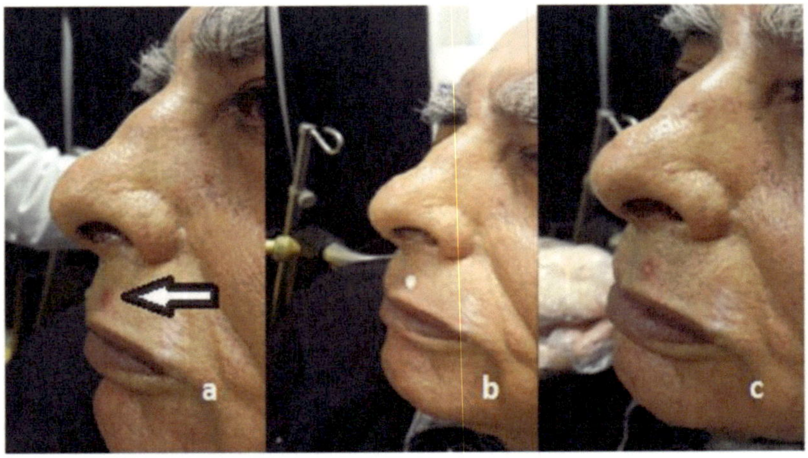

Figure 3. (a) Bowenoid AK lesion on the maxilla, (b) two cycles for 15–20-s freezing time via spray method, (c) before the third session of the treatment, reduction in size, erythema, and hyperkeratosis.

response of the lesion. Especially, the rates were 39% for 5 s, 69% for higher than 5 s, and 83% for higher than 20 s. If they achieved a regression analysis, they suggested the best time for the freezing time to be between 10 and 15 s as mentioned with maximum effect and also with minimum adverse effect. A higher than 30 s damages the dermis and causes scarring tissue and hypopigmentation [16]. As a common sense of clinicians, even though the exact regime does not exist, two cycles are always applied to get more effects.

When cryotherapy was compared with various methods, it has been observed that very different results were obtained. The first retrospective analysis was made in 1999 at 13 centers in 5 European countries by Szeimies et al. As population extended, 699 AK lesions were selected randomly to photodynamic therapy group (367 lesions) and cryosurgery group (332 lesions). They appraised that two modalities have similar complete response rates. Neither cryosurgery has superiorities to photodynamic therapy nor it has better cosmetic results. From this article, the suitability of cryotherapy has begun to be analyzed further [17]. Years later, Kaufman et al. also support this hypothesis in their reports involving more lesions [18]. Freeman et al. collated three groups of AK patients receiving photodynamic therapy (88 patients), cryotherapy (89 patients), and placebo (23 patients). The lesion response rates were found to be 91% in the photodynamic therapy group, 68% in the cryotherapy group, and 30% in the placebo group. As a result, photodynamic therapy has been considered as a better option than cryotherapy for complete lesion response as well as cosmetic outcome [19].

From a point of view, some authors analyzed the other optional modalities. From 1 to 3 years, clinical improvement of patients with 373 AK lesions treated by cryotherapy or 5-fluorouracil per group was investigated in Florida. As a result, cryotherapy was found to be doubly effective than 5-fluorouracil treatment when considering long-lasting comparability and also better cosmetic outcomes [20]. In addition, the efficacies of three different treatment modalities in patients with multiple AK lesions were compared by Krawtchenko et al. Nearly equal number of patients took one cryotherapy session, twice a day topical 5-fluorouracil during 4 weeks and topical imiquimod three times per week for 4 weeks. Patients were analyzed for clinical and histopathological evaluation at the 12th month. They could not determine the correlation between histopathological improvement (32%) and clinical improvement (68%) with the cryotherapy method. According to these values, half of the cases did not cure completely. Despite this, topical imiquimod application was the most effective method, and that also clinical (83%) and histopathological (73%) recovery rates were consistent with each other. Additionally, the patients' satisfaction ratio was found to be significantly higher than the cryotherapy and 5-fluorouracil application. They considered that 5-fluorouracil treatment is not acceptable for AK patients, howbeit topical imiquimod would be the top choice rather than cryotherapy [21].

To get another point of view, authorities have been seeking the correct combined treatment for AK patients for many years. Combination treatment modalities were inquired to manage both the lesion-directed and field-directed therapies. Regarding this, it is logical to combine with frequently used topical therapies including 5-fluorouracil, imiquimod, ingenol mebutate 0.05% gel, and diclofenac gel. All these agents cause some degree of localized inflammatory skin reaction mediated through a variety of biochemical pathways (interference with DNA synthesis, modification of immune response, and increased apoptosis through cyclooxygenase inhibition) and lead to elimination of the AK lesions [9]. Generally, the lowest irritation side effect has been seen with diclofenac gel treatment. As we consider to compare between the utility of combined or monotherapy; Berlin and Digel applicated 3% diclofenac gel two weeks later than the cryosurgery and they had more adequate results than monotherapy [22]. After that, an article made in Italy enrolled 175 patients to configure out the results of monotherapy, cryotherapy, or 3% diclofenac gel, and combined therapy. The first group administered diclofenac gel twice a day for 12 weeks. The second group received two cycles of cryotherapy followed by diclofenac gel for 8 weeks. The last group was administered with two cycles of cryotherapy two times for 1 month. Nearly equal patients followed up for 2 years. They found that the first and third groups showed similar results but the response rate of the first group was slower. Besides that, the second group showed most effective results of nearly 100% of full recovery. That patients answered response for life quality index and so they responded cryotherapy has sufficiently improved the life quality index [23]. Clinicians should choose the modalities that are easy, effective, and not time consuming. Mastrolonardo et al. focused on the difficult recurrent AK lesions in a small group. They applied 3% diclofenac gel for 12 weeks so that the mean number reduced from 8 to 1. After that, they cured cryotherapy each 4 weeks for residual ones. For 10 months, no lesions were observed. They suggested that this combination therapy is remarkable for elder patients who show poor cooperation and recurrent multiple lesions [24]. Hashim et al. examined 16 patients who had cryotherapy; after that, half of them received ingenol mebutate 0.05% gel sequentially for 3 days. Although combined treatment had more side effects profile, which is also tolerable, statistically significant reduction of the lesions had also been observed [25]. In order to promote quantitative analysis for the validity of cryotherapy and 5-flurouracil, combination treatment was made in 2004 firstly. A sample size of 70 patients per treatment group who took 5-flurouracil regime for 1 week and residual lesions are treated with cryotherapy after 4 weeks. Jorizzo et al. calculated the proportion of validity with combined therapy. As a conclusion, they found significant difference between combined therapy and monotherapy for 6 months. They mainly suggested that combined therapy is capable of increasing lesion-free period [26]. In another study, two groups included 30 patients with cryotherapy and 5-flurouracil cream of 0.5%, and combination treatment efficacies were compared. After the application of cryotherapy, they used 5-flurouracil cream once daily for 1 week. Besides that, they followed up for 26 weeks and claimed that no significant difference was found in terms of effectiveness. Despite the fact that adverse effects of 5-flurouracil cream have been more commonly observed [27], recent research has shown that ingenol mebutate 0.05% gel and cryotherapy combination would be the future model for these patients [25]. In conclusion, clinicians should decide case by case due to age, health-care conditions, contraindications, and availability in AK cryotherapy.

4.1.2. Bowen's disease

Bowen's disease is characterized by enlarging well-demarcated erythematous plaque with an irregular border and crusting or scaling surface. It is a form of in situ SCC which behaves differently such as partial progression, minimal invasion, or spontaneous regression [28].

Plaza Lanza et al. compared the freezing ratio through the lesion and found that a single cycle is as efficacious as for two cycles [29]. Another article conducted by Holt found that they also have the same success using single 30-s cycle [30]. Graham and Clark reported one recurrence in 30 patients treated with a single period with the longest time as at least 90 s [31].

The rate of recurrence has been lower than expected. Recurrent lesions have been mostly invaded to dermis and cause SCC. Cox and Dyson demonstrated recurrence in five patients (6%) after a minimum of 1-year follow-up; one of these had a focus of invasive cancer [32]. Additionally, Morton et al. found two (10%) recurrences in the 1-year follow-up period [33].

In order to make shorter total imiquimod bout and milder cryotherapy effects compared with corresponding monotherapies, Gaitanis et al. published a series consisting of eight cases. They used two cycles of cryotherapy along meanly 15 s followed by the application of daily topical imiquimod. No recurrence was seen during the 6-month follow-up [34].

Ahmed et al. aimed to compare two strong options in patients with Bowen's disease, which occasionally mainstays in the lower leg region. Thirty-six patients were treated with cryotherapy via spray method giving two freeze-thaw cycles, each freeze cycle being maintained for 5–10 s. Forty-four patients were therapied with curettage and cautery, the margins beyond least 3-mm of clinically lesion-free skin area. As a result, curettage and cautery is a better modality because of shorter healing time, lesser pain evaluation, and fewer recurrence rates with significant differences [35].

4.1.3. Lentigo maligna

Lentigo maligna is a melanoma in situ which includes malignant cells but do not show invasion. The main reason of that is the long-term sun exposure, which also increased the risk of non-melanoma skin cancers. If middle-aged and elderly patients have larger than 1-cm atypical pigmented *macular* lesions, not in smooth surfaces, mainstays usually on the head and neck should be checked up by the clinicians. There is a risk of conversion to malign melanoma, and patients should be advised to undergo the surgery. As mentioned earlier, the mechanism of extinction between melanocyte of −4 to −7°C has formed the basis of the cryotherapy method in melanoma patients. However, in this method, the inability to scientifically determine the depth limit of the intervention restricts the number of patients. Beyond this reason, it is recommended to implement two cycles, for a long time and at least a distance of 1 cm from the lesion [36].

In a study conducted by Kuflick and Gage, 30 patients who had been diagnosed with lentigo maligna were treated with cryotherapy. At the end of the 3-year follow-up, only two lesions (6%) recurred [37]. In Brazil, 18 patients were diagnosed clinically and histopathologically as lentigo maligna was cured with cryotherapy by Moraes et al. Two freezing cycles were applied for 1 min each separated by thaw cycle of at least 2 min on a single session, and they also used spray method beyond a 1-cm area of vision border. In a 5-year period, they followed up at 6-month intervals. No recurrences or metastases were observed in any patient [38].

A case report is evaluated to propose cryoimmunological treatment of cryotherapy with imiquimod application in lentigo maligna lesions by Bassukas et al. A 78-year-old man who had been denied surgery was treated with 5% imiquimod cream once daily for 3 weeks. When erythema occurs, without cessation of the cream, they continued with cryotherapy via 20 s for two cycles. One year later, a cross check of the lesion was done, and they could not see any malignant cells. The patient became lesion free for 26 months after the treatment. They supposed that this combination therapy could be encouraging for lentigo maligna [39]. However, more research is needed as there are not many studies conducted on a sufficient number of people.

4.2. The use of cryotherapy in malignant skin lesions

4.2.1. Basal cell carcinoma

Basal cell carcinoma (BCC) is the most common cancer worldwide, which belongs to non-melanoma skin cancer group with SCC. BCC behaves as a slow-growing tumor impacting locally destructive cells and causing disfiguration for the metastasis that is very rare. Specifically, renal-transplant patients have an increased risk of developing BCC compared with the general population. Governments should keep in mind that treatment options should be increased to get either health or economic profits. As all you know, the gold standard is Mohs surgery, but as elderly people are not appropriate for this surgery, other methods should be used. The last publications have a few questions. According to the characteristic of the tumor, should elderly people prefer surgery or symptomatic destruction or is screening enough? [40–42].

Superficial and nodular BCCs have relatively well-defined borders, while morpheiform, micronodular, trabecular, infiltrative, and basosquamous BCCs are often irregular borders and are also more aggressive. The most commonly used approach of low-risk BCC (e.g., superficial BCC, nodulo-ulceratif BCC) is cryotherapy. The goal of the treatment is that clinicians should assess the margin of the lesion for complete removal. Because of that, invasion through the dermis, recurrent and aggressive types, larger than 2-cm lesion size and high-risk anatomic positions are contraindications of cryotherapy [43].

Compared with surgery, there are significant missing aspects. The most important ones are higher recurrence rates than surgery, lack of histologic confirmation of malignancy removal, recurrent carcinoma may be seen, hypertrophic scarring, and post-inflammatory pigment changes may occur. Nevertheless, there are some advantages also such as easy to apply, capable for elderly people, postoperative care not required, and life quality not affected [40].

Kuflik managed the widest and longest research in this regard, and overall 30-year cure rate was 98.6%. In this report, the freezing time and lesion width differ from 40 to 90 s and 1–1.5 cm, respectively. The cancer cells have been destroyed in the range of −50 to −60°. The most capable and acceptable procedure achieved satisfactory results. They also had a chance to follow-up the recurrence of lesions, so they declared that a 5-year cure rate of 522 cases was 99.0% [44]. Zacarian et al. reported an overall cure rate of 97.3% in 4228 non-melanoma skin carcinomas [45]. Samain et al. only focused on the mid-face BCC lesions and they investigated the 5-year recurrence ratio. They analyzed 138 patients with 144 BCC lesions and they presented 94% lesion-free ratio for 5 years. With reference to that, morpheiform BCC, which is theoretically a contraindication of cryosurgery, decreases the success ratio. Also, 55 lesions had curettage before cryotherapy that aims to increase the success rate by going deep into the lesion [46]. An article from Egypt used a different technique via intralesional cryoneedle, which had significant response rates and excellent outcomes as minimal or without scarring, erythema, and pigmentation changes for nodular and superficial BCC lesions [47]. Recently, one of the largest, prospective long-term follow-up series was conducted by Lindemalm-Lundstam and Dalenbäck. Like recent reports, they also found 97% complete response and good cosmetic results with the curettage and cryosurgery [48].

Actually in routine clinical practices, two cycles were applied to BCC lesions. Additionally, thaw time is approximately three times longer than freezing time to share out the lesion [13]. According to oncology guidelines, two freeze–thaw cycles with a tissue temperature of −50°C are recommended [49]. In order to estimate the reliability of sequence number, Mallon et al. treated 83 facial lesions with either one thaw 30-s cycle or second thaw 30-s cycle. They found that a double thaw cycle (95.3%) reliability ratio was higher than one cycle (79.4%) but also an interesting point is that one cycle is enough for trunk lesions [50].

Cryotherapy is an old but popular method for BCC treatment; there are some positive and negative value comparisons with other modalities. Kuijpers et al. compared a 5-year cure rate with either cryotherapy or surgical excision with small group, and they did not find statistically significant reduction of lesion number when surgical excision is chosen. Besides that, preferable reason for cryosurgery is better cosmetic outcomes than surgery. Regarding this, cryosurgery wounds generally heal with minimal tissue contraction and atrophy or scarring tissue is not commonly seen, resulting in good cosmetic results [51].

Actually, combined therapies, which were induced by immunological mechanism, are not used in non-melanoma cancers. Some authors worked on cryosurgery combination modalities such as photodynamic therapy or imiquimod cream once daily. Nakuci and Bassukas daily applied 5% imiquimod cream for 5 weeks, and at the second week, they performed cryosurgery. All 24 patients including 36 BCC lesions were satisfied with the cosmetic outcome and expressed their preference for this immunocryosurgery modality again as future choice in the case of a tumor relapse [52]. On the other hand, Wang et al. found that photodynamic therapy and cryosurgery are comparable concerning efficacy but photodynamic therapy has better cosmetic results via assessment of a phase 3 clinical trial [53].

As a result of previous reports, cryosurgery is an effective method for BCC lesions with excellent cosmetic outcomes, causes higher life quality, and also is a practical approach that can implement in office conditions. Especially, superficial and nodular BCC lesions are suitable for this treatment. Future studies should focus on optimization of the treatment strategy for BCCs to administer standard immunocryosurgery.

4.2.2. *Squamous cell carcinoma*

SCC is the second most common cancer in the non-melanoma skin cancer class. SCC originates from keratinocytes due to cumulative sun exposure of skin. The lesions appear as papules or plaques which classified by skin-colored or pink, and smooth or hyperkeratotic. Ulceration may be present. The characteristic of SCC lesions is a high risk of distant metastasis causing higher mortality rates [54, 55].

SCCs are the most common malignancies in organ-transplant recipients. In immunocompromised patients, despite the clinical subtypes, it should be regarded as high-risk lesions. A survey was performed by dermatologists who treated organ-transplant recipients with squamous cell carcinoma. They first choose Mohs surgery among the patients and cryosurgery [56] as the second common therapy.

Curettage and cryosurgery arise from a variation of electrodessication and curettage, and offer a high cure rate for carefully selected superficial non-melanoma skin cancers. Peikert choose four subtypes of facial tumors consisting of superficial BCC (81 lesions), superficial BCC with papillary dermal invasion (2 lesions), SCC in situ (11 lesions), and SCC with papillary dermal invasion (6 lesions) which are smaller than 2 cm. They applied curettage after that one cycle 10-s cryotherapy, which has lesser freezing time for routine practices among the residual tissues. During the 5-year experience, only one recurrence of a superficial BCC on trunk was seen among 100 tumoral lesions [57]. For same samples, Nordin worked on a specific location as an auricula. They performed two sequence cryosurgery and curettage method. For 1-year follow-up, they did not see any metastasis and only one recurrence was determined in 60 non-melanoma skin cancer lesions [58].

Gonçalves described a new method of cryosurgery named as fractional cryosurgery. He dispensed hydrophilic gel between the center of the tumor and caused easing the calorie transfer. A cryoprobe was applied at the center of the tumor and did not require extending safety margin. A normal cryosurgery technique is based on freezing spray, which starts from the peripheral and goes through the center of the lesion. Despite this, they cured nine SCC lesions during the follow-up, which was 1 year for one patient and between 3 and 6 years for the remaining patients. They suggested that no recurrence was statistically significant; due to this, SCC lesions must be treated more aggressively. They also mentioned that larger than 15 mm of lesion width is required for another treatment in non-melanoma skin cancers [59].

It has been mentioned that keratoacanthoma should be accepted as low-risk SCC so that it has to be treated as SCC. The defining characteristic of keratoacanthoma is a symmetric inflammatory nodula with ulcerative debris originating from pilosebaceous glands. Although it has spontaneous regression also over 4–6 months, metastasis risk of SCC is enough to get adequate treatment. Some authors contented that this is a subtype of SCC, also [60, 61].

Chronic radiodermatitis can cause keratoacanthoma in professional physicians who did not protect themselves from the chronic X-ray exposure. Conejo-Mir et al. worked on noninvasive SCC lesions regard as keratoacanthoma which located at the finger. They applied two-cycle 30-s cryotherapy for six patients. During 2 years of follow-up, no recurrence was seen and also the most relevant issue is that finger mobility had been protected in all patients [62].

Lee et al. reported using intralesional cryotherapy technique in four elderly patients with keratoacanthoma. After the local anesthesia, an 18-gauge needle was inserted into the lesion and two cycles were applied beyond 30–60 s. If the residual lesion was presumed, they also used spray cryotherapy for one to three cycles. All lesions had complete remission in 2 months. They argued that small lesions as smaller than 1 cm could have been curable. Intralesional method is superior than the other types due to cosmetic outcomes such as absence of hypopigmentation. However, it would be contraindicated in the anatomic locations where has risk of poor healing due to insufficient circulation [63].

A published case report regards subungual SCC treated first with Mohs surgery after which the residual tissue is destroyed via cryotherapy as two cycles in 90 s. In order to protect tissue integrity and phalanx function, using cryosurgery as an adjuvant may improve cure rates in some cases of SCC [64]. Cryosurgery is one of the suitable options when other options are not appropriate or adjuvant modality for highly invasive non-melanoma skin cancers.

4.2.3. Kaposi sarcoma

Kaposi sarcoma is a vascular tumor that has brownish red to bluish red cutaneous nodules that tended to enlarge into dome-shaped tumors. There are variable modalities used for the treatment of Kaposi sarcoma such as surgery, chemotherapy, cryotherapy, electrosurgery, laser, and radiation therapies.

Kutlubay et al. investigated 30 patients with Kaposi sarcoma in a retrospective cohort study. Nineteen (63%) of them completed response to cryotherapy [65]. In addition, Scheofer et al. and Avilés Izquierdo et al. found cryotherapy to be more effective in superficial and small Kaposi sarcoma lesions [66, 67].

4.2.4. Inoperable malign melanoma metastases

Although the main treatment option for malign melanoma patients is surgery, different alternatives can be used in cutaneous lesions and also metastases as some people could not be operated. Rivas-Tolosa et al. applied cryotherapy and topical 5% imiquimod treatment to 20 patients with locoregional cutaneous metastases of melanoma patients who could not undergo surgery. After an average of five sessions, 13 patients (65%) responded to treatment.

http://dx.doi.org/10.5772/intechopen.70286

Eight (40%) of them have complete remission and the remaining five (25%) patients have partial response [68]. This is the first published pros and cons of the article regarding the life expectancy index of each decision.

5. Conclusion

Cryotherapy is also being discussed as an alternative to surgery in patients with premalignant or malignant skin lesions. The frequency of cryotherapy application has been increased step by step over the years correlated with older ages when such lesions occasionally occur. Response rates usually depend on the clinicians' technique, freezing time, and extended area. Mainly, non-hyperkeratotic lesions have more successful rates due to freezing depth reaching the underlying lesions. It is the first treatment of choice for AK patients. The authors compared the efficacy of modalities and they suggested that topical imiquimod or photodynamic therapy would be better choice rather than cryotherapy. Nevertheless, recent researches have shown that ingenol mebutate 0.05% gel and cryotherapy combination would be the future model for AK patients. Another premalignant lesion is Bowen's disease, which has also a higher risk of converting non-melanoma skin cancer and could be treated by cryotherapy, but cryotherapy-combined modalities (5-fluorouracil cream, curettage, and cautery) showed better results than monotherapy. An interesting point is that lentigo maligna patients are cured by cryotherapy as an alternative for surgery. In non-melanoma skin cancers, cryotherapy is an effective method with excellent cosmetic outcomes, thereby causing higher life quality. It is practical approach for patients who cannot undergo surgery that can implement in office conditions. Negative values of cryotherapy are considered as lack of histologic confirmation of malignancy removal, recurrent carcinoma may be seen, hypertrophic scarring, and post-inflammatory pigment changes may occur. Especially, superficial and nodular BCC lesions are suitable for this treatment. High risk of distant metastasis mostly of SCC lesions have limited the indications of cryosurgery. Regarding this, well-differentiated SCCs such as keratoacanthoma or SCC in situ lesions have benefits for this modality. Besides that, limited study has shown that cryotherapy could be an alternative treatment for Kaposi sarcoma or locoregional cutaneous metastasis of melanoma lesions. Cryotherapy is one of the suitable options when other options are not appropriate or adjuvant modality for highly invasive non-melanoma skin cancers. As a conclusion, future studies should focus on optimization of the treatment strategy in right-selected multitudinous populations to administer standard cryotherapy guidelines.

Author details

Sevgi Akarsu and Isil Kamberoglu*

*Address all correspondence to: isil.kamberoglu@gmail.com

Dermatology and Venerology Department, Dokuz Eylul University, Izmır, Turkey

References

[1] Korpan NN. A history of cryosurgery: Its development and future. Journal of American College of Surgery. 2007;**204**(2):314-324. DOI: 10.1016/j.jamcollsurg.2006.11.006

[2] Gage AA. History of cryosurgery. Seminars in Surgical Oncology. 1998;**14**(2):99-109

[3] Kuflik EG. Cryosurgery for cutaneous malignancy: An update. Dermatological Surgery. 1997;**23**(11):1081-1087

[4] Zouboulis CC. Principles of cutaneous cryosurgery: An update. Dermatology. 1999;**198**(2):111-117. DOI: 10.1159/000018084

[5] Zimmerman EE, Crawford P. Cutaneous cryosurgery. American Family Physician. 2012; **86**(12):1118-1124

[6] Farhangian ME, Snyder A, Huang KE, Doerfler L, Huang WW, Feldman SR. Cutaneous cryosurgery in the United States. Journal of Dermatological Treatment. 2016;**27**(1):91-94. DOI: 10.3109/09546634.2015.1054780

[7] Afsar FS, Erkan CD, Karaca S. Clinical practice trends in cryosurgery: A retrospective study of cutaneous lesions. Postepy Dermatologii i Alergologii. 2015;**32**(2):88-93. DOI: 10.5114/pdia.2015.48048

[8] Akarsu S, Ozbagcivan O, Ilknur T, Semiz F, Fetil E. Influence of demographic and clinical characteristics of actinic keratosis patients on illness perceptions and readiness to increase sun protection behaviours: An exploratory study. Photodermatol Photoimmunol Photomed. 2017 May;**33**(3):143-155. DOI: 10.1111/phpp.12295. Epub 2017 Feb 22

[9] Ceilley RI, Jorizzo JL. Current issues in the management of actinic keratosis. Journal of American Academy of Dermatology. 2013;**68**(Suppl 1):S28-S38. DOI: 10.1016/j.jaad.2012.09.051

[10] de Berker D, McGregor JM, Hughes BR. Guidelines for the management of actinic keratoses. British Journal of Dermatology. 2007;**156**(2):222-230. DOI:10.1111/j.1365-2133.2006.07692.x

[11] Peris PG, Calzavara-Pinton PG, Neri L, Girolomoni G, Malara G et al. Italian expert consensus for the management of actinic keratosis in immunocompetent patients. Journal of European Academy of Dermatology and Venereology. 2016;**30**(7):1077-1084. DOI: 10.1111/jdv.13648

[12] Ianhez M, Miot HA, Bagatin E. Liquid nitrogen for the treatment of actinic keratosis: A longitudinal assessment. Cryobiology. 2014;**69**(1):140-143. DOI: 10.1016/j.cryobiol.2014.06.006

[13] Zouboulis CC. Is cryosurgery less effective that conservative regimens in the treatment of actinic keratoses? Journal of European Academy of Dermatology and Venereology. 2016;**30**(10):e50-e53. DOI: 10.1111/jdv.13294

[14] Goldberg LH, Kaplan B, Vergilis-Kalner I, Landau J. Liquid nitrogen: Temperature control in the treatment of actinic keratosis. Dermatological Surgery. 2010;**36**(12):1956-1961. DOI: 10.1111/j.1524-4725.2010.01804.x

[15] Schmitt AR, Bordeaux JS. Solar keratoses: Photodynamic therapy, cryotherapy, 5-fluorouracil, imiquimod, diclofenac, or what? Facts and controversies. Clinics in Dermatology. 2013;**31**(6):712-717. DOI: 10.1016/j.clindermatol.2013.05.007

[16] Thai KE, Fergin P, Freeman M, Vinciullo C, Francis D, Spelman L, et al. A prospective study of the use of cryosurgery for the treatment of actinic keratoses. International Journal of Dermatology. 2004;**43**(9):687-692. DOI: 10.1111/j.1365-4632.2004.02056.x

[17] Szeimies RM, Karrer S, Radakovic-Fijan S, Tanew A, Calzavara-Pinton PG, Zane C, et al. Photodynamic therapy using topical methyl 5-aminolevulinate compared with cryotherapy for actinic keratosis: A prospective, randomized study. Journal of American Academy of Dermatology. 2002;**47**(2):258-262

[18] Kaufmann R, Spelman L, Weightman W, Reifenberger J, Szeimies RM, et al. Multicentre intraindividual randomized trial of topical methyl aminolevulinate-photodynamic therapy vs. cryotherapy for multiple actinic keratoses on the extremities. British Journal of Dermatology. 2008;**158**(5):994-999. DOI: 10.1111/j.1365-2133.2008.08488.x

[19] Freeman M, Vinciullo C, Francis D, Spelman L, Nguyen R, Fergin P, et al. A comparison of photodynamic therapy using topical methyl aminolevulinate(metvix) with single cycle cryotherapy in patients with actinic keratosis: A prospective, randomized study. Journal of Dermatological Treatment. 2003;**14**(2):99-106

[20] Chiarello SE. Cryopeeling (extensive cryosurgery) for treatment of actinic keratoses: An update and comparison. Dermatological Surgery. 2000;**26**(8):728-732

[21] Krawtchenko N, Roewert-Huber J, Ulrich M, et al. A randomised study of topical 5% imiquimod vs. topical 5-fluorouracil vs. cryosurgery in immunocompetent patients with actinic keratoses: A comparison of clinical and histological outcomes including 1-year follow-up. British Journal of Dermatology. 2007;**157**(Suppl 2):34-40. DOI: 10.1111/j.1365-2133.2007.08271.x

[22] Berlin JM, Digel DS. Diclofenac sodium 3% gel in the treatment of actinic keratosis post-cryosurgery. Journal of Drugs in Dermatology. 2008;**7**(7):669-673

[23] Serena L, Mariateresa C, Maria Grazia F, Claudio L, Anna B, Massimiliano S. Actinic keratosis: Sequential treatment with cryotherapy and 3% sodium diclofenac gel. Clin Exp Dermatol. 2009 Jan;**34**(1):33-5. DOI: 10.1111/j.1365-2230.2008.02783.x. Epub 2008 Jun 25

[24] Mastrolonardo M. Topical diclofenac 3% gel plus cryotherapy for treatment of multiple and recurrent actinic keratoses. Clinical Experimental Dermatology. 2009;**34**(1):33-35. DOI: 10.1111/j.1365-2230.2008.02783.x

[25] Hashim PW, Nia JK, Singer S, Goldenberg G. An investigator-initiated study to assess the safety and efficacy of ingenol mebutate 0.05% gel when used after cryosurgery in the

treatment of hypertrophic actinic keratosis on dorsal hands. The Journal of Clinical and Aesthetic Dermatology. 2016;**9**(7):16-22

[26] Jorizzo J, Weiss J, Furst K, VandePol C, Levy SF. Effect of a 1-week treatment with 0.5% topical fluorouracil on occurrence of actinic keratosis after cryosurgery: A randomized, vehicle-controlled clinical trial. Archives of Dermatology. 2004;**140**(7):813-816. DOI: 10.1001/archderm.140.7.813

[27] Hoover WD 3rd, Jorizzo JL, Clark AR, Feldman SR, Holbrook J, Huang KE. Efficacy of cryosurgery and 5-fluorouracil cream 0.5% combination therapy for the treatment of actinic keratosis. Cutis. 2014;**94**(5):255-259

[28] Cox NH, Eedy DJ, Morton CA. Guidelines for management of Bowen's disease: 2006 update. British Journal of Dermatology. 2007;**156**(1):11-21. DOI: 10.1111/j.1365-2133.2006.07610.x

[29] Plaza Lanza M, Ralphs I, Dawber RPR. Cryosurgery for Bowen's disease of the skin. British Journal of Dermatology. 1980;**103**(Suppl. 18):14

[30] Holt PJ. Cryotherapy for skin cancer: Results over a 5-year period using liquid nitrogen spray cryosurgery. British Journal of Dermatology. 1988;**119**:231-240

[31] Graham GF, Clark LC. Statistical analysis in cryosurgery of skin cancer. Clinical Dermatology. 1990;**8**(1):101-107

[32] Cox NH, Dyson P. Wound healing on the lower leg after radiotherapy or cryotherapy of Bowen's disease and other malignant skin lesions. British Journal of Dermatology. 1995;**133**(1):60-65

[33] Morton CA, Whitehurst C, Moseley H, McColl JH, Moore JV, Mackie RM. Comparison of photodynamic therapy with cryotherapy in the treatment of Bowen's disease. British Journal of Dermatology. 1996;**135**(5):766-771

[34] Gaitanis G, Mitsou G, Tsiouri G, Alexis I, Bassukas ID. Cryosurgery during imiquimod cream treatment ("immunocryosurgery") for Bowen's disease of the skin: A case series. Acta Dermato-Venereologica. 2010;**90**(5):533-534. DOI: 10.2340/00015555-0896

[35] Ahmed I, Jones B, Holmes C, O'Callaghan C, Ilchyshyn A. Comparison of cryotherapy with curettage in the treatment of Bowen's disease: A prospective study. British Journal of Dermatology. 2000;**143**(4):759-766. DOI: 10.1046/j.1365-2133.2000.03772.x

[36] Kasprzak JM, Xu YG. Diagnosis and management of lentigo maligna: A review. Drugs Context. 2015;**4**:212281. DOI: 10.7573/dic.212281

[37] Kuflick EG, Gage AA. Cryosurgery for lentigo maligna. Journal of American Academy of Dermatology. 1994;**31**:75-78

[38] Moraes AM, Pavarin LB, Herreros F, Aguiar Michelman F, Velho PE, Souza EM. Cryosurgical treatment of lentigo maligna. Journal der Deutschen Dermatologischen Gesellschaft. 2007;**5**(6):477-480. DOI: 10.1111/j.1610-0387.2007.06331.x

[39] Bassukas ID, Gamvroulia C, Zioga A, Nomikos K, Fotika C. Cryosurgery during topical imiquimod: A successful combination modality for lentigo maligna. International Journal of Dermatology. 2008;**47**(5):519-521. DOI: 10.1111/j.1365-4632.2008.03562.x

[40] Ceilley RI, Del Rosso JQ. Current modalities and new advances in the treatment of basal cell carcinoma. International Journal of Dermatology. 2006;**45**(5):489-498. DOI: 10.1111/j.1365-4632.2006.02673.x

[41] Linos E, Chren MM. Is screening for basal cell carcinoma worthwhile? Too soon to tell. British Journal of Dermatology. 2016;**174**(6):1181-1182. DOI: 10.1111/bjd.14706

[42] Telfer NR, Colver GB, Morton CA. Guidelines for the management of basal cell carcinoma. British Journal of Dermatology. 2008;**159**(1): 35-48. DOI: 10.1111/j.1365-2133.2008.08666.x

[43] Martinez JC, Otley CC. The management of melanoma and nonmelanoma skin cancer: A review for the primary care physician. Mayo Clinical Proceedings. 2001;**76**(12):1253-1265. DOI: 10.4065/76.12.1253

[44] Kuflik EG. Cryosurgery for skin cancer: 30-year experience and cure rates. Dermatological Surgery. 2004;**30**(2 pt 2):297-300

[45] Zacarian SA. Cryosurgery of cutaneous carcinomas: An 18-year study of 3,022 patients with 4,228 carcinomas. Journal of American Academy of Dermatology. 1983;**9**:947-956

[46] Samain A, Boullié MC, Duval-Modeste AB, Joly P. Cryosurgery and curettage-cryosurgery for basal cell carcinomas of the mid-face. Journal of European Academy of Dermatology and Venereology. 2015;**29**(7):1291-1296. DOI: 10.1111/jdv.12798

[47] Weshahy AH, Abdel Hay RM, Metwally D, et al. The efficacy of intralesional cryosurgery in the treatment of small- and medium-sized basal cell carcinoma: A pilot study. Journal of Dermatological Treatment. 2015;**26**(2):147-150. DOI: 10.3109/09546634.2014.906037

[48] Lindemalm-Lundstam B, Dalenbäck J. Prospective follow-up after curettage-cryosurgery for scalp and face skin cancers. British Journal of Dermatology. 2009;**161**(3):568-576. DOI: 10.1111/j.1365-2133.2009.09310.x

[49] Avci G. An Overview on Basal Cell Carcinoma,. Skin Cancer Overview Edited by Yaguang Xi, ISBN 978-953-307-746-8, 226 pages, Publisher: InTech, Chapters published December 16, 2011 under CC BY 3.0 license DOI: 10.5772/2440

[50] Mallon E, Dawber R. Cryosurgery in the treatment of basal cell carcinoma. Dermatological Surgery. 1996;**22**:854-858

[51] Kuijpers DIM, Thissen MRTM, Berretty PJM, Ideler FHLB, Nelemans PJ, et al. Surgical excision versus curettage plus cryosurgery in the treatment of basal cell carcinoma. Dermatological Surgery. 2007;**33**(5):579-587. DOI: 10.1111/j.1524-4725.2007.33117.x

[52] Nakuci M, Bassukas ID. Office-based treatment of basal cell carcinoma with immunocryosurgery: Feasibility and efficacy. Acta Dermatovenerologica Alpina, Pannonica et Adriatica. 2013;**22**(2):35-38

[53] Wang I, Bendsoe N, Klinteberg CA, Enejder AM, Andersson-Engels S, et al. Photodynamic therapy vs. cryosurgery of basal cell carcinomas: Results of a phase III clinical trial. British Journal of Dermatology. 2001;**144**(4):832-840

[54] Sapijaszko M, Zloty D, Bourcier M, Poulin Y, Janiszewski P, Ashkenas J, et al. Non-melanoma skin cancer in Canada chapter 5: Management of squamous cell carcinoma. Journal of Cutaneous Medical Surgery. 2015;**19**(3):249-259. DOI: 10.1177/1203475415582318

[55] Alam M, Ratner D. Cutaneous squamous-cell carcinoma. New England Journal of Medicine. 2001;**344**(13):975-983. DOI: 10.1056/NEJM200103293441306

[56] Clayton AS, Stasko T. Treatment of nonmelanoma skin cancer in organ transplant recipients: Review of responses to a survey. Journal of American Academy of Dermatology. 2003;**49**(3):413-416

[57] Peikert JM. Prospective trial of curettage and cryosurgery in the management of non-facial, superficial, and minimally invasive basal and squamous cell carcinoma. International Journal of Dermatology. 2011;**50**(9):1135-1138

[58] Nordin P. Curettage-cryosurgery for non-melanoma skin cancer of the external ear: Excellent 5-year results. British Journal of Dermatology. 1999;**140**:291-293. DOI: 10.1111/j.1365-4632.2011.04969.x

[59] Gonçalves JC. Fractional cryosurgery for skin cancer. Dermatological Surgery. 2009;**35**(11):1788-1796. DOI: 10.1111/j.1524-4725.2009.01292.x

[60] Manstein CH, Frauenhoffer CJ, Besden JE. Keratoacanthoma: Is it a real entity? Annals in Plastic Surgery. 1998;**40**(5):469-472

[61] Gleich T, Chiticariu E, Huber M, Hohl D. Keratoacanthoma: A distinct entity? Experimental Dermatology. 2016;**25**(2):85-91. DOI: 10.1111/exd.12880

[62] Conejo-Mir JS, Moreno JC, Camacho F. Cryosurgical treatment of professional chronic radiodermatitis. Dermatological Surgery. 1997;**23**(6):483-486

[63] Lee CN, Pan SC, Lee JY, Wong TW. Successful treatment of cutaneous squamous cell carcinoma with intralesional cryosurgery: Case report. Medicine (Baltimore). 2016;**95**(39):e4991. DOI: 10.1097/MD.0000000000004991

[64] Ruiz Santiago H, Morales-Burgos A. Cryosurgery as adjuvant to Mohs micrographic surgery in the management of subungual squamous cell carcinoma. Dermatological Surgery. 2011;**37**(2):256-258. DOI: 10.1111/j.1524-4725.2010.01860.x

[65] Kutlubay Z, Küçüktaş M, Yardımcı G, Engin B, Serdaroğlu S. Evaluation of effectiveness of cryotherapy on the treatment of cutaneous Kaposi's sarcoma. Dermatological Surgery. 2013;**39**(10):1502-1506. DOI: 10.1111/dsu.12285

[66] Scheofer H, Ochsendorf FR, Hochscheid I, Milbradt R. Facial Kaposi's sarcoma. Palliative treatment with cryotherapy, intralesional chemotherapy, low-dose roentgen therapy and camouflage. Hautarzt. 1991;**42**(8):492-498

[67] Avilés Izquierdo JA, García-Andrade CR, Gómez-Cornejo LP, Lazaro Ochaíta P, de Portugal Alvarez J. Characteristics of Kaposi's sarcoma. A retrospective study in a reference hospital. Anales de Medicina Interna. 2003;**20**(4):170-174

[68] Rivas-Tolosa N, Ortiz-Brugués A, Toledo-Pastrana T, Baradad M, Traves V, Soriano V et al. Local cryosurgery and imiquimod: A successful combination for the treatment of locoregional cutaneous metastasis of melanoma: A case series. Journal of Dermatology. 2016;**43**(5):553-556. DOI: 10.1111/1346-8138.13197

[69] Wood LD, Stucki JK, Hollenbeak CS, Miller JJ. Effectiveness of cryosurgery vs curettage in the treatment of seborrheic keratoses. JAMA Dermatology. 2013 Jan;**149**(1):108-9. DOI: 10.1001/2013.jamadermatol.275

[70] Gupta S, Sharma VK. Standard guidelines of care: Keloids and hypertrophic scars. Indian Journal of Dermatology, Venereology and Leprology. 2011;**77**(1):94-100. DOI: 10.4103/0378-6323.74968

[71] Levy LL, Zeichner JA. Management of acne scarring, part II: A comparative review of non-laser-based, minimally invasive approaches. American Journal of Clinical Dermatology. 2012;**13**(5):331-340. DOI: 10.2165/11631410-000000000-00000

[72] Pagliarello C, Fabrizi G, Feliciani C, Nuzzo S. Cryoinsufflation for Hurley stage II hidradenitis suppurativa: A useful treatment option when systemic therapies should be avoided. JAMA Dermatology. 2014;**150**(7):765-766. DOI: 10.1001/jamadermatol.2014.430

[73] Laosakul K, Juntongjin P. Efficacy of tip cryotherapy in the treatment of idiopathic guttate hypomelanosis (IGH): A randomized, controlled, evaluator-blinded study. Journal of Dermatological Treatment. 2016;**23**:1-5. DOI: 10.1080/09546634.2016.1221498

[74] Labandeira J, Vázquez-Osorio I, Figueroa-Silva O, Pereiro M Jr, Toribio J. Tolerability and effectiveness of liquid nitrogen spray cryotherapy with very short freeze times in the treatment of xanthelasma palpebrarum. Dermatological Therapy. 2015;**28**(6):346-350. DOI: 10.1111/dth.12254

[75] Andrews MD. Cryosurgery for common skin conditions. American Family Physician. 2004;**69**(10):2365-2372

Chapter 3

Application of Cryogenic Methods in Skin Diseases of Different Etiology

Tatyana Gennadyevna Kotova,
Sergei Nikolaevich Tsybusov,
Vladimir Ivanovich Kochenov and
Maksim Igorevich Tcyganov

Additional information is available at the end of the chapter

http://dx.doi.org/10.5772/intechopen.70509

Abstract

The modern demand for effective treatment options in dermatology was successfully addressed by the invention of cryogenic method. By 2009, Dr. V.I. Kochenov had developed and patented cryogenic set of instruments based on 30 years of his personal clinical experience. The set includes a number of instruments, which could be used independently. It allows implementing a wide range of therapeutic and surgical procedures and has no commercially available alternatives. The main applications of the set include cryogenic revitalization, and treatment for such common dermatological ailments as psoriasis, warts, acne, hypertrophic scars, purulent diseases of the skin and subcutaneous fat, epithelial cysts, skin hemangiomas, precancerous skin lesions, and even malignant melanoma of the skin. A brief overview of etiology, classification and pathogenesis of these maladies is presented alongside with the step-by-step guidelines to cryo-exposure procedures. Not only guidelines but also comprehensive theoretical and practical training is provided to physicians at the center which was established at Nizhny Novgorod State Medical Academy. Physicians at Scientific Clinical Center of Medical Cryology "OnKolor" have been using the set, which proved to be effective even in the most difficult and otherwise costly cases. The procedures that have pronounced cosmetic effect, leaves no scars and dark spots.

Keywords: cryosurgery, cryotherapy, premalignancy, melanoma, acne, hemangioma, treatment dermatologic diseases

1. Introduction

Today, cryogenic treatment method is worth being applied much more widely than it occurs in reality. Paradoxically, cryosurgery has its opponents, despite the fact that this method has almost no complications, and its high efficiency in many situations based deeply in physiology and immunology puts it above traditional treatment methods. Cryodestruction differs favorably from all known methods of active treatment by properties such as, for example, complete ablasticity in the treatment of malignant tumors, natural immunostimulating effects, and organotypic regeneration.

The main objective of the cryosurgical method can be defined as the absolute destruction of pathological cells in a given volume of living tissue without damaging the normal, healthy cells around this tissue.

The effectiveness of cryosurgery has been demonstrated primarily in such areas of medicine as dermatology. In 1938, the first in-depth clinical study was published—a book by M.A. Beridze "About the use of cryotherapy in dermatology," where the method was described imaginatively and in detail and the long-term treatment outcomes were presented. The author noticed that the removal of skin neoplasms with dry ice does not leave scars, and made recommendations on the proper use of cryotherapy.

Cryosurgery studies were carried out in almost all areas of medicine. Among these new technological developments in medical cryology, the most notable are cryogenic treatment methods patented by Scientific Clinical Center of Medical Cryology "OnKolor," which have a very diverse range of medical applications. In Nizhny Novgorod State Medical Academy (Rector—Prof. B.E. Shakhov) and Scientific Research Institute of Applied and Fundamental Medicine (Director—Prof. S.N. Tsybusov), cryogenic methods of treatment are applied in otorhinolaryngology, gynecology, dermatology, oncology, and proctology (implemented by the medical team under the leadership of Prof. S.N. Tsybusov and Dr. V.I. Kochenov).

A "Set of instruments for medical cryology by Dr. V.I. Kochenov" was developed and approved by the Ministry of Health of the Russian Federation in 2009. This invention allows implementing all the available and a number of new treatment technologies in medical cryology in any area of clinical medicine. A center for theoretical and practical training was established at Federal State Budgetary Educational Institution of Higher Education "Nizhny Novgorod State Medical Academy," Ministry of Health of the Russian Federation, where physicians of any clinical specialty relevant to medical cryology can take comprehensive training including new patented technologies using this set of instruments.

The set of instruments for medical cryology was developed upon 30 years personal experience of Dr. V.I. Kochenov, holder of second-level doctorate degree in Medical Sciences, certified physician of highest category, Co-chairman of All-Russian cryosurgical society, ISC member, inventor, and Director of Scientific Center of Medical Cryology "OnKolor." All components of the set passed long-term clinical testing. This set of instruments for medical cryology is unique (never manufactured previously), all cryo-instruments have the original design and each is protected by the RF patent. Its composition is ample for diverse applications in medical cryology: cosmetology, dermatology, otolaryngology, stomatology, surgery, proctology, gynecology, oncology and other areas of clinical medicine.

Patented cryo-exposure techniques are based on the phenomenon of liquefaction of the ambient oxygen fraction, which creates the effects of cryo-oxygen saturation, cryo-oxygenation in pathologically altered tissues, as well as cryo-oxy-cavitation and cryo-ozone destruction of neoplasms, and have contributed significantly to the treatment of visually localized tumors.

The set includes: cryoclamps of various modifications—their design allows for the radical elimination of pathologically altered tissues; a cryospray unit with various nozzles; ring-shaped cryoapplicators with different ring opening and a tube; ring-shaped magnets with an opening; cryotrocar; Dr. V.I. Kochenov's cryogenic device "Ledok" (Icelet) with cannulas of different diameters; tampons for deep cryogenic massage with a meshed-cellular elastic surface and inserted thermal accumulators; a roller placed on the handle for cryosurgical massage; cryosticks with different configurations of the working surface; and a device for columnar cryobiopsy of the frozen tissue.

These instruments were developed for the purposes of medical cryology and have no commercially available alternatives. The set allows for implementing multiple new techniques of cryotherapy and cryosurgery, which expands the horizon of possibilities of medical cryology. An essential advantage of the set is that all instruments can operate independent of the power supply, that is, in a standalone mode.

2. Cryogenic revitalization in cosmetology

It is indisputable that treating any pathological process on the skin and especially the facial skin should be performed with cosmetic method. First and foremost, these requirements are adequately met by cryogenic therapy methods. However, cosmetologists should not take them simplified and consider cryogenic exposures as the basic techniques having only functional mechanisms of medical effect.

A great mistake in the activity management of beauty salons is to give charge over implementation of cryogenic procedures to the hands of nursing staff and such approach should be absolutely avoided. Cryogenic techniques intended for skin exposure are exclusively medical procedures.

When working with cryo-exposure techniques, we need to remember that liquid nitrogen is not the same piece of ice like a chamomile infusion frozen in a domestic refrigerator, which can hardly injure the facial skin look. Only the non-contact volatile exposure to liquid nitrogen vapors can be absolutely safe. Any skin application, even very brief (especially if done with cotton wool soaked in liquid nitrogen), if applied in the presence of skin moisture or sebaceous secretions, in case of sensitive or aging skin, will lead to adhesion, uncontrolled heat transfer, glaciation in the form of a solid spot and can end eventually with the formation of bubbles, necrosis, hyper- and hypopigmentation, and subsequently to hyperplastic scars.

To avoid such implications and create deep regenerative pulses in the skin through the actual formation of interstitial ice, the best proven technique is used and tested in clinical practice for many years—a technique of deep rejuvenation by cryo-kneading with special tampons with mesh embossed surface ("Method of cryogenic treatment of skin," a technique developed by Dr. V.I. Kochenov). It prevents the accidental creation of a drain freezing zone on the skin, which would have ended in the development of cryonecrosis and complications are almost excluded. The objectives can vary very widely, from mild stimulation of blood supply and reviving complexion during the day or before going to the theater, to the elimination of hyperpigmentation and superficial keratoses, elimination of fine mesh of wrinkles, and skin smoothing in 3–4 weeks after the procedure. It depends on the degree of exposure, velocity of skin kneading performed with the tampon chilled in liquid nitrogen, and the number of cryo-exposure repetitions at a particular site.

Therapeutic effects come even from a very short-term skin freezing: exfoliation of the upper skin layer is facilitated; skin pores are reduced; blood vessels' tone is increased, and production of the innate skin collagen is stimulated. Longer freezing destroys viral manifestations and pathogenic microbial associations.

To provide a focused local effect, any cryo-spray device is suitable, if the distance to the tissue surface is increased and manipulation is performed in a pulse mode with close visual inspection of the treated surface.

The workplace of cryo-cosmetologist should be equipped not only with cotton sticks and a vacuum flask. To perform any cryological therapeutic intervention, destroying pathological tissue with a wadding stick is simply careless in our days.

The objective of the suggested method of cryogenic skin exposure described in this book is to provide a pronounced and persistent medical cosmetic effect without the risk of complications. The proposed method ensures:

- marked and long-lasting therapeutic cosmetic effect;
- possibility to control the treatment quality and effectiveness, due to the available clear criteria for assessing the zone and timing of cryo-exposure;
- excluded formation of skin vesicles and bullae;
- individual and differentiated approaches to treatment;
- rapid and non-traumatic freezing of the upper skin layers;
- dosed, with the possibility of precise localization and, ultimately, uniform and deep skin freezing;
- creation of discrete linear, non-merging freezing zones, with the direct formation of interstitial ice;
- complete cryosurgical destruction (cryodestruction) of individual minor pathological, exophytic and diffuse formations, and pigmentary changes; and
- possibility of multiple actual skin freezing without the risk of complications and cosmetic defects after the procedure.

A beauty salon that offers cryological procedures in its list of services needs an accessible set of devices to implement medical cryology techniques for facial skin rejuvenation. To perform cryoablation of pathological formations, cryo-cosmetologists are recommended to use "Ledok" (Icelet) unit with cannulae of different diameter.

The proposed set of spherical cotton tampons retain their elasticity at liquid nitrogen temperature and are encapsulated in natural fabric (textile—cotton, wool—with a checkered relief (waffle) structure, or braided, netlike, perforated leather). Capsules should have cells of different size, for example, a structure where the wall thickness between the cells does not exceed $^1/_{10}$ and the cell depth—$^1/_5$ of the cell side, respectively. Diameter of applicators can be correlated conveniently with the known morphological features of the human face, for example, the size of the optic fissure. The set should include tampons of at least three sizes, with diameters corresponding to the entire length, $^1/_3$ and $^1/_5$ of the patient's optic fissure. Capsules for three tampons of the same diameter are selected in such a way that the cell size for each tampon makes $^1/_{10}$, $^1/_{20}$, and $^1/_{30}$ of its circumference, and this pattern is kept for tampons of all three diameters, as follows from their practical use. A cotton wad is tightly crumpled, covered with a piece of textile under tension to form a ball-shaped tampon. The tampon is fixed, for example, by capturing the gathered textile elements in the proximal part of the tampon with a surgical clip on a thermally nonconductive handle.

2.1. Cryo-exposure procedure

Before starting treatment, the patient's skin is treated with an alcohol-free facial cleanser. Then a moisturizer is applied to the skin and gently rubbed in a circular motion. Wait for 10–15 minutes.

The first step is the pointwise cryodestruction of pigmented spots and minor benign skin tumors (papillomas and hemangiomas) by special applicators.

Then all tampons are immersed in the working container with liquid nitrogen. When rapid boiling of liquid nitrogen is stopped, tampons are ready for use.

Next, the tampon of the largest diameter and the largest cell size is taken from the liquid nitrogen and its excess is removed from the tampon. This tampon is used for test applications on the places, where the skin surface is the smoothest: the forehead or the chin. The tampon is rolled with its lateral surface, applying a gentle pressure on it and stretching the skin. The handle should be oriented at a very acute angle to the skin surface, thus making the rotation of the tampon archwise, almost by 180°,. Thus, the tampon is rolled by a distance approximately equal to the half of its circumference. The average time of the tampon move is selected from 2–3 to 3–5 seconds depending on the skin type (sensitive or oily skin). After completing rotational rolling, the tampon leaves behind it an ellipsoidal relief imprint—the freezing zone. The surface of this zone is examined using a binocular magnifier and fiber optic lighting, and its characteristics are evaluated.

Next, two to three test applications are performed in the same way, rolling the tampon at different velocity, changing the angle of the handle and under control of thawing time, which should not exceed 1–3 seconds. Then the visual characteristics of the resulting zones are compared and the optimal rolling speed is selected, for which the freezing zone structure fully corresponds to the characteristic pattern of the tampon capsule. Upon completed cryomassage, the imprint fully disappears from the skin surface, due to the natural heat uptake.

Cryomassage of the face, neck, and décolleté is performed with the optimal selected velocity, following the basic rules:

- a single, one-time selected tampon is used for three to five applications; then it must be cooled by immersing in liquid nitrogen for 5–10 seconds, squeezed out and used further;
- the rolling direction during the cryo-exposure on the same section of the skin surface is changed along the line of visible skin folds and in short movements perpendicular to them.

When all the desired skin areas are subjected to cryo-exposure with a tampon of $^1/_{10}$ circumference cell size, the same areas are treated with tampons of $^1/_{20}$ and then $^1/_{30}$ circumference in the same way. As a result, a marked skin hyperemia appears 5–10 minutes after exposure, which is manifested in elongated spots on the places that were first subjected to cryo-exposure. During repeated massage of cryoapplications on hyperemic skin areas, the rolling velocity should be slightly reduced, and the freezing time in each point of the skin surface should be increased, respectively. Subsequent cryo-massage applications are oriented to those areas, where the hyperemia is less pronounced or has not yet developed.

Cryomassage for the less accessible facial skin areas (parotid region, nose bridge and wings, around the nostrils, around the lips, upper and lower eyelid, and eye corners) should use applicators as follows.

First, cryo-manipulations are performed with tampons of the large cell size: a tampon with a diameter of $^1/_3$ of the optic fissure is applied to the skin in the superciliary region, the nose bridge, the parotid region, and around the lips; a tampon with a diameter of $^1/_5$ of the optic fissure is applied to the skin around the nose wings, the nostrils, eyelids, and the internal and lateral angle of the eye; cryo-manipulations along the line of the most pronounced skin folds are performed with the same tampon. In doing so, the skin is stretched preliminarily with the other free hands in the direction perpendicular to the tampon rolling line, smoothing the wrinkled tissues and opening the skin folds for cryo-exposure. Ensure that the checkered relief freezing zone is formed on the stretched skin areas. Then cryomassage applications are repeated with tampons of the smaller cell size in the same way.

The relief zones of cryo-exposure performed with tampons of different sizes should overlap with no absolutely distinct boundary between them. Continuous "checkered" microfocal real freezing ensures repeated cryo-exposure on the same skin area without risk of blisters appearing after the procedure. A clinical sign of an adequate cryo-exposure is the development of persistent and uniform skin hyperemia. A high-quality cryomassage of face, neck, and décolleté lasts from 40 minutes to 1 hour.

Immediately after completion of the procedure, nourishing and regenerating products in the form of cream or gel should be applied on the hyperemic skin and relevant medications—to the sites of pathological diffuse lesions (acne). Skin cryo-session can be repeated not earlier than in a month.

Currently, cryolifting techniques for the interstitial correction of manifestations of gravitational ptosis on the facial skin by linear subcutaneous cryo-exposure are under development. The outcome of treatment is presented in **Figure 1**.

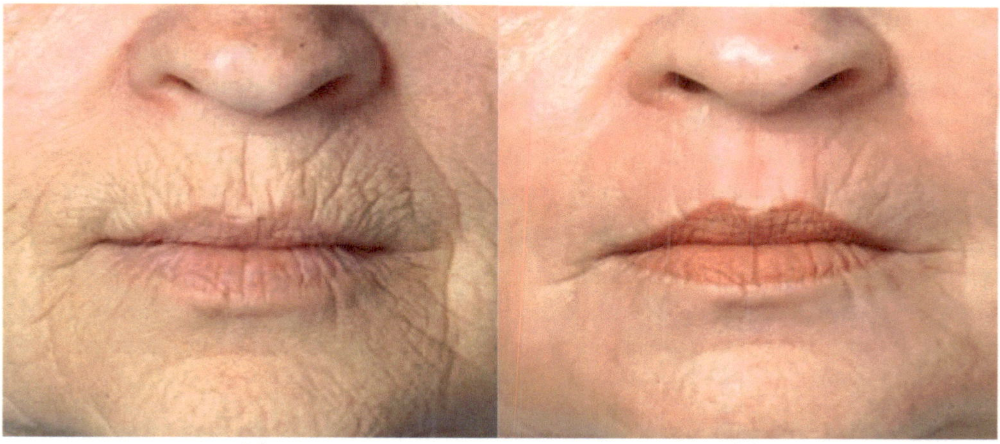

Figure 1. Facial skin in a female patient (a) before and (b) after cryogenic revitalization.

3. Multiple cryogenic treatment for psoriasis

Psoriasis is a chronic multifactorial systemic disease characterized by epidermal-dermal papular rashes. It occurs with equal frequency in males and females and persists over the years with alternating periods of remission and relapses. It is one of the most common, refractory, and often severe dermatoses. The effective treatment of psoriasis requires considerable efforts but in many cases it comes untenable.

When treating mild forms of psoriasis, dermatologists tend to use the least toxic medications and treatment methods with the lowest risk of possible side effects. If the treatment goals are not achieved, other potentially more effective treatments can be tried but those are more toxic and have a higher risk of serious side effects. Such methods are typically reserved for severe cases resistant to other, less toxic treatment methods for psoriasis. This is referred to as "therapeutic intervention ladder."

The etiology and pathogenesis of psoriasis is not yet fully identified. Currently, there are two main hypotheses about the nature of the process leading to the development of this disease. According to the first hypothesis, psoriasis is a primary skin disease, when normal processes of maturation and differentiation of skin cells are interrupted and the excessive proliferation of these cells is observed. The defenders of this hypothesis view psoriasis as a disrupted function of the epidermis and its keratinocytes. The second hypothesis assumes that psoriasis represents an immunopathological or autoimmune disease, where the excessive growth and reproduction of skin cells and, particularly, keratinocytes are secondary in regard to various mediators of inflammation, lymphokines, and cytokines produced by the immune cells and/or in relation to the autoimmune damage of skin cells causing the secondary regenerative response.

Genetic determination of psoriasis has never been disputed by medical experts and the extensive clinical experience proves it. Many genes associated with or directly involved in the emergence of psoriasis are discovered but it still remains unclear, how these genes interact in the development of the disease. The majority of genes known to be associated with psoriasis affect the immune system in one way or another, particularly, the function of T lymphocytes and for the major histocompatibility complex (MHC).

So far, the viral theory of the origin of psoriasis is controversial and gives rise to a number of scientific publications, both in favor of this theory, and against it. According to V.I. Kochenov, it is the viral nature of psoriasis, with its patterns of development of clinical manifestations similar to those for papillomavirus that justifies the exclusive adequacy of cryogenic treatment for multiple benign foci of psoriasis.

Indeed, the cryogenic technique allows sparing devitalization of psoriatic lesion, attribute antigenic properties to it, with spontaneous natural phagocytosis, rejection of modified cells and the immunostimulatory effect. At the same time, it provides a possibility of simultaneous radical cryodestruction for the large number of foci on a large area of skin surface without the negative reactions of the entire organism. Moreover, cryogenic treatment stimulates immune activity against the modified cells by performing cryotherapy of the lymphoid pharyngeal ring and the total extreme aerocryotherapy.

The cornified cells in the superficial skin layers form the *stratum corneum*. It is particularly pronounced in the psoriatic lesion and this explains for its considerable elasticity and low thermal conductivity. Special cryoablation techniques are needed for the efficient cryotherapy of psoriatic foci and to stimulate the regeneration of the normal skin cover.

3.1. Cryo-exposure procedure

A full course of successful cryogenic treatment for psoriasis was developed in "OnKolor" Scientific Clinical Center of Medical Cryology. It is important to keep in mind that local cryogenic exposure needed for the complete elimination of the psoriatic focus cannot be referred to as cryotherapy. This should be a proper cryosurgery performed in line with the rules of tumor cryodestruction but less deep penetration of the freezing zone into the pathological tissue.

Therefore, a combination of techniques is applied in cryoablation of psoriatic foci (even if a single focus is treated):

1. Continuous cryo-irrigation with liquid nitrogen until a stable, visible for 5–10 seconds, icing of the entire surface of the psoriatic focus occurs, with two to three iterations of the freeze-thaw cycle at each site during one procedure.
2. Prolonged exposure, with a slow rolling of the cotton wool tampon with braided mesh-like surface chilled in liquid nitrogen on the focus, until a stable, persistent for 4–5 seconds, visible freezing of the psoriatic lesion occurs.
3. Cryoapplication without adhesion performed with passively or actively chilled cryo-instruments by straightening the focal surface and consecutive stops of the applicator for 2–5 seconds at each site.

4. Stepwise freezing of the entire lesion surface by touching with a drop of atmospheric oxygen passively liquefying on the lateral side of the non-thermally insulated cannula and flowing down to "Ledok" cryoapplicator.

It should be noted that in the first two cryodestruction options, psoriatic lesions reveal an increased rate of the surface freezing.

To enhance cryodestruction and increase the cooling rate prior to the cryo-exposure, a mixture of glycerol and dimexidum 40% solution or soft magnetic dosage forms (SMDFs) should be applied to the focal surface and in this case, a permanent magnet is placed around the freezing area.

Thus, one psoriatic lesion is subjected to three freeze-thaw cycles, in line with the above described cryodestruction techniques. Repeated cryo-exposure procedures should be continued until the complete elimination of psoriatic plaques. Complete persistent elimination of dermal psoriatic manifestations can be reached after three to four adequate cryodestruction operations for all psoriatic lesions but may require 5–7 sessions.

The course of general extreme aerocryotherapy (GEACT) included in the cryogenic treatment complex for psoriasis is carried out in "Krion" cryosauna, as follows:

- three procedures per day, simultaneously with the start of the local treatment;
- next, four procedures every other day;
- then one procedure once a week for three weeks; and
- then one procedure per month, up to a year.

Usually GEACT course includes 10–15 sessions.

By the end of a combined treatment course, the remaining minor psoriatic lesions should be impregnated with a mixture of glycerol-dimexidum 40% before the GEACT session. Cryogenic treatment is well tolerated by all patients and has no contraindications.

To enhance the activity of the immune status, local cryodestruction of psoriatic plaques should be supplemented by cryotherapy of the lymphoid pharyngeal ring.

Subject to compliance with these cryogenic treatment recommendations for psoriasis, the patient's skin stays clean for the period of 1–3 years. However, if there is a slightest tendency to recurrent psoriatic lesion, this site should be immediately subjected to the superficial cryoablation. The outcome of treatment is presented in **Figures 2** and **3**.

4. Cryosurgical treatment for warts

Warts are benign skin tumors based on the proliferation of the epidermis and papillary dermis. Warts are caused by the human papillomavirus, which is passed only between humans.

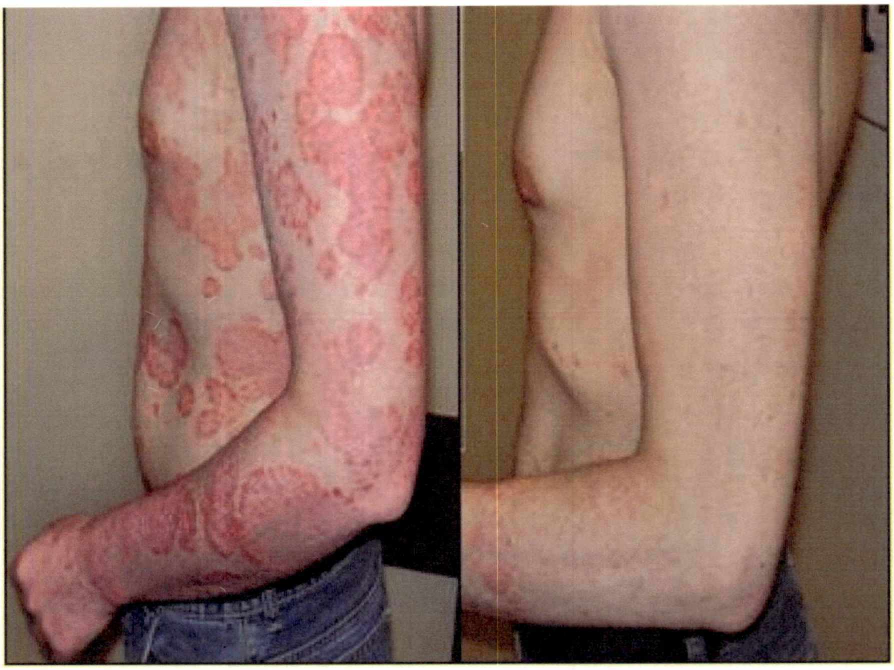

(a) (b)

Figure 2. Plaque psoriasis vulgaris: (a) before and (b) after combined cryogenic treatment.

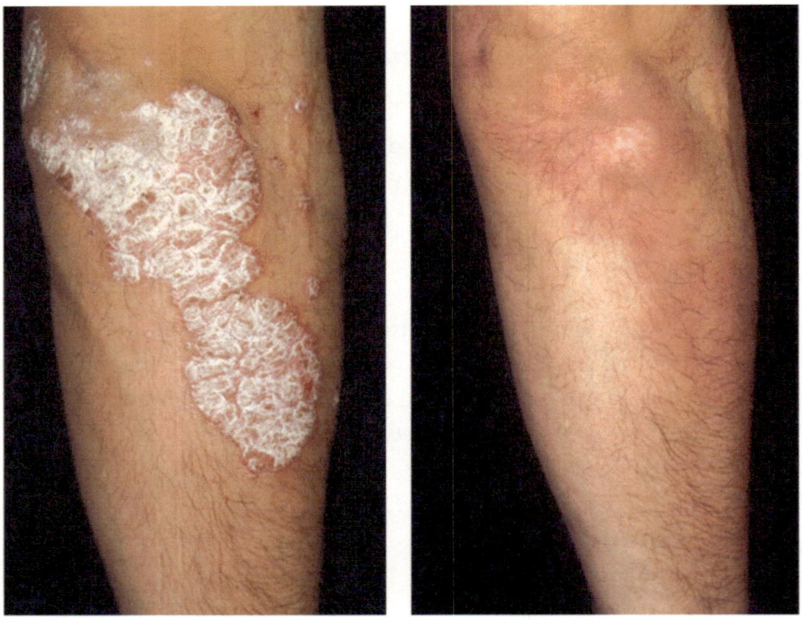

(a) (b)

Figure 3. Palmoplantar psoriasis: (a) before and (b) after combined cryogenic treatment.

http://dx.doi.org/10.5772/intechopen.70509

There are more than 600 HPV strains. According to some estimates, 60% of human population carries this virus.

The following types of warts are distinguished: common, flat, genital, and senile. Common, flat, and genital warts are caused by a single virus. Common warts (*verruca vulgaris*) are the most widespread and contribute to over 70% of the total number of warts. For this reason, we will discuss cryodestruction techniques for this type of warts in detail.

Being the most reliable destruction mechanism damaging all pathological tissues along with preserving cosmetic result, cryosurgery is the best suitable method for the elimination of warts. A very important effect in the treatment of warts by deep freezing is ablastics of cryodestruction that blocks all the elements of the pathological focus and prevents the spread of newly formed wart viruses in the body. They remain in the exfoliated cryonecrotic scab and are removed mechanically from the body.

However, the wart structure is very peculiar, which puts a number of obstacles and complicates cryogenic destruction of this skin formation. Its base goes deep into the tissue and its surface diameter makes always only a portion of the root depth. The wart capsule is dense and dry; the surface is cornified and tuberous, which prevents the proper heat transfer between the cryoapplicator and the pathological tissue.

Thus, the cryoablation technique for the common wart is the same as in the case of a malignant tumor.

Wiping the wart surface with cotton wool soaked in liquid nitrogen does not refer to the radical cryosurgical techniques; such exposure is just too superficial. According to our experience, incomplete cryogenic destruction of wart tissue often stimulates its rapid growth and proliferation.

4.1. Cryo-exposure procedure

First, the wart is prepared by steaming its surface and the *stratum corneum* is removed mechanically to the greatest possible extent. Warts located on the hand back, foot, and the lateral surface of the finger are subjected to cryocompression destruction by capturing with transformation of the affected area into a fold using cryo-clamps with spatial heat accumulators. The exposure time is needed to get the entire surface of the pathological focus and the area of 1–3 mm beyond its borders fully covered by the freezing zone.

This technique is absolutely nonapplicable on the palmar surface and the feet. The basic manipulation for cryodestruction of common warts in these locations is the applicative freezing with adhesion using "Ledok" apparatus. Cryogenic treatment is continued until complete icing of the entire pathologically modified site within its borders.

Icing comes instantly together with the full-rate adhesive effect and freezing-in the working tip into the wart tissue. Therefore, mechanical contact and heat transfer are maintained at all absolute values of the subzero temperature, even after the true adhesive effect disappears. It persists even after the start of passively condensing ambient oxygen flow to the frozen surface via the lateral open surface of the cannula. This phenomenon is used at freezing temperature of −182°C.

The exposure is continued until complete icing of the entire pathologically changed site and the creation of the freezing zone that extends beyond the borders of the skin formation, at a distance equal to its diameter. Only under such excess over the size of freezing zone, the pathological wart tissue is expected to be covered by destructive temperatures.

Freeze-thaw cycles for each wart are repeated three times, regardless of the cryoablation technique.

Another option for additional deep local cooling, appropriate for large-size common warts, is cryo-irrigation of the wart surface with the same parameters of freezing expansion area, which is carried out at the final stage. Cryo-irrigation as a single freezing method cannot be recommended for eliminating warts.

Genital warts, flat warts, and senile warts are subjected to cryo-compression destruction as described above, by using a cryo-instrument with spatial heat accumulators of the most appropriate size.

5. Cryosurgical treatment for purulent diseases of the skin and subcutaneous fat using SMDF in a magnetic field

Purulent diseases of the skin and subcutaneous fat account for about 70% cases in surgeon's outpatient reception. The most common causative agent of these diseases is the staphylococcal flora (70–90%).

The main purulent diseases of the skin and subcutaneous tissue include furuncle, carbuncle, hydradenitis, and abscess. Diseases complicated by lymphangitis and lymphadenitis take a particularly severe course. In addition to surgery, treatments of purulent diseases of the skin and subcutaneous fat use an intensive combined treatment: antibacterial, detoxification, and immunomodulation.

Following the rejection of a rod consisting of necrotic tissue and pus, ulcer-like skin defect is formed, is rapidly replaced with granulation tissue and healed by secondary intention, leaving a deep inverted scar. A cosmetic skin defect is often formed at the site of surgical wound.

In recent decades, active development of cryosurgery attracts particular attention, due to the creation of uncomplicated, reliable, and inexpensive cryogenic devices. An important factor is the elimination of the causative agent of purulent infection in the inflammation focus subjected to freezing, with subsequent fixation of purulent focus by swelling of the underlying tissues and vascular thrombosis.

Currently, the cryogenic treatment for purulent diseases of the skin and subcutaneous fat is almost unused, despite its proven success, as described in some published works.

Obviously, difficulties arise during freezing pathological cavities. This situation can be addressed by the creation of heat-conducting liquid layer between the cryoapplicator tip and the freezing tissue, providing adhesion and congruence of surfaces. Traditional use of aqueous layers, which are characterized by low thermal conductivity, impairs the main characteristics of the cryo-instrument, while oil- and alcohol-based layers have even lower heat conductivity and adhesion capacity.

Furthermore, healing under cryonecrotized biological tissue occurs in two main stages. First, necrotic tissue is transformed into long-drying moist cryonecrosis. Due to the fact that cell membranes are damaged by ice crystals formed during freezing, the intracellular fluid exudates to the surface of cryonecrotic tissue, thus preventing the secondary infection of cryonecrosis. When the exudative process concludes, moist cryonecrosis turns into a solid dry scab—dry cryonecrosis. During this period, the epidermal cells regenerate from the periphery to the center. The time length of regeneration correlates with the focal diameter of the cryogenic lesion and its depth. During this period, the dry cryonecrosis covers the wound surface and acts as an antiseptic dressing.

Since the dry cryonecrosis has a much lower elasticity, as compared to the skin, it tears away during the healing process. This process is promoted by the natural partial exfoliation of dry cryonecrosis from the periphery as regeneration proceeds.

If purulent diseases of the skin and subcutaneous fat are subjected to superficial cryo-exposure, microbial associations are often preserved in the pathological cavity. To avoid this situation, cryodestruction should be performed more intensively. An increase in the depth and area of cryo-exposure will inevitably result in a more extensive damage to healthy tissues and will significantly lengthen their recovery.

Such problems as an insufficient depth of cryo-exposure or a significant surface expansion of the freezing zone on healthy tissues in an attempt to increase the depth of the freezing area, the lack of effective heat transfer and the duration of postoperative period remain yet unresolved and restrict the application of the cryogenic method in the treatment of purulent diseases of the skin and subcutaneous fat.

A new class of pharmaceuticals that appeared in recent years includes preparations that have high thermal conductivity and are capable of penetrating into small cracks, pores, caverns, ducts, and various cavities in the presence of magnetic field, which enables a wider use of the advantages provided by the cryosurgical treatment.

SMDF is a pharmaceutical form containing fine particles of magnetized ferromagnetic (Fe_2O_3–Fe_3O_4, $SrO{\cdot}6Fe_2O_3$, Nd–Fe–B, FeB). SMDF consistency, viscosity, and fluidity depend on concentrations of ferromagnetic and the base substance. As the strength of magnetic field increases, SMDF thermal conductivity approaches that of the metal, i.e., SMDF is in fact a soft metal body. It comes important with regard to the fact that thermal conductivity increases in cryo-exposed pathological tissue and subsequently, the destructive effect of cryoablation is enhanced.

Moreover, SMDF applied locally has pronounced antiseptic and dehydrating effects, which are essential in the postoperative period to reduce the moist necrosis phase and accelerate the regeneration under dry cryonecrosis. These effects can be supplemented, if necessary, by the introduction of anesthetic, hemostatic, vasoconstrictive and other medications into the SMDF composition.

5.1. Cryo-exposure procedure

Cryosurgical treatment of patients with purulent diseases of skin and subcutaneous fat does not include the general antibacterial therapy.

Antibacterial agents are applied only locally in ointment. To enhance skin susceptibility to penetration of all SMDF components, dimexidum (dimethyl sulfoxide, 40% solution) is included in the ointment composition.

During the *infiltration stage*, SMDF is applied to the entire zone of hyperemia, the cryoapplicator is brought into contact with the magnetic ointment, and cooling is performed until the freezing zone is spread to the uninflamed skin. Under such short-term cryo-exposure, superficial cryonecrosis is formed, not deeper than 1.2 mm (**Figure 4**).

A sharp pain in the inflammation focus perceived by patients prior to the cryo-exposure therapy is arrested. Edema and hyperemia of the infiltrate that develop within hours after cryoablation disappear in the first 2–3 days. Necrotic tissue has an intense dark brown color, due to the admixture of ferromagnetic particles.

In the postoperative period, magnetic ointment should be replaced daily, simultaneously by applying magnetic fields to the focus of inflammation. The thin cryonecrotic layer is rejected within 7–10 days, depending on the area of cryonecrotized tissue.

During the *necrosis stage*, cryo-exposure is performed until the freezing zone is spread on the healthy tissue, then the edema of subcutaneous fat in the entire depth of the abscess is developed in 20–30 minutes. When swelling is observed below the focus of purulent inflammation, the pyogenic abscess is dissected. Pus and necrotic content are removed from the furuncle cavity by washing with 0.9% isotonic solution. Then, SMDF is injected in the abscess cavity with a syringe.

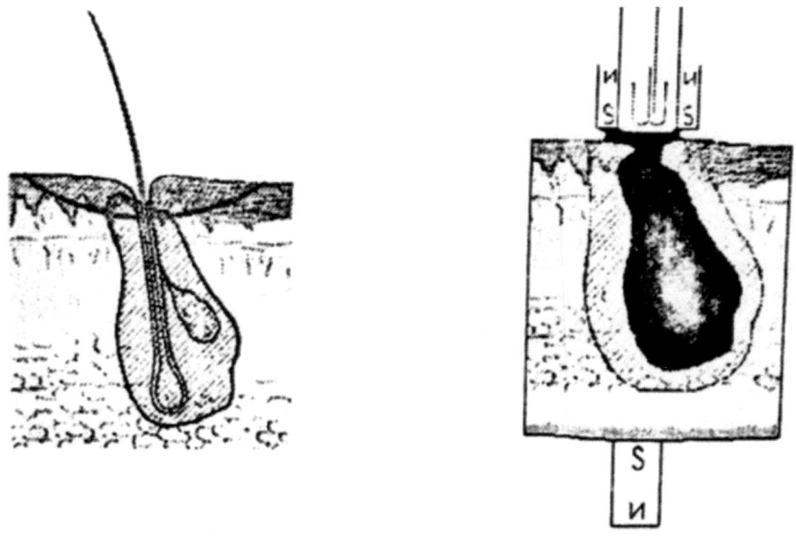

Figure 4. Spread of the freezing zone produced by the traditional cryoablation and by SMDF in a magnetic field.

Magnetic fields generated by the permanent magnets promote the maximum penetration of the ointment into the abscessed cavity. A cryoapplicator is brought into contact with a ferromagnetic ointment on the abscess surface and it starts cooling. Thus, the cavity is frozen inside by using SMDF as a thermally conductive material. At the same time, the effect of magnetic field should not be interrupted, in order to enhance thermal conductivity of the ointment.

In the postoperative period, most ointment is removed spontaneously together with the exudate. The ointment residues are removed from the abscess cavity with a cotton tampon and a permanent magnet, and then fresh ointment is introduced with a syringe. During the wound healing, ointment containing the antibacterial agent should be applied on the surface of the cryonecrotic tissue. As regeneration goes, the wound healing occurs by the day 7–10, without scar formation.

In the *open abscess stage,* the cavity is flushed with 0.9% aqueous solution of sodium chloride to evacuate necrotic masses, with the subsequent cavity filling by SMDF, performing cryo-exposure and maintaining the postoperative period in line with the above described procedure.

The experience of magnetic ointment applications proved that SMDF allows for establishing a tighter thermal contact between the cryo-instrument and the tissue, to accelerate cooling and increase its depth, due to higher thermal conductivity of SMDF, and to intensify frost penetration into the deep tissue, due to the active SMDF penetration into the pathological substrate.

Applying additional SMDF on the abscess surface in the postoperative period reduces the periods of moist and dry cryonecrosis, due to the stimulation of regenerative processes.

The postoperative use of magnetic ointment makes possible exclusion of systemic antibiotic therapy, eliminates formation of cosmetic defects on the skin and prevents the development of complications.

It is particularly important that the cryosurgical method using SMDF provides absolute elimination of pyogenic bacteria, particularly, methicillin-resistant *Staphylococcus aureus* (MRSA) resistant to traditional methods of antibacterial treatment.

6. Cryosurgical treatment for epithelial cysts

Epithelial cyst is a cavitary lesion developed from the epidermis; its capsule produces the mass filling of the cyst. Epithelial cysts of the skin are classified into several types depending on their microscopic structure: epithelial (epidermal), dermoid, and trichilemmal cysts.

Epithelial cysts are traditionally treated with surgical methods. Cystectomy implies the excision of the entire cyst capsule together with the intact surrounding tissue through cuts outside of the cyst. Under pyogenesis, the cyst is first subjected to oncotomy only and cystectomy is performed when inflammation decreases. This treatment leads to a cosmetic defect in the form of scar and pyogenesis poses another problem—completeness of the capsule removal, when its remains to create conditions for disease recurrence.

Cryosurgical treatment for epithelial cysts eliminates the occurrence of relapse and improves cosmetic result of the operation. A set of instruments for medical cryology suggested by Dr. V.I. Kochenov is intended for the efficient implementation of various techniques of deep local cryoablation of various cysts localized visually. Instruments and methods should be used differentially at different stages of the operation depending on the cyst size and its location/depth.

6.1. Cryo-exposure procedure

Prior to the start of cryo-exposure, the surgical field is treated with antiseptic and the skin is irrigated with 10% lidocaine solution.

For *cysts of less 8 mm in diameter*, with their content visible through the skin or mucosa, cryo-compression destruction is performed by capturing pathological tissue in the fold with cryo-grasp accumulators cooled passively in liquid nitrogen. After the first freeze cycle, the cyst cavity is perforated by a pointed cryostick cooled in liquid nitrogen during spontaneous thawing phase. In the next cryocompression freeze cycle, the cyst content should be evacuated by bringing together cryoaccumulators to the closest possible position. Thus, two freeze-thaw cycles are performed under tight pressing of collapsed cyst walls to each other and with the time of cryo-exposure equal to 3–5 seconds.

For *cysts of up to 1.5 cm in diameter* and transparent contents, cryodestruction with adhesion is performed with "Ledok" cryodevice with active supply of liquid nitrogen. The exposure is continued until the freezing zone extends 1–2 mm beyond the projection of the cyst diameter from all sides. During spontaneous thawing and some softening, a linear incision, 4–6 mm long, is performed with a scalpel, with penetration into the cyst cavity and its content is removed with a Volkmann spoon. Then a warm rounded applicator sized to the diameter of the cyst cavity is inserted through the produced hole, as if the cystic bag is put on the cryo-applicator. The operation is carried out in two to three freeze-thaw cycles, cryo-exposed for 5–10 seconds and under palpation control.

For *cysts of up to 1.5 cm in diameter* and nontransparent content, cryo-exposure is performed through applications with active cryoapplicator adhesion or by pulse cryo-irrigation onto the projection of the cyst center with 2–3 mm extension of the freeze zone beyond its borders. Without waiting for complete thawing, incision is made with a warmed scalpel (or focused radiation CO_2 of laser/RF scalpel) in the projected cyst center with penetration into the cavity, in order to evacuate its content during the thawing phase. In the process of thawing, the cyst is emptied and then dried. Next goes cryo-insufflation of the cavity using the cryo-spray device. Cryodestruction is completed by cryocompression freezing under tight pressing of the collapsed cyst walls. The exposure is continued until the freezing zone is established at 2–3 mm beyond the cyst borders.

For *cysts with a thin capsule* and provided that the rounded cyst shape is not regained after compression, the operation is finalized at this stage and pressure dressing is applied.

For *cysts with a dense capsule*, multidirectional cryo-irrigation is carried out within the cystic cavity prior to its icing. After thawing, a warm cryoapplicator with a protective insulating element with axial displacement is introduced into the cyst cavity. The free distal tip of the applicator is placed into contact with the cavity bottom and liquid nitrogen is applied briefly until adhesion appears. Then traction is performed with a cooled cryoapplicator in rotational clockwise motion, thus reaching full excision of the epithelial cyst capsule, and the operation is completed.

In the presence of inflammation or purulence, the cyst is dissected with a cryo stick chilled in liquid nitrogen, its content is evacuated, the cavity is washed with chlorhexidine 0.05% aqueous solution and dried. Then, a warmed "Ledok" cryoapplicator of the appropriate size and with active supply of liquid nitrogen is inserted into the cyst cavity and the cystic capsule is subjected to cryodestruction with adhesion, performing three freeze-thaw cycles, with an exposure time of 5–10 seconds and under palpation control.

When the cavity diameter is larger than the cryoapplicator, it is filled with the soft ferromagnetic heat-conducting ointment or gel (a 20% mixture of nano-ferromagnetic particles of carbon iron in antiseptic ointment or gel base) and then the applicator is dipped into it. A ring-shaped permanent magnet should be placed around the cyst projection. Freezing with adhesion is carried out until the freezing zone is spread 2–3 mm beyond the cyst capsule in all directions, in three freeze-thaw cycles.

When the cyst cavity diameter is much larger than the applicator, it should be moved with pressing to different sites of the walls until icing, in order to ensure at least triple freezing of each site of the cyst capsule and surrounding soft tissues.

Cryosurgical treatment for epithelial cysts allows to:

- guide surgical interventions directly onto the cyst projection and into its cavity, rather than around it, thus reducing the width of the surgical field and the incision;
- ensure radical treatment through the absolute destruction or complete and quality removal of the entire capsule;
- eliminate the cause of recurrence;
- perform cryo-exposure in a differentiated mode depending on the size, depth of the cyst location, as well as the capsule thickness;
- provide ice fixation of the cyst capsule at the moment of its dissection;
- prevent formation of a scar and cosmetic defects; and
- achieve the absolute elimination of pathogenic flora under inflammation and purulent dissolution of the cyst content, simultaneously with its removal.

Thus, cryosurgical treatment for epithelial cysts is acceptable both in non-inflammatory and purulent conditions. A thin cyst capsule is easily subjected to the total cryoablation, whereas thick capsules of larger cysts are better treated by cryo-excision. This technique allows for a radical treatment, which excludes relapse in the long term. In addition, cryosurgical treatment of epithelial cysts provides a good cosmetic effect. In the course of the epithelial recovery, the cryo-necrotic scab is rejected gradually layer-by-layer, without scarring.

7. Cryosurgical treatment for skin hemangiomas

Hemangioma is the most common benign tumor formed by blood vessels. This tumor develops, due to the unrestrained growth of defective blood vessels, which are arranged randomly, fail to perform blood circulation in tissues and organs, and form a tumor [1, 2].

The results of various treatments for skin hemangiomas are not always satisfactory for the patients and doctors. Relapses and cosmetic defects are observed commonly after the treatment.

Application of cryogenic treatment to skin hemangiomas was limited by the lack of adequate cryo-instruments needed for the effective cryoablation. The available cryogenic equipment was used in the treatment for extensive large hemangiomas located in the parenchymal organs, whereas there were no targeted developments for the treatment of cutaneous hemangiomas. Previously, application techniques were widely used for this purpose. However, recent developments made a step forward to the use of cryosurgical methods for treating skin hemangiomas of any localization and of different sizes.

The instrument, which proved the most optimal in cryosurgery of hemangiomas, was manufactured by the order of Cryology laboratory, Department of operative surgery and topographic anatomy, Nizhny Novgorod State Medical Academy, and was included in the Medical Cryology Set proposed by Dr. V.I. Kochenov [3].

The instrument is made of a metal alloy with high heat capacity allowed to be passively cooled in liquid nitrogen. It comprises movably connected jaws with ring-shaped handles; their working parts, from the place of joint to the distal tip, are made spatial, with the possibility of closing the working surfaces relative to each other. When closing, the outer surfaces of the jaws' working parts are oval-shaped; the distal tip is sharpened at an angle of 30–35° to the closing plane; the length of each is 30 mm (can range up to 40 mm). The greatest convex extension of jaws corresponds to the middle of the oval and makes $^1/_5$ of its length. Capillary slit-like grooves for penetration of liquid nitrogen are made in the deep working part of jaws and are directed to its distal parts. All instrument surfaces are polished.

7.1. Cryo-exposure procedure

When performing cryoablation, the internal surfaces of working parts of jaws act as applicators and the exophytic part of hemangioma is clamped between them. If the hemangioma is flat, i.e., is located deep in the skin, it is captured in a skin fold, so that the entire formation is fixed between the jaws and the slit grooves are directed up and down. Liquid nitrogen flows via grooves to the hemangioma and enhances freezing. When performing cryo-exposure, the hemangioma is compressed by $^1/_2$–$^1/_3$ of its diameter; then, it is slightly retracted and rotated to an angle of up to 45° to the skin surface. When the freezing zone is expanded to 5 mm beyond the perimeter of the tumor base, the contact is ceased and the instrument is removed. After complete spontaneous thawing of the hemangiomas, all manipulations are repeated thrice in the same order. After freezing of the hemangioma tissue, cryobiopsy for histological examination should be taken.

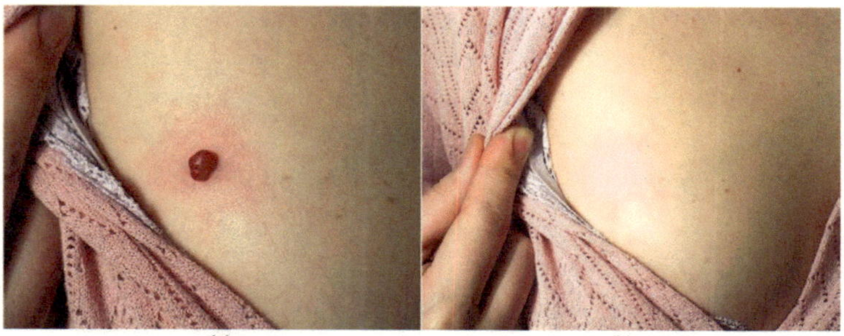

Figure 5. Hemangioma on the breast skin: (a) before and (b) after cryodestruction.

The time of cryo-exposure to liquid nitrogen may be different in each case; the average value is 60 seconds. All capillary skin hemangiomas of any location, sized up to 3 cm^2, regardless of their number, are recommended to cryo-exposure in a single session.

The advantages of cryosurgical treatment for hemangiomas are as follows:

- wide range of indications (no restrictions on age, number, location, size, and morphological type of hemangiomas);
- no limitations on the volume and number of hemangiomas subjected to simultaneous cryoablation; and
- good cosmetic results after treatment (rehabilitation of the normal skin color and structure without scarring and depigmentation). The outcome of treatment is presented in **Figure 5**.

8. Cryosurgical treatment for precancerous skin lesions

The term "precancer" was introduced by the French dermatology researcher N. Dubreuilh over a hundred years ago. This term denotes the processes that precede the development of a malignant tumor but not always result in cancer formation. Further in 1933, S.C. Becks suggested the division of precancerous conditions into the obligate and facultative.

Under obligate precancerous diseases, skin changes are characterized by the oppositional type of growth and their reverse development is not observed. In the current world literature, local malignant processes that do not spread beyond the skin cover are described commonly as carcinoma *in situ*.

Under facultative precancerous conditions, cornification of the mucous membrane and stromal inflammation are observed. The greatest significance in the genesis is attributed to the cell hyperplasia, which differs from regeneration by the fact that it goes beyond the physiological needs and transforms into dysplasia. Dysplasia has three stages—strong, medium, and weak; of those, the first represents a reversible process already with some signs of morphological anaplasia, the second comes close to a tumor, and the third sometimes cannot be distinguished from it. All these clinical signs should raise cancer alertness.

According to WHO experts, the recent and predicted increase in the incidence of malignant skin tumors is explained by the characteristics of the skin being the most exposed to unfavorable exogenous factors organ. The foci of superficial dyskeratosis very often contain human papillomavirus of strains HVP-16, HVP-31-35, HVP-51-54, and others. Histological examinations of precancerous skin lesions reveal inflammatory and hyperplastic processes.

The number of skin and mucosal tumors increases with high malignant potential and this confirms the current need in methodological improvements in early detection technologies, timely and adequate treatment of patients with visually localized tumors with a high tendency toward malignant transformation.

In this context, such advantages of cryosurgery as affordability, effectiveness, minimal invasiveness, possibility of geriatric application, ablastics, organotypic regeneration, as well as triggering the general immune-stimulating antitumor effect by preserving nativity of pathological protein and nucleic acid structures of the rejected tumor are particularly important.

Unlike the most common minimally invasive treatment techniques—electrocoagulation and laser destruction—cryoablation features the delayed necrosis development, which allows obtaining a section of the frozen, i.e., non-viable tissue suitable for morphological examination.

The antitumor immunostimulatory effect is triggered against the neoplasm subjected to cryoablation and preserved at the time of cryonecrosis formation. According to Dr. V.I. Kochenov, the effective induction of specific antitumor immunity is achieved by introducing a natural immune stimulation into the mechanisms of the general therapeutic and prophylactic antitumor effect during cryoablation.

However, cryoablation is often applied to neoplasms diagnosed by inspection only, without morphological examination. This situation complicates the problem of their quality treatment. In dermatology, morphological examination plays an important role in dyskeratosis diagnostics, whereas cancer diagnosis lacking morphological verification is considered nonvalid.

Special attention should be paid to the eczema-like skin lesions accompanied by itching, burning and pain, unevenly colored spots with scaling phenomena, focal plaques with moist velvety surface and areas of hyper- and hypopigmentation, focal changes with erosions, ulcerations and nodules, plaques covered with dry rough scales resembling psoriatic plaques, focal skin lesions with blurred contours, and a tendency to peripheral growth. Such focal transformations of the skin should never be subjected to an intervention without morphological diagnosis and they require radical treatment. Histological examination of these tissue fragments should be conducted after preliminary cryoablation.

The quality of histological examination, clinical and histological diagnoses, as well as selection of further treatment and the overall cosmetic result depend on a properly performed biopsy. However, the potential of morphological diagnosis for cryology is underutilized by dermatologists and cosmetologists. To solve this problem, cryodestruction should be combined with biopsy that would improve significantly the quality of diagnostics and treatment of precancerous skin conditions.

The temperature regimes of cryoablation are not yet standardized; the applicator's temperature ranges from −60 to −180°C in different devices, which affects the cryoablation quality and prevents comparing cryoablation results obtained for similar pathological changes by different authors. In some cases, treatment of precancerous skin conditions is attempted by applying cotton wool soaked in liquid nitrogen, despite the fact that this technique is inapplicable even for superficial therapeutic cryo-exposures, since the temperature in the contact zone (cotton-pathological tissue) does not fall below −20°C. Therefore, in cryosurgery of precancerous skin diseases, we need to find a way for standardization, in regard to the intensive destructive effect and visualization of the lowest temperature of cryoapplicator used for tumor destruction.

Another unresolved cryoablation problem is how to determine the completeness of cryo-destructive effect at early stages. Today, the completeness of cryo-destructive effect is most often determined visually by the presence of a tumor residue, 1–1.5 months after the full cryonecrosis rejection, which is absolutely unacceptable in case of malignant neoplasia. During the period of cryonecrosis rejection, the tumor can grow significantly and even spread metastases.

The current recommendation in cryosurgery is to achieve the expansion of the freezing zone 2.5 cm outside the visible tumor borders is only a safety net when the cryoapplicator in use has an insufficiently low temperature and contains no objective productivity criteria for cryo-destruction in any pathological focus. There are no available literature references about the early criteria for localization of the prospected cryonecrosis rejection line to be defined morphologically in the first days after cryodestruction.

To address these objectives and in order to improve the quality of treatment for precancerous skin diseases, the major conditions should be implemented:

- to develop visualized standardization for the intensity of cryogenic destruction of the pathological tissue; and
- to ensure monitoring of early adequacy of cryodestruction volume for various tumors, along with defining the projected borders of the deep cryonecrosis zone.

These objectives are achieved through the following steps. Cryoablation is performed in at least two freeze-thaw cycles with adhesion and cover all clinically defined tumor volume by the freezing zone. The working part of the instrument should be cooled to below −182°C, as can be evidenced by visible liquefaction of atmospheric oxygen fraction. The next step is excision of the pathological tissue for morphological examination within 6–12 hours after cryoablation. The fragment is removed with a warmed scalpel (or CO_2 laser, RF-scalpel) via oval cuts in the direction of possible infiltrative growth. The cut is made in a single block that includes the frozen tumor tissue and non-frozen ambient healthy tissues surrounding the freezing zone.

After that, local freezing for hemostasis is performed in the defected area of the tumor bed and then a series of column biopsies is carried out along the tumor radius line, in the direction of the most probable latent growth, with access to the clinically healthy tissue in depth and to the periphery.

Histological examination of the excised tissue fragments and in a series of column biopsies involves morphological identification of tumors and comparison between the boundary of pathological changes and the boundary of small blood vessels thrombosis on the surface and in depth. If the zone of pathological changes does not extend beyond the borders of thrombosis, the cryogenic destruction of a tumor is considered complete, otherwise additional, deeper and broader cryodestruction is performed and cryo-extirpation is applied to the transformed site. Additional cryodestruction is carried out in such a way that the freezing zone overlaps the borders of pathological changes identified by histological examination.

In 6–12 hours after additional cryodestruction, the tissue fragments are excised for repeated morphological examination using the same methodology as earlier. Then a series of biopsies is taken along the radius line of the tumor in the direction of the latent growth detected histologically, with access to clinically healthy tissues. After removing the column tissue fragment and if hemostasis is needed, cryo-exposure is performed inside the channel by cryo-insufflation or by inserting the cryoapplicator of appropriate diameter into the channel.

When the pathologically changed tissues are absent beyond the borders of thrombosis, cryodestruction is considered as radically complete. In the postoperative period, antiseptic care for the cryonecrosis zone is carried out until its rejection.

According to physics studies, the temperature of liquid oxygen is −182°C. The phenomenon of ambient oxygen liquefaction on metal objects cooled with liquid nitrogen occurs due to the difference between the temperature of liquid nitrogen (−196°C) and the temperature of oxygen liquefaction at normal atmospheric pressure. Physical and chemical experiments demonstrated that the atmospheric fraction liquefied passively with the most chilled instruments represents molecular oxygen.

The optimal time for histological sampling was identified by the experimental studies on animals with grafted skin tumors. It turned out that the minimum period for the emerging first signs of localization of the future demarcation line is 6 hours, and this sign is a line of ingression of solid thromboses in all blood vessels in the tissue. 12 hours is a period when necrotic changes do not complicate morphological identification of the tumor after cryoablation.

Moreover, the experiment shows that a clearly established border of the future cryonecrosis and tissue rejection at the border of solid thromboses occurs within the specified time period only after the most intensive applicative cryodestruction performed with adhesion and against the temperature of cryoapplicator, which visualizes the ambient oxygen liquefaction on the cryo-instrument. Cryodestruction performed at less values of negative temperatures does not provide a clear boundary for the future demarcation line in 6 hours and the cryonecrosis border does not coincide with the boundary lines for thromboses and freezing but lies within this zone, because cryoablation process at temperatures less than −182°C proves less effective.

The proposed cryosurgical method of treatment ensures the following positive effects:

- radical therapeutic effect for all precancerous diseases of visual localization;
- standardization of the most intensive destructive effect from cryoablation, due to the stabilization of the lowest temperature value for cryoapplicator;

- visualization of the lowest possible temperature on the cryo-instrument, under ambient conditions;
- emergence of a stable, well-defined under visual and histological examinations, change in the tissues, which coincides with the line of the future tissue rejection—solid thrombosis of small blood vessels that appears in a clearly defined time frame and depends on the intensity of cryoablation;
- simultaneously provided morphological verification of the diagnosis of skin tumor to be removed and the evaluation of radicality of cryogenic destruction;
- possibility to confirm the completeness of the destructive effect underway within the first day after cryoablation and to identify the need for additional cryogenic exposure;
- ensuring the absence of relapses, even in malignant tumors at early stages;
- robust hemostasis during manipulations; and
- histotypic tissue regeneration, without the formation of rough scar.

9. Cryo-circular excision in treatment of skin melanoma

Along with squamous cell and basal cell skin cancers, melanoma refers to the malignant tumors and represents one of the most dangerous skin cancers in humans, which is often recurrent and metastasizing into almost all organs via lymphatic and hematogenous pathways. Its characteristic feature is a weak or even absent response of the body, so melanoma often progresses rapidly [4–6].

In the opinion of medical cryology community of Nizhny Novgorod, the major advantages of cryosurgery are best manifested in treating the skin melanoma, such as ablastics, due to the tissue reactions that develop immediately after freezing (swelling around the focus with an increase in the interstitial pressure, lymphostasis, compression, and thrombosis of blood vessels), and feasibility of application in hard-to-reach areas of tumor location. Studies conducted by the national and foreign researchers have proved that cryogenic exposure creates conditions for rapid fixation of melanoma cells with their subsequent devitalization and thus can prevent the dissemination of tumor cells as much as possible [3, 7, 8]. The cryogenic method is a choice of priority in treating skin melanomas located in anatomically inaccessible places, such as the external ear, angle of eye, nose wing, etc., where traditional surgical intervention is associated with the formation of a cosmetic defect.

Diagnosing melanoma is distinguished by an absolute ban on aspiration, incisional or excisional biopsy. Such intervention gives an impetus to the intensive tumor growth, metastasizing, and hematogenous dissemination of the process [8–10]. In regard to melanoma, only complete removal within the healthy tissue is permissible, with subsequent histological examination. In all cases of the emerging pigmented skin tumor or rapidly changing pigmented formation against the absent clinical signs of cutaneous metastasis, diagnosis and treatment should be started with the cryogenic exposure. During this procedure, a column biopsy is taken and a part of pathological tissue is forwarded for complete morphological examination. Sampling for histological examination should include two tumor fragments—for urgent and routine examination. Such approach ensures the absolute ablasticity and high diagnostic accuracy, despite the conventional view that cryodestruction of melanoma is not applied, due to the impossibility to reliably determine the level of invasion into the underlying tissues [11].

One of the reasons for the unsuccessful radical cryodestruction of malignant tumors is the inclination to visually correlate the clearly defined (usually, ultrasonic-aided) freezing zone with a hypothetical tumor boundary. However, malignant tumors are distinguished from the benign ones by lacking clear boundaries. Variable prediction of tumor infiltrate boundaries is possible only at early stages, and they are highly individual for each type of a malignant tumor and its localization, which stipulates the urgent search for the boundaries of the latent spread of the primary focus of neoplasia. The computerized microdermoscopy systems available to date improve early melanoma diagnosis from 60 to 90%, but often under experimental conditions only. Therefore, if cryodestruction is applied solely with a radical purpose, even with localized, externally small malignant tumors, it should be performed within the frame of generally accepted rules of surgical radicality.

No less surprising is the faulty trend to issue indications for cryodestruction only after unsuccessful treatment outcomes from all other methods or during relapses. Obviously, combining radio- and chemotherapy technologies with cryodestruction are expedient in conditions of the disseminated process. Such combination has logic and sense when planning deep freezing of the entire neoplasm prior to radiotherapy, regional or systemic chemotherapy, since under this condition, cryodestruction brings the effect of potentiation and initially provides ablasticity to the whole treatment schedule.

A string requirement in applying the cryogenic method is the availability of appropriate cryo-applicators capable of creating complete and irreversible necrosis of the entire volume of tumor tissue within the surrounding healthy ones [3].

9.1. Cryo-exposure procedure

The most adequate instrument for deep freezing of the skin melanomas is an applicator with a ring-shaped working surface and an open tube mounted on it. The applicator is placed on the healthy tissue around the tumor. Cryodestruction is performed with a continuously cooled ring-shaped cryoapplicator until the freezing zone expands 1–2 mm beyond its boundaries. Deep cooling with adhesion allows for freezing melanoma with simultaneous and all-round preblocking of blood supply, which excludes mechanical contact with the tumor. The tube accelerates the freezing process, due to the simultaneous direct exposure of the exophytic part of the neoplasm to liquid nitrogen. Cryobiopsy is taken via the tube opening without breaking contact between the instrument and the frozen tissue.

When the diagnosis of skin melanoma is confirmed by the urgent histological test, cryolaser excision of the tumor is performed in a single frozen block. Focused radiation of the CO_2 laser is directed along the frozen tissue surrounding the applicator, preferably around −20°C isotherm. Additional cryo-irrigation along the incision line is carried out using "Ledok" apparatus. Such excision may also be performed using ЭХВЧ-500 electrosurgical apparatus (electrocautery). The control biopsy is taken from the sides and the bottom of the resultant wound defect, as well as around its circumference, stepping 0.5–2.5 cm from all sides (depending on the tumor thickness). The postoperative wound is closed in layers.

Application of this technique in patients with skin melanoma (operated using tumor cryofixation, cryobiopsy, and cryo-extirpation) can reduce significantly (twofold to threefold) the volume of surrounding healthy tissues removed during surgery, as compared with the traditional surgery. Another advantage of this technique is the fact that preradiation therapy is not required. When used properly, this technique demonstrates 100% 5-year survival rate of patients.

If the absence of metastases is confirmed, cryoablation may be applied without removing a single block of the frozen pathological tissue, in order to provide the immunostimulatory effect by prolonged preservation of the devitalized frozen tumor tissue in contact with the body. In such cases, a ring-shaped applicator or "Ledok" cryoapparatus (with nonvacuum cannula of 10–12 mm diameter, opened at the working end) are used.

To enhance heat transfer and encapsulation properties, magnetic gel is used in cryo-circular excision, applied as a sealing layer to the healthy skin at the site of the expected cryoapplicator placement and a ring-shaped magnet placed at the applicator. Radical cryoablation for the skin melanoma is performed in five to seven freeze-thaw cycles depending on the size of neoplasia.

When implementing cryoablation with "Ledok" device, a cotton ring impregnated with dimexidum 40% solution should be tightly placed around the applicator at the distal part of the cannula. This ring provides adhesion and, being passively soaked by the liquefied ambient oxygen flowing down along the cannula wall, represents an active cryoapplicator continuation when its temperature is stabilized at below −182°C, and surrounds gently the tumor tissue of any configuration.

At the first stage, the tumor is frozen up to its visible borders; then the cannula is warmed actively and retracted. After that, cryobiopsy is taken via a hole in the frozen cotton ring. Urgent morphological confirmation of the melanoma diagnosis qualifies for the extensive cryosurgery, upon the same methodology, providing a visible spread of the freezing zone beyond the tumor border not less than 1.5 cm in all directions, overlapped freezing zones and five to seven freeze-thaw cycles repeated for each point of the visible pathological tissue.

All manifestations of facultative precancerous skin diseases (in particular, all exophytic pigmented lesions) are subjected to cryoablation in the same or the next day.

At the stage of clearly marked demarcation line and gradual dehydration of the top cryonecrosis layer (3–5–7 days after the first cryoablation), cryo-destruction procedure is repeated, in order to accelerate mummification of the pathological tissue. It is preceded by the removal of exophytic part of cryonecrosis and repeated column cryobiopsy, multiple by the tumor radius, 1.0 cm indented from the primary focus to underlying healthy tissues (the first underlying fascia) is taken.

If foci of neoplasia are detected, additional cryodestruction of the tumor bed should be performed by the method of interstitial linear freezing with needle flow applicators or the cryolaser destruction is applied.

To evaluate the immunostimulatory therapeutic effect, we have examined the immunological status before and after treatment, once in every 2 months during the first year and once in every 3 months for 5 years starting from the second year. Humoral and cellular immunity was evaluated using monoclonal antibodies CD_3, CD_{16}, CD_4, CD_8, CD_4/CD_8.

Application of cryosurgical treatment for skin melanoma was accompanied by twofold increase of CD_4/CD_8, as compared with the baseline value; in 6 months, the CD_4/CD_8 level averaged 1.5 ± 0.2. Thus, the cryosurgical treatment provides an immunostimulating effect, while the consolidating effect lasts approximately 48 months, depending on the reactivity of the immune system.

It should be particularly noted that the mummified cryonecrosis sites on the skin larger than 4–5 cm^2 require active mechanical removal within 1–1.5 months after cryoablation, otherwise the epithelialization process is delayed and the dried cryonecrosis site displays itself as a foreign body, thus becoming an activator of the secondary inflammation. Complete rejection of the damaged melanoma tissue occurs within 2–3 months.

Filling the defect with local tissues or a displaced skin flap after cryo-circular excision of skin melanoma is not required. The retracted scar can remain in the cryoablation zone but it is incomparably smaller and has less cosmetic defect than that after traditional surgical excision of such tumor. Local recurrence is not observed provided that all requirements for this technique are met.

Specific features of the cryo-circular excision method for skin melanoma make it advantageous for outpatient practice of oncologists. The outcome of treatment is presented in **Figure 6**.

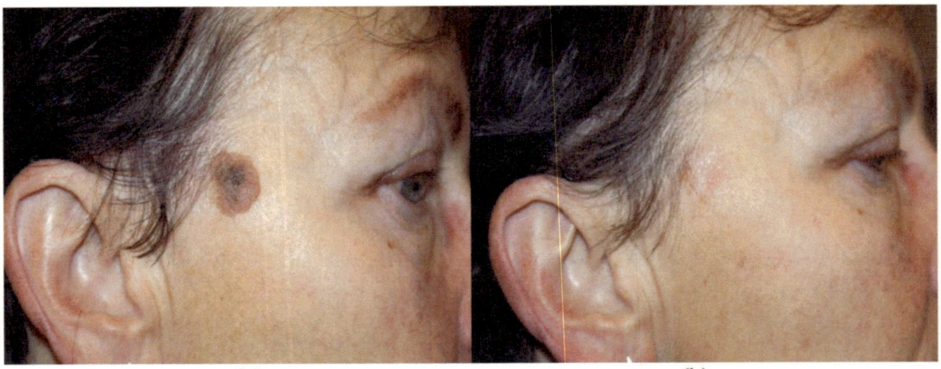

(a) (b)

Figure 6. Superficial spreading melanoma T_{3a} N_0 M_0 (stage IIA, according to AJCC classification): (a) before cryodestruction and (b) after cryosurgical treatment.

http://dx.doi.org/10.5772/intechopen.70509

10. Cryolipolysis

Cryolipolysis or cryo-liposuction is a method of cold destruction of adipocytes and the elimination of gynoid lipodystrophy. Current studies are aimed at determining the mechanism of cryolipolysis but the scientific evidence is still insufficient. At the meeting of the American Society for Laser Medicine and Surgery (ASLMS) in 2012, Dr. Christine C. Dierickx introduced the theory that decreasing temperature in the subcutaneous fat causes energy starvation in adipocytes, which triggers the process of programmed cell death followed by their excretion from the body via the blood and lymph. As the number of fat cells in the hypodermis reduces, its thickness declines from 20 to 25% in 2–3 months after the procedure. This explains the fact that the first result is obtained in a few weeks.

Today, the principle of cryolipolysis is implemented in CoolSculpting ZELTIQ (USA) equipment. This device is approved for use in the Russian Federation. The procedure can be performed on any part of the body except the face, neck, and décolleté. The main condition of the cryolipolysis procedure is the presence of the fat layer 1–2 cm thick. The major advantages of the cryolipolysis method are: liposuction performed without punctures and cuts; the absence of rehabilitation period; and painless procedure and minimum side effects. The indication for the procedure is the local destruction of the excessive fat deposits under obesity of various etiologies.

10.1. Cryo-exposure procedure

Before conducting cryolipolysis, the size and thickness of the fat fold is evaluated and an appropriate nozzle is selected depending on its thickness. Then, a gel is applied to the desired exposure area. A handpiece is placed on the exposure area and the skin fold together with subcutaneous fat is sucked into it. A vacuum is created. Cryo-exposure is performed for 60 minutes. The power and speed of exposure are controlled by the device software. To maintain the normal blood circulation in tissues, vibratory massage starts simultaneously with the local cooling.

After removing the applicator, the skin hyperemia in the "capture" area can be active and passive; its manifestations are terminated after 20–30 minutes. At that time, the patient can perceive chills and hypoesthesia of the skin surface subjected to cryolipolysis. These phenomena are terminated spontaneously within 20–30 minutes and they do not require medical correction.

Possible complications include persistent manifestations of venous hyperemia and prolonged hypoesthesia of the local skin area.

The result can be seen 4 weeks after the procedure. The amount of fat tissue in problem areas is reduced by 2–4 cm in volume. The thickness of the fat fold is reduced by 3–5 cm. As a rule, three to four treatment sessions of 1 hour each are needed for the maximum effect 3 months after conducting cryolipolysis.

The most significant disadvantages of this method are: high cost of the procedure; delayed result; low efficiency in slack skin; one-step reduction of adipose tissue can be performed only for one area of the body; destruction of the excess fat deposits is possible on the localized areas only; a wide range of contraindications for cryolipolysis procedure: obesity grade II and III; electric cardiac pacemaker in the body; pregnancy and lactation; vascular diseases; blood diseases; renal and hepatic failure; diabetes; and Raynaud's syndrome.

Thus, the advantages of the local cryolipolysis method compare poorly with its disadvantages against the wide range of contraindications and a number of significant drawbacks, which sharply limit the implementation of this method into wide practice.

11. Treatment for hypertrophic scars

Reparative processes (postsurgery, or after thermal, chemical, or mechanical injury) that take place in the skin and develop against disturbed local processes of proliferation and differentiation, with an excessive growth of scar tissue, result in the formation of a keloid or a hypertrophic scar.

Hypertrophic scars expand up to 3 mm above the skin surface. The scar growth is initiated immediately after healing, which distinguishes it from keloids. The color of hypertrophic scars may be of pinkish or reddish shade. A mature hypertrophic scar ceases its growth and turns pale within the same time interval as a normotrophic scar. The primary clinical sign of keloid scars (or keloids) is their capacity for continuous growth. Regardless of the scar age, keloids can be active (proliferating) and inactive (stabilized), with alternating periods of rest and of increased growth. An active scar elevating above the level of the skin considerably, becomes palpably dense and red with a cyanotic shade. Keloids and hypertrophic scars can appear not only from the skin injury but also from the resolution of certain dermatoses. The incidence of keloid and hypertrophic scarring, complexity, and duration of their treatment, as well as predisposition to relapse determine the urgency of the problem considered in this monograph.

Emergence of the posteruptive keloids and hypertrophic scars at the sites of resolved acne is not uncommon. A number of authors mention that this cosmetic defect leads to psychoemotional disadaptation of patients manifested by a decreased self-esteem, various psychological, and in some cases, psychosomatic disorders. Therefore, elimination of cosmetic defects plays an important role in the social and interpersonal adaptation of such patients.

Multiple attempts to find a method for effective scar correction were undertaken throughout the twentieth century. The most significant and numerous were the methods concerned with the local influence upon the excessive keloid tissue. Thus, the core of the problem lies in the frequent scar recurrence after their "successful" elimination at the sites of primary occurrence, rather than the lack of methods for their destruction or removal. Despite the extensive armamentarium of surgical, radiotherapy, and medication treatment methods, the proportion of recurrence remains quite high, since none of the suggested methods suppresses keloid growth zones, as evidenced by a number of studies.

http://dx.doi.org/10.5772/intechopen.70509

Keloid and hypertrophic scars bear clinical similarities but differ by their morphology and pathogenetic mechanisms of development. The major differences relate to the structure of the microvasculature, type of collagen that forms connective tissue, cellular composition, and the structure of intercellular substance [12].

The presence of immature connective tissue is typical for keloid scars; it is characterized by an increased content of hyaluronic acid and collagen type III, both possessing high hydrophilic properties. Poorly differentiated (immature) cells, juvenile and atypical giant fibroblasts are predominant. "Young" and "old" keloid scars also have morphological differences. The structure of a "young" keloid is characterized by the presence of four zones: epidermis, subepidermal zone, growth zone, and deep zone. The growth zone represents keloid tissue. This is a young connective tissue, where numerous young fibroblasts are identified, 92 ± 35 cells in the visual field. The presence of giant forms of fibroblasts is typical. The deficit of blood capillaries was detected (0–1 capillary in 1–3 visual fields) in the "young" keloid tissue. "Old" keloids are characterized by the appearing signs of maturation. The growth zone is partially reduced, fibrosis increases, the number of fibroblasts declines and vascularization expands (0–3 capillaries in a single visual field), and the zones of dystrophic and necrotic modifications emerge. At the same time, the signs of activity (foci of young connective tissue) are present.

Hypertrophic scars have another morphological structure. The zones of epidermis and scar tissue are identified there. The number of fibroblasts is less than that in keloid tissue (59 ± 2 in the visual field), with the predominance of mature forms. Vascularization in the hypertrophic scar tissue is increased (3–5 capillaries in the visual field), which determines the biosynthetic activity of mature fibroblasts and the excessive growth of collagen type I.

In this aspect, the cryogenic method of scar treatment is the most advantageous, because the mechanism of cryogenic destruction is correlated with the specifics of subsequent reparative processes in tissues. The treatment for hypertrophic scars is targeted at microcirculatory vessels of the skin, and for keloids—at both the capillaries and the hydrophilic immature connective tissue, rich in fibroblasts that are extremely sensitive to ultra-low temperatures.

Thus, the mechanism of local cryo-exposure is justified pathogenetically and includes two stages. At the first stage, the cells are destroyed directly through the action of ultra-low temperatures, while at the second, destruction of tissues occurs, due to hemodynamic disturbance.

The morphological study of cryobiopsy samples taken from scar tissue 30 minutes after the three-cycle cryo-exposure demonstrated the presence of degenerative changes in all zones, including the growth zone. Fibroblasts had necrotic modifications and the blood capillaries were under destruction. The microhemodynamics blockade increases destructive changes in the tissue. The study of scar tissue samples collected after cryogenic exposure indicates that this method allows to completely destroy the mass of scar tissue (keloid or hypertrophic scar). This is evidenced by the destruction of microcirculatory vessels and the total necrosis of fibroblasts identified in all areas of the keloid scar and in the hypertrophic scar tissue. In 3–4 months, a regenerate is formed at the site of the former scar, which has the appearance of a normal skin and the structure similar to that of organotypic regenaration.

11.1. Cryo-exposure procedure

Prior to performing cryodestruction, we determined the linear dimensions and the projected area of the scar, as follows. First, he colorant was applied to the skin surrounding the scar deformation using the coloring rod. Then the scaled millimeter paper was imposed on the stained surface in such a way that one of the mapping directions coincided with the greatest length of the scar. Linear dimensions were determined on the obtained imprint, according to the millimeter grid, as the distance between the two most distant points located on the long axis of the unstained spot and the length of the perpendicular to this axis corresponding to the scar section in the region of its greatest width. In case the scar is not stretched relative to the skin surface, its diameter is taken as its linear dimension and the scar area is calculated by the formula:

$$S = a + b/2 \quad (1)$$

where, S is the area of pathologically modified skin site, a is the number of totally unstained millimeter squares within the unstained spot, b is the number of partially unstained millimeter squares within the unstained spot.

At first glance, this step may seem tedious and useless but actually it has great practical importance for the choice of cryodestruction method. Treatment for keloid and hypertrophic scars should involve a sufficiently deep cryogenic destruction of pathological tissue and be always accompanied by the subsequent formation of multiple vesicles and/or bullae at the site of exposure.

When the scar area is up to 20 mm², cryo-exposure without adhesion is applied by cryoinstruments chilled passively or actively, by smoothing the scar surface and stopping the applicator for 2–5 seconds at each site.

When the scar area is 20–35 mm², a stepwise freezing of the entire scar surface is applied by touching it with a drop of atmospheric oxygen passively liquefying on the lateral side of the non-thermally insulated cannula and flowing down to the "Ledok" cryoapplicator.

When the scar area is 35–55 mm², a prolonged exposure is applied, a slow rolling of the cotton wool tampon with braided mesh-like surface, chilled in liquid nitrogen, along the scar until a stable, visible for 4–5 seconds freezing of the scar tissue occurs.

When the scar area is over 55 mm², a prolonged cryo-irrigation with liquid nitrogen is applied until a stable, visible for 5–10 seconds, icing of the entire scar surface occurs, with two to three iterations of freeze-thaw cycle at each site during one procedure.

When scar deformities are extensive, a combination of methods is recommended. In order to smooth the surface of atrophic scar, cryotherapy with liquid nitrogen is performed as topical applications.

Along with the destruction of hypertrophic and keloid tissues, cryo-exposure aids in restoration of skin sensitivity and elimination of functional disorders caused by pathological scars.

http://dx.doi.org/10.5772/intechopen.70509

In this case, the effect is determined by a direct damage to pathological cells and modified microcirculation under the influence of extremely low temperatures.

In conclusion, it needs to be emphasized that four main goals should be pursued in developing the plan and schedule for keloid and hypertrophic scar treatment: functional rehabilitation of the affected anatomical segment, reduced manifestation of local symptoms, improved esthetic appearance and prevention of relapse. The absence of a relapse within 2 years represents a guarantee of successful treatment.

12. Treatment for acne

Acne is a polymorphic disease and one of the most common skin dermatoses with characteristic clinical manifestations in the form of non-inflammatory (open and closed comedones) and inflammatory (papules, pustules, nodes) elements. The lesions are mainly localized in seborrheic zones: face, neck, shoulders, chest, and upper back.

Consensus conference organized in 1990 by the American Academy of Dermatology (AAD) discussed the challenges of developing a standardized and reproducible system for acne classification, with special reference to high polymorphism of lesions, diverse combinations of acne elements, variability in the course of the disease, severity and density of inflammatory lesions at different localizations in the same patient. In accordance with the AAD recommendations adopted in 1991, grading acne severity is evaluated by the number and nature of lesions, distinguishing between the mild, moderate, severe and very severe grades. However, the lack of precise quantitative gradation complicates their practical application. According to the classification adopted at the 20th World Congress of Dermatology [13], acne disease is classified into the mild, moderate and severe grades, where the comedonal and papulopustular (up to 10 elements) forms are referred to as "mild," papulopustular (more than 10 papulopustules and up to 5 nodes) and nodular (more than 5 nodes)—to "moderate," and the abscessed and conglobate forms—to "severe" grade.

Despite the large number of dedicated studies, acne still persists as the most common dermatoses in young people. The most widespread clinical variety is *acne vulgaris,* which peaks at the age of 14–17 years old. This draws special attention to the treatment of this dermatosis in adolescents. By quoting Sulzberger [14], "There is probably no other disease that causes more mental stress, misunderstanding between children and parents, the greater overall lack of self-confidence, as well as a lot of mental suffering, as acne," we can unhesitatingly agree that this statement reflects expressively the problems of relationship between the acne and the psyche.

With view of such facts that lesions are localized on the face skin and that the face represents the major link in interpersonal communication, there is no doubt that acne affects the emotional status of any patient. Hautmann and Panconesi [15] refer the acne to the group of dermatoses, which trigger somatopsychic resonance due to the actual or perceived esthetic discomfort. Both Russian and foreign researchers indicate that skin problems, if accompanied by psychological fixation on the disease, come as a psychotraumatic factor. Thus, acne has a negative effect on self-esteem and self-perception of patients, interpersonal interactions, and social functions.

These observations demonstrate the formation of such patterns as avoidance behavior, social phobias, anxiety, depression, sensitive reactions, hypochondriacal disorders, suicidal thoughts and attempts, due to acne. The authors agree unanimously that all mental disorders developing against acne cause maladaptation in the social, professional, family life and are able of disrupting compliance with the treatment for skin pathology.

The study performed by Volkova and Glazkova [16] involved collection, interpretation, and integration of clinical data derived from the patients' communications and observations of specialists. Their findings indicate that the overall prevalence of anxiety-depressive mental disorders among outpatients with diagnosed acne amounts to 35.2%, of which anxiety makes 24.2%, depression—26.2%, and mixed anxiety-depressive disorder—43.74%, respectively. Anxiety-depressive disorders reduce greatly the quality of life in patients suffering from acne. The linkage between the Dermatology Life Quality Index (DLQI), Assessment of the Psychological and Social Effects of Acne (APSEA) and mental disorders reflects the relationship between the skin processes and the development of anxiety and depression. Moreover, the objective status of a patient does not necessarily coincide with his/her subjective perception of this disease. Welp and Gieler [17] confirmed this statement in their experimental study by observing patients with a pronounced discrepancy between the objective picture of the disease diagnosed by the physician and the subjective severity of mental suffering.

Moreover, as noted by Bosse and Hunecke [18], the subjective severity of suffering is affected by such factors as localization and visibility, chronic course and skin changes, gender and age, complaints against personal looks, and self-esteem. The subjective perception of ugliness can reduce self-esteem until the paranoid reevaluation the disease's significance. Due to the revaluation of the somatic phenomenon, the person becomes morose, minimizes communication with surrounding people and tries to avoid external contacts, up to the social isolation. According to Bosse [19], a patient with skin disease is granted only a limited approved social right to make claims; the author calls it "the hypothesis of non-fastidiousness." The role of negative evaluation of one's subjective attractiveness is described in a large number of works, which can be summarized vividly by Bosse's [20] quotation: "Pimples on the face – scars on the soul." Cases of dysmorphophobia are common even with the minimal acne lesions.

Resolution of dermatosis is often accompanied by the development of persistent posteruptive keloid and/or hypertrophic, atrophic scars, which leads to an uneven skin texture. At the same time, postinflammatory pigmentation disorders make common cases with acne. Emergence of the secondary persistent dyschromia is observed at the sites where dermatosis elements were resolved. Melanin hyperchromia, or local hypopigmentation, in combination with posteruptive scars, makes a persistent cosmetic defect. Acne disturbs the esthetic effect of the skin and thus has a pronounced effect on the psycho-emotional sphere of the patient and his/her social adaptation. This determines the urgency of developing new adequate treatment modalities for acne to address effectively the healthcare and social problems. Undoubtedly, all the above mentioned factors underline the need for a novel method of treating acne with a good cosmetic effect, to ensure the esthetic comfort and recover the psychoemotional health. Moreover, treatment should be a short-term and highly effective, in order to avoid psychosocial consequences.

Several important factors are identified in the pathogenesis of acne: hyperplasia and hyperfunction of sebaceous glands, follicular hyperkeratosis, microbial colonization, and inflammation of the sebaceous gland. Inflammation can be both superficial and deep, which brings about a variety of clinical manifestations. A vast number of national and international works is devoted to studying skin micro-landscape in patients with acne. In 1983, V.M. Kovalev studied the microflora of acne elements; 668 strains were isolated and identified, where staphylococci communities and *St. aureus* strains prevailed. This was apparently associated with the presence of excoriations in the area of localized pathological elements, which preconditions higher *St. aureus* incidence under this pathology. Microbial associations were found to be inoculated more often than monocultures. To date, it is commonly believed that acne is closely associated with the excessive colonization of the skin and its appendages by *Propionibacterium acnes (R. Acnes*), the dominating follicular resident organism. There exist other opinions but these are in minority.

Given the key role of pathogenic microorganisms in the pathogenesis of acne, the applied treatment modalities become obvious.

Antibiotics have been used for over 40 years until now and they represent a fundamental part of modern acne therapy, as confirmed by the recommendations of the International Union of Acne Treatments (Paris, 2002). The limiting factor to the topical antibacterial therapy is its time length. A lasting positive effect can be achieved only when applied permanently for 4–6 months, because such medications should exercise their curative effect through several periods of the epithelial renewal. Unfortunately, these terms of use involve a high risk of developing resistance. According to Kar [21], the first clinically significant changes in *P. acnes* sensitivity were found in the USA in the late 1970s. Later, in the late 1980s- early 1990s, the comprehensive studies revealed clinically significant resistance to antibiotics and identified strains with multiple antibiotic resistance, as reported by Del Rosso [22]. Moreover, Rivera [23] emphasized that resistance was developed not only by the skin surface bacteria but also microbial populations in the nasal cavity, which is a permanent reservoir of microflora and can reduce the effectiveness of antibiotic therapy. Kirichenko [24] pointed out the fact that microorganisms are characterized by natural and acquired resistance to antibiotics; they survive successfully and retain their virulence, especially in microbial associations. Eady [25] emphasized that patients with developed resistance to local forms of antibiotics were also unresponsive to systemic antibiotic therapy. Moreover, it should be kept in mind that prolonged use of topical broad-spectrum antibiotics can lead to the appearing gram-negative rods on the facial skin that are uncharacteristic of its natural microflora and can eventually result in the development of gram-negative folliculitis, untreatable by traditional methods.

Despite the available abundance of antibacterial drugs, all those have diverse side effects. We will not list in detail the side effects that occur during systemic antibiotic therapy. The most significant complications, such as dysbiosis of various localization, hepatotoxicity, hematologic reactions, or toxic epidermal necrolysis are known to every physician since student's years. When appointing a certain drug to the patient, a full list of complications and contraindications can be viewed in the national medication registry.

Here, we will only mention that many antibacterial preparations included in the standard treatment plans cause photosensitization and, therefore, an increased risk of dermatoses based on photodynamic reactions. In addition, there is a high risk of medical melanodermia, against the prolonged intake of drugs with pigment-forming properties, which presents an additional cosmetic problem. Moreover, antibiotic treatment can be considered as a major risk factor for scarring, especially in the presence of papules or pustules, since antibiotics trigger the intensified scarring processes in the lesions.

Burkhart and Gottwald [26] indicated the need to develop new technologies in acne treatment aimed at minimizing the use of antibiotics and thus to prevent the development of microflora resistance. We fully share the opinion stated by Zainullina [27] concerning the modern demand for a totally new approach to the effective treatment of various forms of acne.

In 2009, by the decision of the Global Alliance for the Treatment of Acne (GA), retinoids were introduced into the list of drugs of the first choice, in addition to topical antibiotics. The adverse effects of retinoid therapy include xerophthalmia, conjunctivitis, cheilitis, irritative dermatitis, skin xerosis, erythema, nasal hemorrhage, pyogenic granuloma, impetigo, allopathy, Achilles tenosynovitis, hyperostosis, myalgia and arthralgia, hepatotoxicity, neutropenia, benign increased intracranial pressure. However, the most significant complication is teratogenicity. According to Racine [28], 50% of pregnant women under isotretinoin treatment developed grave intrauterine fetal anomalies in the first trimester of pregnancy including pathologies of the cardiovascular system, central nervous system, skeleton and sensory organs.

A trend towards increasing resistance of etiologically significant microorganisms to basic antibiotics used in the standard treatment regimens determines the urgent imperative to find the effective acne treatment. Treatment of various clinical forms of acne is still a challenge, despite the already available algorithms and protocols for patient management. Thus, for example, the effectiveness of antibiotic therapy depends not only on sensitivity, but also on the ability of medications to be delivered to the target organ. Poor skin permeation presents a limiting factor for some antibiotics that have proven high sensitivity of pathogenic microflora. In addition, it is established that *P. acnes* secretes glycocalyx biofilms impermeable to antibiotics. For this reason, topical medications are applied mostly as components of fixed dose combination. Recommendations of the European Dermatology Forum (EDF) for the treatment of acne (2011) emphasized the fundamental importance of combined therapeutic approach to all pathogenetic components in the topical acne treatment, taking into account full diversity of pathogenetic factors.

Resistance of various groups of microorganisms to antimicrobial drugs stated in the treatment algorithms has been studied extensively since 1979 by Russian and foreign authors. Their findings demonstrated the general long-term trend toward increasing resistance of the main microbial agents of pathogenetic significance to the basic antibiotics. Development of resistant strains and, consequently, reduced effectiveness of antibacterial treatment determine the need for monitoring the microflora of skin biota, together by identifying the sensitivity of cause-significant groups of microorganisms to antibacterial drugs. There is no possibility to perform antibiotics sensitivity tests in routine clinical practice. In this regard, new approaches to the treatment of acne are needed, which would prevent the emerging resistance in cause-significant microorganisms.

The complex nature of pathogenesis dictates the need to affect all pathogenic factors of acne, particularly for local therapy, as confirmed by the EDF recommendations (published in 2016), which reaffirmed the importance of combined therapeutic approach to all pathogenetic components in the topical acne treatment.

However, cryotherapy fully meets all these requirements. We have considered the opinion of Konchugova [29] and developed a non-drug technology for the treatment of acne. The therapeutic effect is based on the normalized microflora of the facial skin and its appendages, improved microcirculation in the foci of dermatosis, eliminated follicular hyperkeratosis, and improved sebum evacuation. Local cryo-exposure causes the destruction of differentiated keratinocytes, intensifies desquamation of epidermal corneocytes and facilitates exfoliation of the epidermis.

The species composition of microbial community and the antibiotic sensitivity of its dominant component can be analyzed endlessly. We have already mentioned the vast amount of relevant studies, which bring only one conclusion – the increasing resistance of microbial associations to the antibiotics. For this reason, we did not investigate the facial microbial landscape with the subsequent determination of antibiotic sensitivity. Sharing the opinion of E. Rivera, we studied the antimicrobial effectiveness of cryotherapy on microbial populations in the nasal and oral cavities under the ENT pathology. Our findings were published in a number of other papers and here we would only notice that there are no microorganisms or microbial associations that are insensitive to ultra-low temperatures.

Skin smoothness was evaluated by the computer analysis of facial skin replicas in patients with severe late acne after cryogenic treatment and in similar patients after traditional treatment. A silicone-based replica reflects all irregularities of the skin microrelief. According to our results, it can be stated unequivocally that cryogenic treatment for acne smoothes the skin micro-relief considerably, thus improving greatly the esthetic posttreatment effect on the facial skin. Due to the labor-intensive process of manufacturing skin replicas, the analysis of images obtained directly with high-resolution digital cameras has become very popular in today's practice.

Evaluation of the immune status in patients with moderate to severe acne prior to treatment demonstrated a decrease in the absolute content of CD3, CD4, CD8, and an increase in CD72. A decrease in the relative and absolute content of T suppressors with the CD4 + and CD8 + markers, B-lymphocytes with the CD72 + marker was characteristic of the patients with papulopustular form. In some cases, a decrease in the absolute content of the total T-lymphocytes with a CD3 + marker and T-helpers with the CD4 + marker was found against the normal values of the total leukocyte and lymphocyte counts.

The immunomodulating effect of cryo-exposure on parameters of the cellular and humoral components of immune system was translated into an increase of conventionally low baseline values for the absolute content of lymphocyte subpopulations with CD4+, CD8+, CD72+ markers and IgA serum content. In patients with low baseline levels, there was a trend towards an increase in CD4+, CD8+, CD16+, and a substantial increase in CD72+, IgA and IgG in the blood. As regards the humoral component of immune system, IgA and IgG concentrations significantly decreased and IgM concentration increased; these parameters were in direct correlation with CD 72. IL-1 concentration in the blood of patients with acne increases with the increasing disease severity and is increased twice under "severe" grade. These disturbances indicate the inhibition of innate and adaptive immunity and the depletion of reserve capacity of the body.

12.1. Cryo-exposure procedure

Our practice of cryogenic treatment for acne relies upon the AAD classification (modified Russian version), which enables the most adequate selection of the tentative cryo-exposure method:

- Grade I is characterized by the presence of comedones (open and closed) and up to 10 papules;
- Grade II is characterized by the presence of comedones, papules, and up to 5 pustules;
- Grade III is characterized by the presence of comedones, papulo-pustular rash, and up to 5 nodes;
- Grade IV is characterized by a pronounced inflammatory reaction in the deep dermal layers, along with soreness and ulceration, formation of fistulae and nodulocystic elements.

Inverse acne (*acne inversa*), conglobata-cystic acne (*acne conglobate*), and resistant acne are subjected to cryogenic treatment in line with our method developed for the Grade IV acne severity, according to the above classification. To implement these techniques, we use a set of instruments for medical cryology developed by Dr. V.I. Kochenov. Prior to the start of cryo-exposure, the facial skin is wiped with a cotton tampon moistened with 3% salicylic acid alcohol solution and a drop of 10% glycerol solution is applied to each acne element. Given the high polymorphism of lesions, diverse combinations of acne elements, and to improve the effectiveness of treatment, we apply a combination of cryogenic methods.

Acne severity Grades I and II: cryodestruction of each acne element with cryostick chilled in liquid nitrogen. Cryo-exposure is continued until the complete icing of the pathological element. Each cryo-manipulation consists of three freeze-thaw cycles. Then, a prolonged cryo-exposure is performed by rolling a cotton wool tampon with a woven mesh surface, cooled in liquid nitrogen, over the entire face skin (and/or other site with signs of dermatosis), until a stable, persistent for 4–5 seconds, visible freezing track occurs.

Grade III: cryo-irrigation with liquid nitrogen of each acne-element using a nozzle for interstitial linear freezing, until a stable, visible for 5–10 seconds icing of the entire surface of the pathological element occurs, with two to three iterations of the freeze-thaw cycle at each site during one procedure.

This is followed by the facial cryomassage (and/or other site with signs of dermatosis), according to the technique described above.

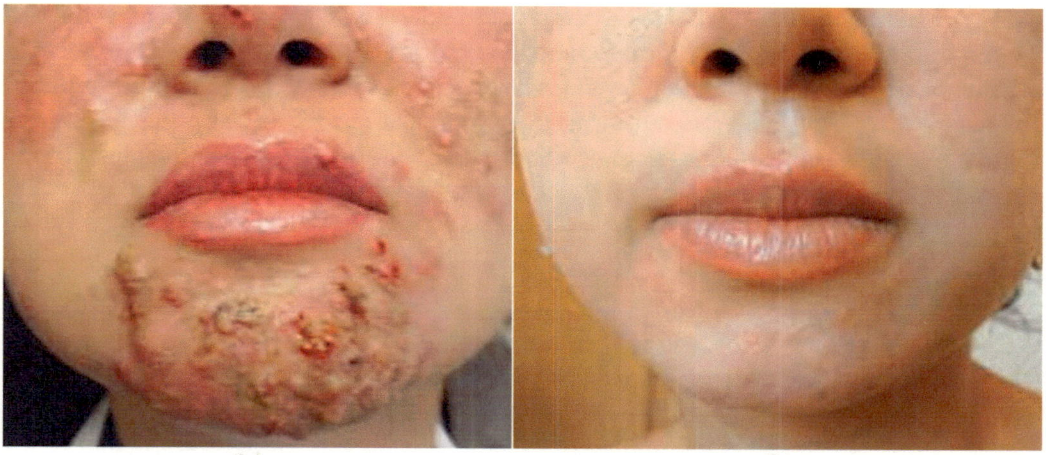

(a) (b)

Figure 7. Facial skin in a female patient with acne disease, severe grade (a) before and (b) after completed treatment course.

Grade IV: consecutive freezing of pathological acne elements by applying a drop of atmospheric oxygen liquefied passively on a cannula (4 mm), using "Ledok" cryoapparatus with an oval pointed applicator. Each acne element is subjected to cryo-exposure three times. Then, cryomassage of facial skin (and/or other site with signs of dermatosis) is performed with a roller cooled in liquid nitrogen, until a visible white freezing trace is formed.

Our treatment method for *provoked acne* (*acne artificialis*, acne mechanica, acne venenata, contact acne, acne toxica, acne de la brilliantine, acné excoriée des jeunes filles) and Gram-negative folliculitis involves topical application using an applicator with the meshed-cellular elastic surface, 7–10 cm long, fixed to the handle. The applicator is moistened with liquid nitrogen, placed parallel to the treated surface and is slid in continuous rotational movements, under light pressure from the operating hand, over the affected surface until the minute skin whitening is formed.

Cryo-sessions are conducted once or twice per week. Depending on the acne severity, the course includes 10–15 procedures.

Cryogenic treatment for acne affects successfully three key components of pathogenetic significance through normalizing the sebum evacuation and destroying microbial associations and thus it arrests inflammation. At the same time, cryo-exposure triggers a pronounced immunomodulatory effect. The clinical effectiveness of cryotherapy is translated into the shorter time of treatment, the longer remission period, as well as the prevention of posteruptive scarring and persistent dyschromia.

Its high efficiency is based on the marked compensation of the initial microcirculatory disturbances and the immunocorrecting effect on both the cellular and humoral immunity, which is manifested in the normalized ratio of immunoregulatory subpopulations of T-lymphocytes, increasing their functional activity, and recovery of serum immunoglobulins A and G up to their normal level. Moreover, ultra-low temperatures destroy melanocytes, thereby preventing traumatic pigmentation and local melanodermy. Additionally, the obtained morphological data prove that cryodestruction provides an effective treatment method for posteruptive keloids and hypertrophic scars, ensuring their complete destruction and the subsequent skin regeneration, similar to that organotypic regeneration. The outcome of treatment is presented in **Figure 7**.

13. Conclusion

Dermatoses, in particular, acne and psoriasis, can provoke sensitive reactions and hypochondriac disorders. Obviously, formation of secondary (in relation to the somatic pathology) mental disorders depends on a number of social and demographic factors, specifics of the primary disease, and premorbid properties of the person, but eventually they only emphasize the significance of this problem. In addition, the internal picture of the disease, as the major complex of secondary psychological symptoms, can complicate the course of the disease in certain cases, hinder the success of therapeutic measures, and slow down the rehabilitation. Treatment for dermatoses is in need and the effective treatment is in double need. Treatment of all dermatological pathologies can not be described just in one chapter and for this reason the priority was given here to the most common dermatoses. Our current work includes development of a guideline for physicians "Cryogenic treatment methods in dermatology" (the tentative title).

Author details

Tatyana Gennadyevna Kotova[1*], Sergei Nikolaevich Tsybusov[2], Vladimir Ivanovich Kochenov[3] and Maksim Igorevich Tcyganov[1]

*Address all correspondence to: 261126.79@mail.ru

1 Scientific Clinical Center of Medical Cryology "OnKolor", Nizhny Novgorod, Russia

2 Nizhny Novgorod State Medical Academy, Scientific Research Institute of Applied and Fundamental Medicine, Nizhny Novgorod, Russia

3 Nizhny Novgorod State Medical Academy, Nizhny Novgorod State Medical Academy, Scientific Clinical Center of Medical Cryology "OnKolor", Nizhny Novgorod, Russia

References

[1] Burrows PE, Mason KP. Percutaneus treatment of low flow vasculae malformations. Journal of Vascular and Interventional Radiology. 2004;**1**(5):431-445

[2] Chen H, Lin X, Jin Y, et al. Patients with intralesional hemonhage in venous malformations: Diagnosis and embolosclerotherapy. Journal of Vascular Surgery. 2009;**49**(2):429-433

[3] Kochenov VI. The future of the cryogenic treatment method. Medical Cryology. – Nizhny Novgorod. 2001;**7**(1):200-205 (in Russian)

[4] Algazi AP, Soon CW, Daud AI. Treatment of cutaneous melanoma: Current approaches and future prospects. Cancer Management and Research. 2010;**2**:197-211

[5] Besser MJ, Treves AJ, Itzhaki O, et al. Adoptive cell therapy for metastatic melanoma patients: Pre-linical development at the Sheba Medical Center. Israel Medical Association Journal. 2006;**8**(3):164-168

[6] Dummer R, Robert C, Chapman PB, et al. AZD6244 (ARRY142886) vstemozolomide (TMZ) in patients (pts) with advanced melanoma: An openlabel, randomized, multi-center, phase II study. Journal of Clinical Oncology. 2008;**26**(Suppl. Abstr):9033

[7] Paches A.I. Tumors of the head and neck – Medicine 2000;245-251. 480 p (in Russian)

[8] Whiteman D, Green A. Melanoma and sun exposure: Where are we now. International Journal of Dermatology. 2000;**38**:481-489

[9] Markel G, Seidman R, Cohen Y, et al. Dynamic expression of protective CEACAM1 on melanoma cells uring specific immune attack. Immunology. 2009;**126**(2):186-200

[10] Schallmach E, Sareli R, Besser MJ, et al. Collection of large-scale expanded lymphocyte cultures for adoptive immunotherapy using a COBE spectra apheresis machine. Journal of Immunotherapy. 2008;**31**(6):563-568

[11] Taghizadeh R, Noh M, Huh YH, et al. CXCR6, a newly defined biomarker of tissuespecific stem cell asymmetric self renewal, identifies more aggressive human melanoma cancer stem cells. PLoS One. 2010;**5**(12):e15183

[12] Borkhunova EN. Characteristics of reparative regener ation of tissues after cryodestruction, SHF cryodestruction, and SHF destruction, wxtended abstract of doctoral (Biol.). Dissertation, Moscow, 2004

[13] 20th World Congress of Dermatology: 1st to 5th July 2002, Paris, Masson, 2002

[14] Sulzberger MB. Year Book of Dermatology and Syphilology. Chicago: Year Book Publishers; 1949. p. 14

[15] Hautmann G, Panconesi E. European Guidelines for the Treatment of Dermatological Diseases. EDF. 2008

[16] Volkova NV, Glazkova LK. Psychosomatic aspects of acne. Russian Journal of Dermatovenereology 2013;3

[17] Welp K, Gieler U. Acne vulgaris: Morphologic, endocrinologic and psychosomatic aspects. Zeitschrift für Hautkrankheiten (German). 1990 Dec;**65**(12):1139-1145

[18] Bosse K, Hunecke P. Entstellung-Erleben und Verarbeitung der äußeren Erscheinung. In: Whitlock FA. (Hrsg.) Psychophysiologische Aspekte bei Hautkrankheiten. Erlangen: Perimed; 1980

[19] Bosse K, Fassheber P, Hunecke P, Teichmann AT, Zuaner J. Social situation of persons with dermatoses as a phenomena of interpersonal perception. Psychotherapie, Psychosomatik, Medizinische Psychologie. 1976;**21**:3-61

[20] Bosse K. Psychosomatic criteria in the treatment of atopic neurodermatitis. Zeitschrift für Hautkrankheiten. 1986 Apr 15;**61**(8):543-545

[21] Kar BR, Tripathy S, Panda M. Comparative study of oral isotretinoin versus oral isotretinoin + 20% salicylic acid peel in the treatment of active acne. Journal of Cutaneous and Aesthetic Surgery. 2013;**6**(4):204-208

[22] Del Rosso JQ. The changing face of challenges in the management of acne and rosacea. Journal of Drugs in Dermatology. 2014 Jun;**13**(6):649

[23] Rivera AE. Acne scarring: A review and current treatment modalities. Journal of the American Academy of Dermatology. 2008 Oct;**59**(4):659-676

[24] Kirichenko IM. Modern approaches for infectious skin diseases therapy. Dermatology. 2006;01 (in Russian)

[25] Eady EA, Farmery MR, Ross JI, Cove JH, Cunliffe WJ. Effects of benzoyl peroxide and erythromycin alone and in combination against antibiotic-sensitive and -resistant skin bacteria from acne patients. British Journal of Dermatology. 1994 Sep;**131**(3):331-336

[26] Burkhart CN, Gottwald L. Assessment of etiologic agents in acne pathogenesis. SKINmed. 2003 Jul-Aug;**2**(4):222-228. Review

[27] Zainullina ON, Khismatullina ZR, Khairetdinova TB. Correction of dysbiotic intestinal microflora imbalance in patients with acne. Eksperimental'naia i Klinicheskaia Gastroenterologiia. 2012;(1):38-42

[28] Racine A, Cuerq A, Bijon A, Ricordeau P, Weill A, Allemand H, Chosidow O, Boutron-Ruault MC, Carbonnel F. Isotretinoin and risk of inflammatory bowel disease: A French nationwide study. The American Journal of Gastroenterology. 2014 Apr;**109**(4):563-569

[29] Konchugova TV. Aspects of acne treatment. Plastic surgery and cosmetology. 2010;(1): 73-80

Section 2

Advanced Skin Surgical Procedures

Chapter 4

Simultaneous Excisions and Extemporary Skin Plastics: New Reconstructive Techniques after Tumor Surgery

Paolo Boggio, Benedetta Miglino,
Federica Veronese, Rossana Tiberio and
Paola Savoia

Additional information is available at the end of the chapter

http://dx.doi.org/10.5772/intechopen.71691

Abstract

Occurrence of two or more skin tumors closely situated to each other is not so rare in clinical dermasurgical practice. Excision of multiple contiguous skin lesions can represent a major dermasurgical problem that can be solved in different surgical times. However, in our opinion, the best therapeutic solution is to carry out the removal in a single surgical session; this choice allows saving time, an easier plastic reconstruction, and better esthetic results. Many different reconstructive procedures can be designed and applied, to achieve the best result. The simplest Burow's triangle flap permits excision of two contiguous lesions with less tension compared to two fusiform cuts, but many other plastic solutions can be chosen to satisfy the needs of different anatomical sites and according to skin features. In the author's personal experience, of about 8000 patients who have undergone dermatologic surgery over the past 20 years, the presence of multiple contiguous lesions occurred in about 200 cases. In all of these, triangle, rotation, advancement, or transposition flaps allowed simultaneous removals, saving time and money and giving better esthetic results compared to multiple direct excision carried out at successive times. In this chapter, the different techniques are described and illustrated in detail.

Keywords: dermatologic surgery, multiple skin tumors, plastic skin reconstruction techniques, simultaneous excisions, Burow's triangle

1. Introduction

The aim of this chapter is to focus on a new way to employ traditional techniques when skin tumors present themselves as multiple and contiguous. In fact, the occurrence of two or more skin lesions closely situated to one another is not so rare in dermatologic surgery daily practice [1]. The frequency of this condition can be greatly influenced by the grade of attention given to the problem; in our personal experience over the last 20 years, this event was observed and treated in 3% of cases. This problem can be solved by multiple excisions in different surgical times after choosing, for the first ablation, the lesion most clinically malignant or localized in the more difficult anatomical site [1–3]. However, in our opinion the best choice is to find a solution allowing a unique surgical time, giving time-sparing, easier plastic reconstruction, and good esthetic results. This goal can be achieved with a twisted suture line and less skin traction. Many reconstructive possibilities can be found and applied for the best and easier result according to the anatomical disposition [5]. The theory of random pattern flaps can be applied to multiple simultaneous excisions, with all types of flaps.

In the following paragraphs, we present some theoretical considerations on the use of flaps for plastic reconstruction after multiple simultaneous excisions and numerous practical examples. In particular, we describe (i) advancement flaps, (ii) rotation flaps, and (iii) transposition flaps (**Figure 1**).

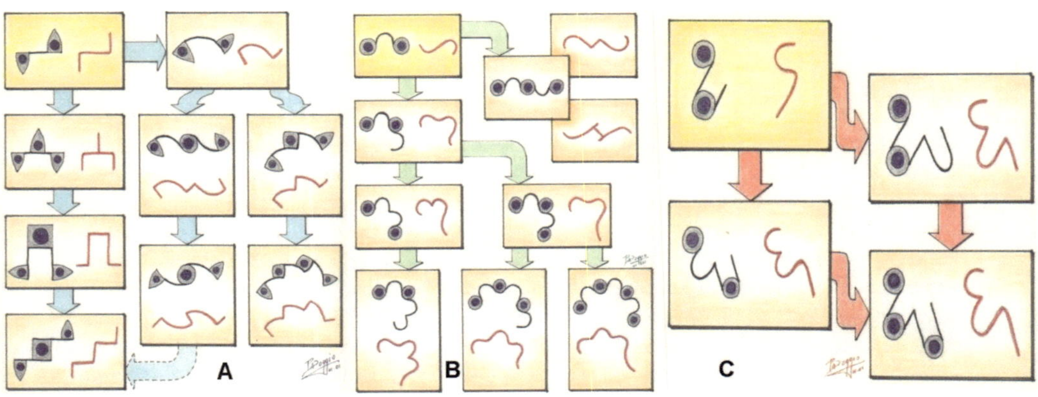

Figure 1. The different types of flaps (simple or elaborated) that can be used after simultaneous excision of multiple lesions. (A) Advancement and rotation flaps, (B) interposed transposition flaps, and (C) coaxial transposition flaps.

2. Advancement flaps

The advancement flap is one of the most basic and versatile flaps available for the dermatologic surgery. Despite its apparent straightforwardness, the advancement flap, which simply involves the linear advancement of the tissue in one direction, can be used to close a variety of defects, ranging from small defects on the scalp or extremities to large, complicated defects involving multiple cosmetic units on the face. A great deal has been written about advancement flaps, including new and innovative ways to use them [6].

Some of these ways are hereby described. All these flaps give the possibility to perform simultaneous and easier reconstructions with a single plastic, after the removal of multiple contiguous lesions of the skin. We discuss the fundamental principles underlying the advancement flap, as well as the potential uses, advantages, and disadvantages of the various types of advancement flaps in different situations of multiple lesions.

http://dx.doi.org/10.5772/intechopen.71691

2.1. Burow's flap

The simplest way to remove cutaneous lesion is the elliptical excision, because it is simple and fast and it leaves a smaller wound than any other technique [5]. When two contiguous lesions cannot be removed with a single elliptical excision, due to the excessive tension that would result from direct suture, it is possible to use two Burow's triangle advancement flaps. This technique is a variant of the single Burow's triangle flap [1], in which the secondary triangle (the so-called Burow's wedge) contains one of the lesions.

In the case of two very close lesions, it is possible to draw two triangle flap variants, as two possible tangential incisions are available. The direction of the tangential incision should be chosen so that it fits well with the creases, folds, and skin tension lines (**Figure 2**).

The Burow's triangle advancement flap is functional only when the distance between the lesions does not exceed 2 "diameters" (width of the hypothetical elliptical excision needed to resect a lesion). The resulting suture line is in this case longer than the sum of the two potential elliptical incisions, but the more esthetic Z-shaped incision and the decreased tension are shown in **Figure 3**. In this case, the distance between the lesions is 1 "diameter," and the resulting suture line is as long as the sum of the two elliptical excisions; so, the absolute tension is the same as that obtained with a single elliptical excision. However, when the distance between the two skin lesions exceeds 2 diameters, the use of this technique is not recommended, because of the need for extensive undermining and the length of the final closure.

Overall, this technique is excellent for the simultaneous removal of two lesions that are closely approximated, as the resulting tension is comparable to that of two elliptical incisions, with acceptable esthetic results.

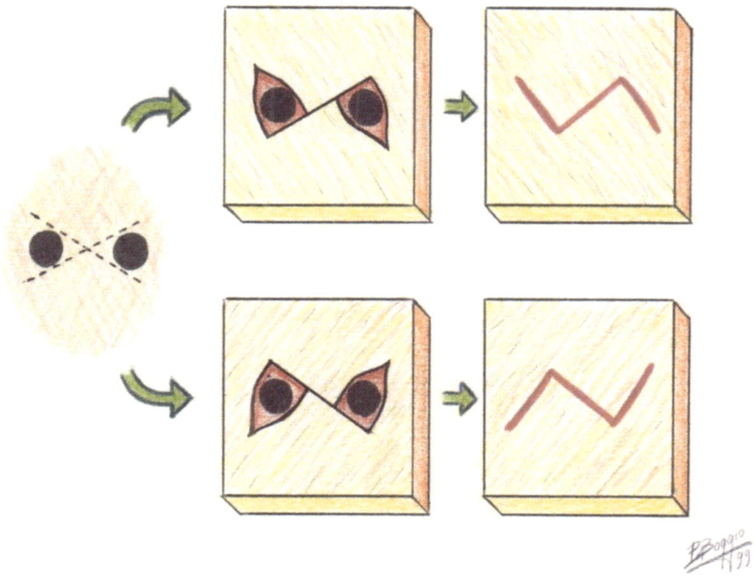

Figure 2. Burow's flap.

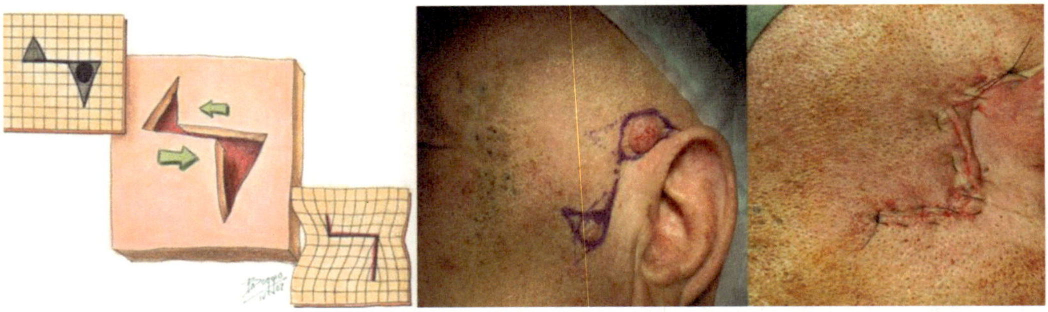

Figure 3. The graphic representation and a clinical example of a Z-shaped incision and the excision of two lesions, with a good esthetic result.

2.2. A-T flap

The A-T flap, also known as the O-T flap, can be thought as half of a double advancement flap. The basic technique for an A-T flap involves the construction of a triangular or A-shaped defect, superimposed over the primary circular or elliptical wound to be closed. The flap is constructed by making an incision along the base of an ideal triangular defect and then joining the two basal tips of the triangle with the midpoint of the base. This results in an inverted, T-shaped closure (i.e., the "T" is inverted with respect to the "A") (**Figure 4**).

Obviously, dimensions of the imaginary triangle that guides the formation of this flap are variable, depending to the size of the wound and of the standing cutaneous cone that is formed and to the proximity of adjacent structures. However, in the absence of any such limitations, some authors [6, 7] determined that, in order to minimize the closure tension, the optimal design for an A-T flap includes a height that is twice the defect diameter, a base extension corresponding to one defect diameter on each side, and three defect diameters (measured from the center of the wound) of undermining. The A-T flap should be considered to avoid

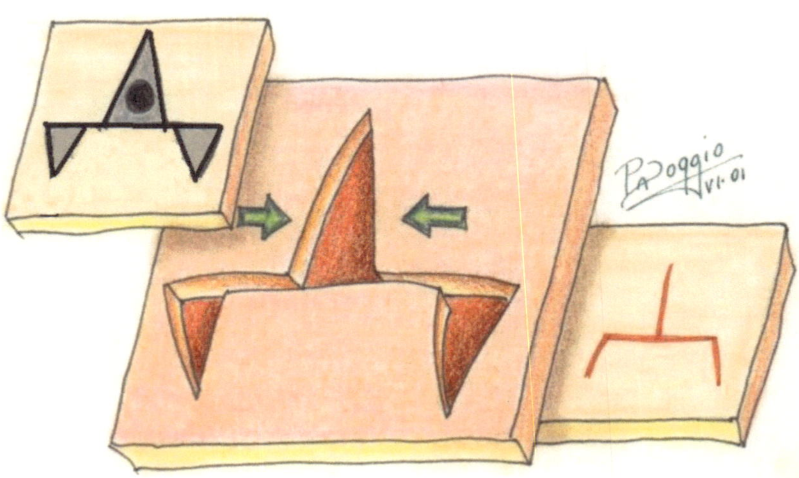

Figure 4. The A-T flap scheme.

distortion of anatomical structures near the wound edge. When this condition is needed, the base of the flap should be placed along the border of the structure to be preserved. The A-T flap prevents the damage of important anatomical structures and leads to the formation of esthetically acceptable scars. This flap is particularly useful: (i) on the forehead, where the base incision can be concealed along the eyebrow or hairline; (ii) on the chin, where the base incision can be concealed along the mental crease; (iii) on the lip, where the base incision can be concealed along the vermilion border.

The A-T flap also allows to use Burow's triangles (that are created at the base of the triangular flaps to facilitate sliding), inserting any contiguous lesions inside them. In this way it is possible to carry out a single reconstructive plastic. This technique is described in **Figure 4**.

2.3. Rectangular flap

The rectangular advancement flap is realized by tracing a rectangle contiguous to the breach to close. The direction of this triangle is chosen on the basis of the best possible esthetic results, along the lines of Langer or in the direction of greater skin distensibility. The ideal length ratio of the rectangular flap width is from 2:1 to 3:1.

Single advancement flaps are useful to repair defects on the forehead.

Single and double advancement flaps are also advantageous because the resulting scars can be camouflaged within normal anatomic boundary lines (e.g., forehead scalp junction or vermilion border).

One of the major drawbacks to constructing advancement flap is represented by the need to build two Burow's triangles to eliminate standing cones of redundant tissue. It should be remembered that the removal of each standing cone creates an extra scar. Standing cones can be sometimes eliminated or diminished simply by sewing them out using the "law of halves." However, this is not always possible. Some authors [4–7] described a fine modification of the basic advancement flap which prevents the formation of standing cones. A curvilinear incision can be performed along the limb of the flap, to redistribute the redundant tissue along the length of the incision. The result is an advancement without Burow's triangle. This modification results in a more desirable final scar; however, it has some minor limitations, including a slight narrowing of the flap pedicle and the relinquishment of the additional tissue movement gained by Burow's triangle excision. When constructing larger flaps, attempts to avoid the excision of Burow's triangles may lead to extensive stretching and subsequent thinning of the flap. It should be kept in mind that an excessively thinned flap has a poor cosmetic outcome and is more susceptible to necrosis. Hence, avoiding standing cone is not necessarily the best possible approach.

The choice to draw two Burow's triangles at the base of the rectangular flap to facilitate its advancement is often the best one. Also, this choice allows to remove three lesions with a single rectangular flap as shown in **Figure 5** (this figure shows the skin tension lines), when such triangles coincide with other skin lesions.

This theoretical principle can be adapted to the disposition of the contiguous lesions, giving rise to trapezoidal shapes other than rectangular (**Figure 6**).

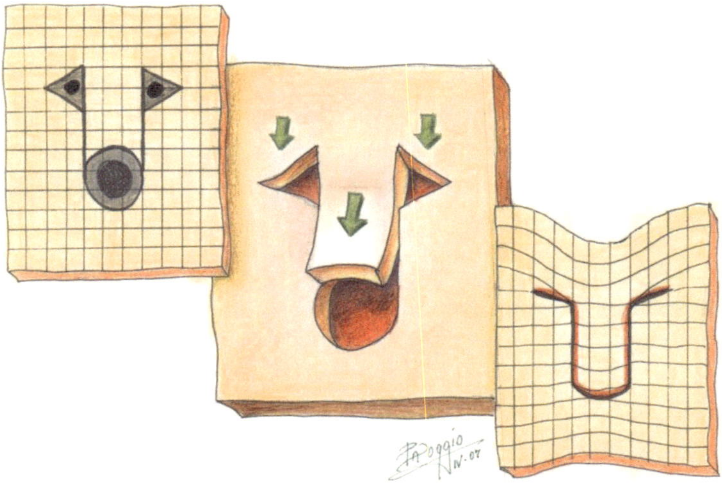

Figure 5. Rectangular flap scheme.

2.4. Opposite triangular flap

Triangular flap is a useful variant to close a surgical breach through advancing the two opposite sides, when one-on-one advancement is difficult. Sometimes, the two opposite advancements can be obtained with two rectangular flaps (**Figure 7**).

However, to reduce the number of surgical cuts, the two flaps can be transformed into two Burow's opposite triangles, cutting one side and using Burow's triangle on each arm. If the two

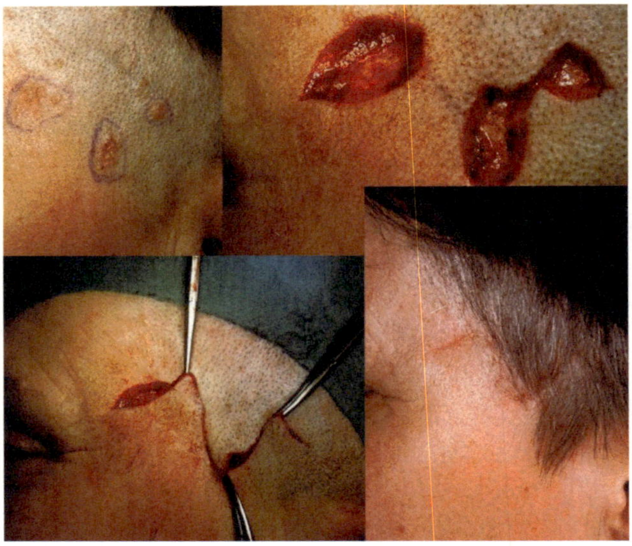

Figure 6. Clinical examples of contiguous lesions.

Burow's triangles can result in other two cutaneous lesions, we will obtain the excision and the simultaneous reconstruction of three injuries with a single broken suture line (**Figure 8**).

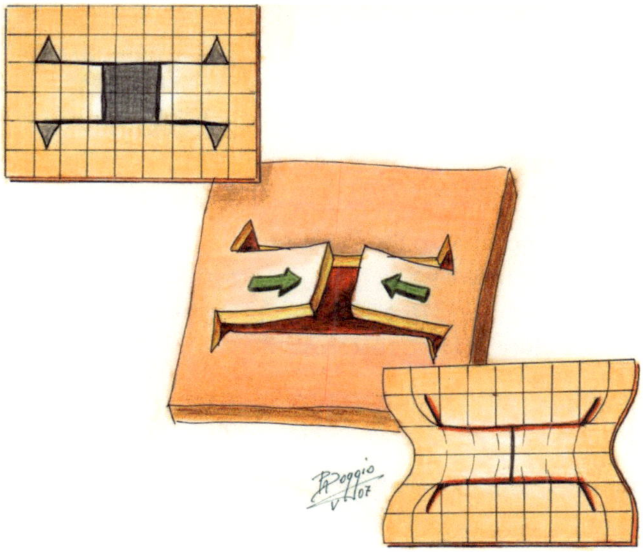

Figure 7. Opposite triangular flap graphic scheme.

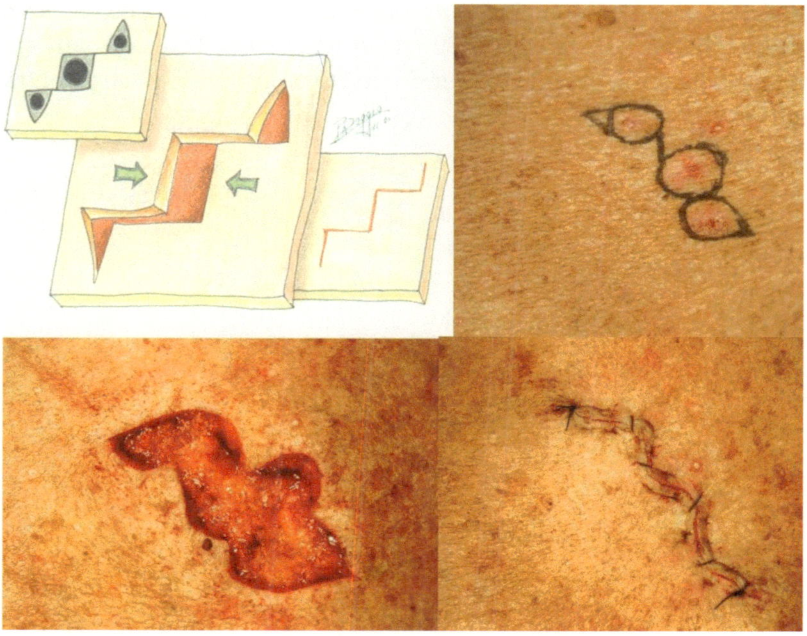

Figure 8. A clinical example for multiple lesions.

3. Rotation flaps

3.1. Fan flap

A rotation flap is usually taken from more resilient skin regions to fill losses of the tissue from adjacent less-resilient regions. It is usually fan-shaped up to two to four times wider than the excision area, and Burow's triangle is catted out at its base, to facilitate rotation. In the case of two close lesions, it is possible to obtain a simultaneous excision circumscribing one of them with Burow's triangle. This technique is similar to that adopted for Burow's triangle flap (**Figure 9**).

Four different variants are possible in this specific situation, allowing the choice of four corresponding types of the final suture based to cosmetic needs. The distance between the lesions can reach a width of 3–4 "diameters" (the width of the hypothetical rhomboid exercise needed to eradicate the lesion) (**Figure 10**).

A practical example of application of the rotation flap to removal two contiguous lesions from the eyebrow and temporal region is shown in **Figure 10**.

If the distance between the lesions is about 1 diameter, this rotation flap becomes a variant of the Dufourmentel transposition flap (a flap whose length is 1.5 times longer than the width of the lesion gap) [7]. It is possible, in fact, to cut out a flat between the lesions, whose length-width ratio is 1:1; the rotation of this flap and whose rotation is facilitated by the direct suture of one of the two gaps. In this case, all the four direction variants mentioned above are possible. The wide base makes the flap very vital, and, in contrast to the Dufourmentel flap, only a mild torsion of the peduncle occurs, with a better vascularization. It is noteworthy that this flap variant, although structurally and conceptually similar to the rotation flap, can be more appropriately considered to be a very simple type of transposition flap (**Figure 11**).

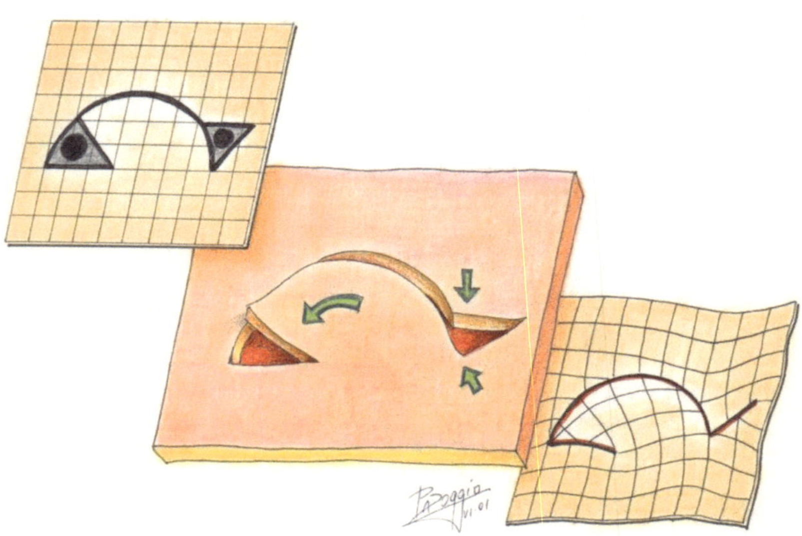

Figure 9. Fan flap scheme.

http://dx.doi.org/10.5772/intechopen.71691

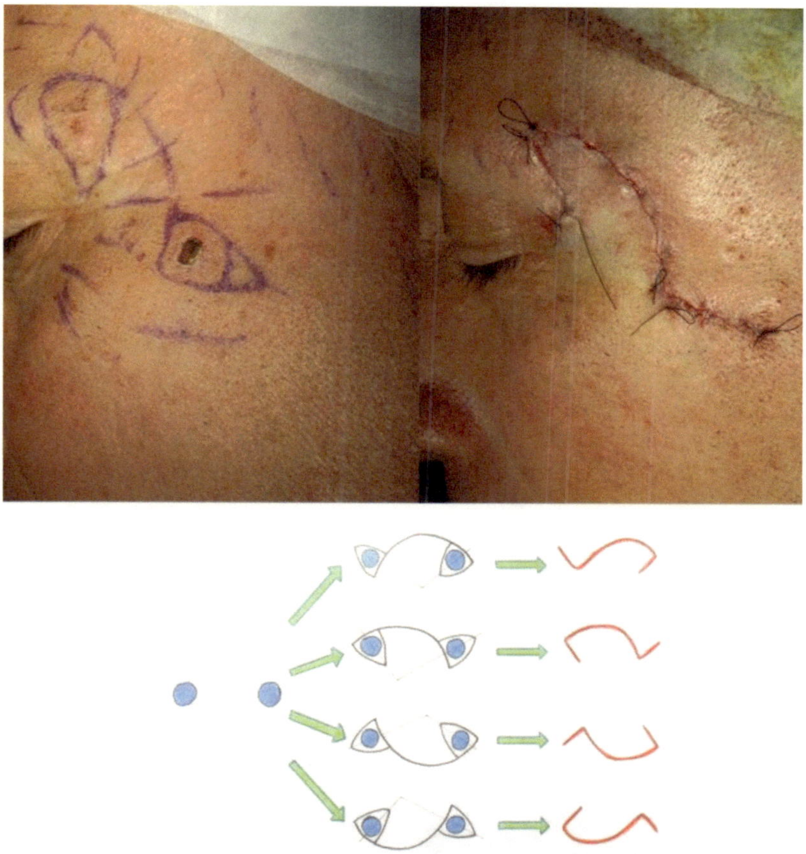

Figure 10. Clinical application of fan flap.

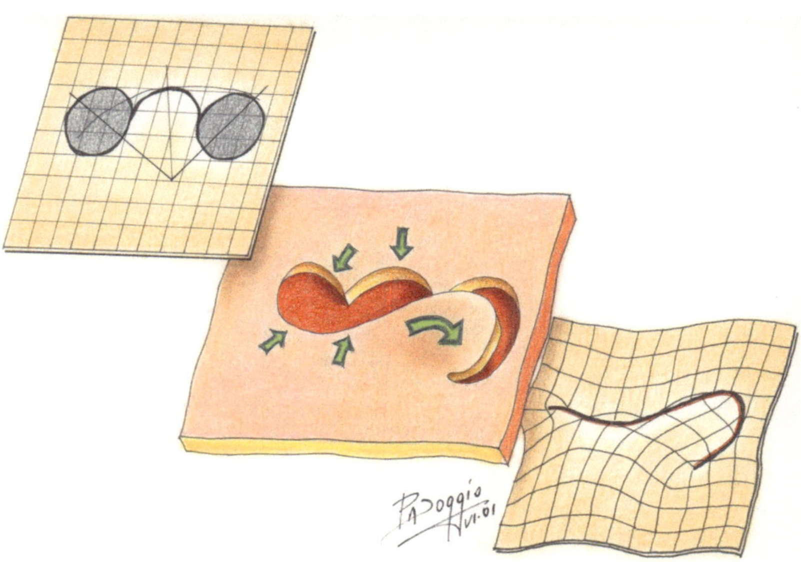

Figure 11. The scheme of the variant of fan flap.

3.2. Opposite rotation flap

Considerations similar to those reported in Section 2.1 for the double triangular advancement flap can be made for opposing rotational flaps. In this variant, the contour of the flap is curved, and the advancement movement becomes a rotation. At the base, two Burow's triangles are drawn to facilitate convergent movement. If in these triangles there are two other lesions, we can obtain the simultaneous excision of three lesions (**Figure 12**).

However, the rotation of the flaps may be divergent, taking advantage of the central breakaway as facilitating the lateral movement of the flaps; in this way a final suture according to the anatomical areas can be easily obtained, with a good esthetic result (**Figure 12**).

3.3. Multidentate rotation flaps

A multidentate rotation flap can be easily modified to fit many defects, including multiple lesions localized along an ideal arcuate line.

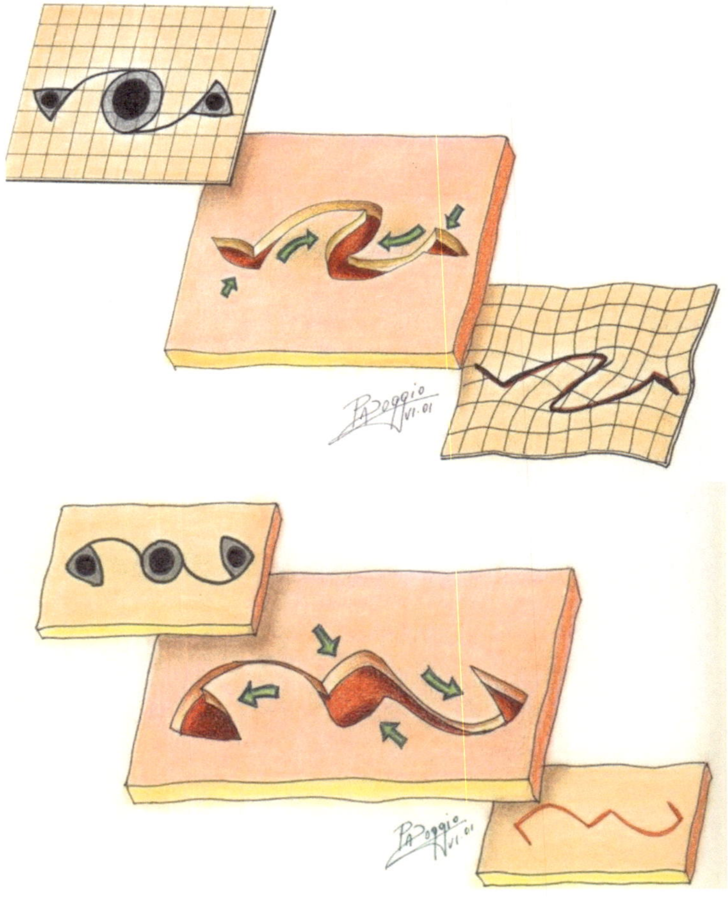

Figure 12. Opposite rotation flaps schemes.

http://dx.doi.org/10.5772/intechopen.71691

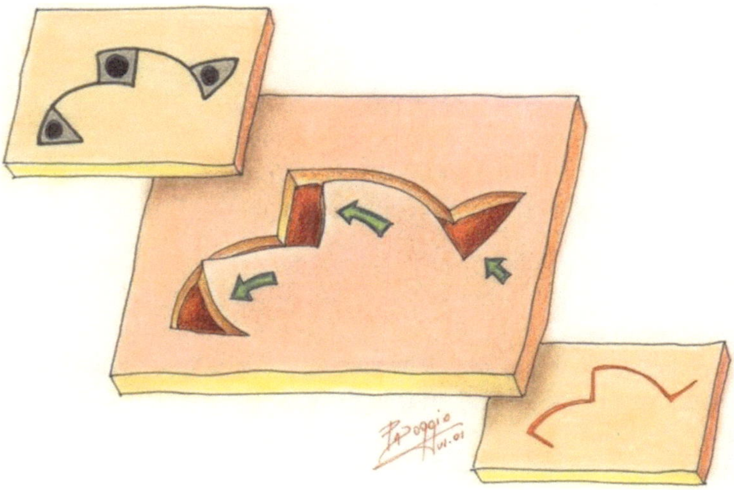

Figure 13. Multidentate rotation flap scheme.

It represents the mix of multiple fanlike rotation flaps, each of which facilitates the rotation of the previous: this is possible by using the last excision area as Burow's triangle and by closing the donor areas directly; the technique diagram is shown in **Figure 13** for the excision of three lesions and can also be applied to remove four lesions.

Obviously, the adoption of this flap should be evaluated in each individual case. When this technique is possible, it gives a very good outcome, due to the curved suture lines; a significant portion of the skin is saved, and there is a reduction of the overall surgical time.

The practical application of multidentate flap for four lesions excision is shown in **Figure 14**.

Also, in multidentate flaps, it is possible to choose between two different directions of rotation, depending on the skin distention and on the desired final esthetic result.

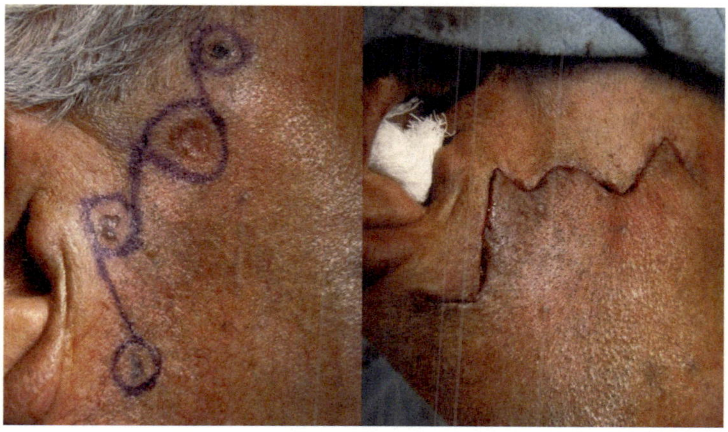

Figure 14. A clinical application of a multidentate rotation flap.

4. Transposition flaps

The transposition flap is realized by completely removing the flap from the donor area and transporting it to the receiving site by rotating it on its peduncle and overcoming a portion of healthy skin. The simplest transposition flap is Dufourmentel's flap; in this case, the flap length is about 1.5 times its width that is equal to the width of the surgical defect that must be covered (**Figure 15**).

A transposition flap can be used when the surgical wound is localized in low-resilient areas, where it is impossible to perform a direct suture. It is obtained by cutting out distant resilient donor areas that can easily be sutured. The rotation of this flap allows the surgeon to skip over the skin, although its base corresponds to the gap. The rotation angle of the flap axis can reach an angle of up to 180° (a limit to the peduncle torsion degree angle), but the rotation is usually not more than about 90°.

In the case of two close lesions, this type of plastic can be used when one of the two gaps is localized in a fairly resilient region. In this case, the flap is cut out with the gap localized in the more resilient area, in order to create a unique gap that is directly suturable, making the flap rotation to the gap easier in the low-resilient area.

In this case, it is a coaxial flap with a surgical breach. Otherwise, if the breaches are spaced apart about one in diameter, the flap can be made between the two ones and rotated to cover one of them, while the other breach (located in the denser skin zone) acts as a rotating facilitator (according to the principle of Burow's triangle). In this case, the flap can be defined as an interposed transposition flap.

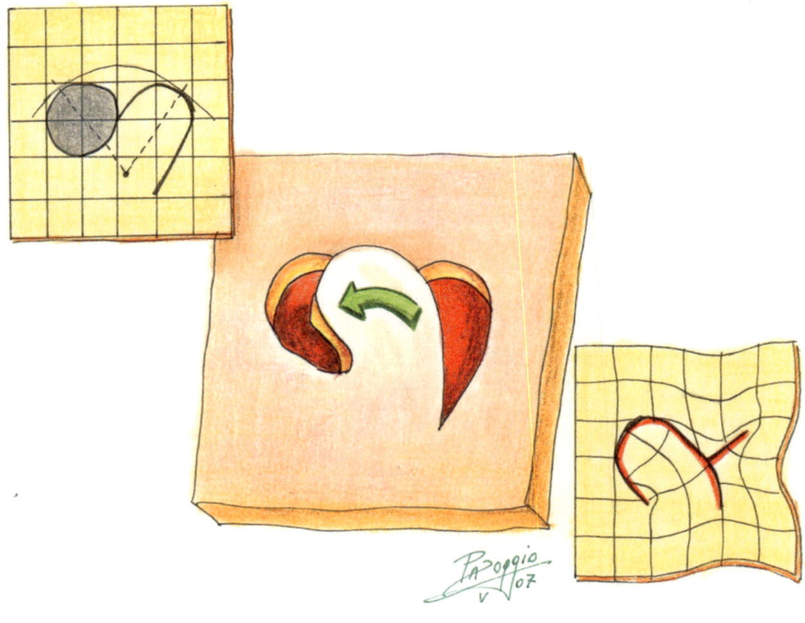

Figure 15. A transposition flap scheme.

The adoption of this technique depends on the distance between the lesions, which should not exceed 1.0–1.5 diameters, because the length of the flap must be proportional to the receiving wound so as to avoid waste-redundant skin.

4.1. Interposed transposition flaps

4.1.1. Simple transposition flap

This is the simplest form of transposition flap, useful for the closure of two contiguous surgical breaches; it is performed when the distance between the breaches is about 1 diameter (**Figure 11**). This simple plastic technique can be adapted according to local needs and to different skin drifts in the two breaches; at least two different types of scar can be obtained depending on the direction of flap rotation (**Figure 16**).

The options may even become four by flipping the cutting direction of the flap, as already described above about the simple rotation flap (see Section 3.1 and **Figure 10**).

A practical excursion of this plastic is summarized in **Figure 16**.

Starting from this simplest form of flap, it is possible to develop surgical solutions that can solve situations with multiple breaches located in very different ways.

4.1.2. Bilobed flap

When the second breach is not placed in a sufficiently drifting area, an accessory lobe can be required in the transposition flap; so, a bilobed flap is created. In this case, the donor area for

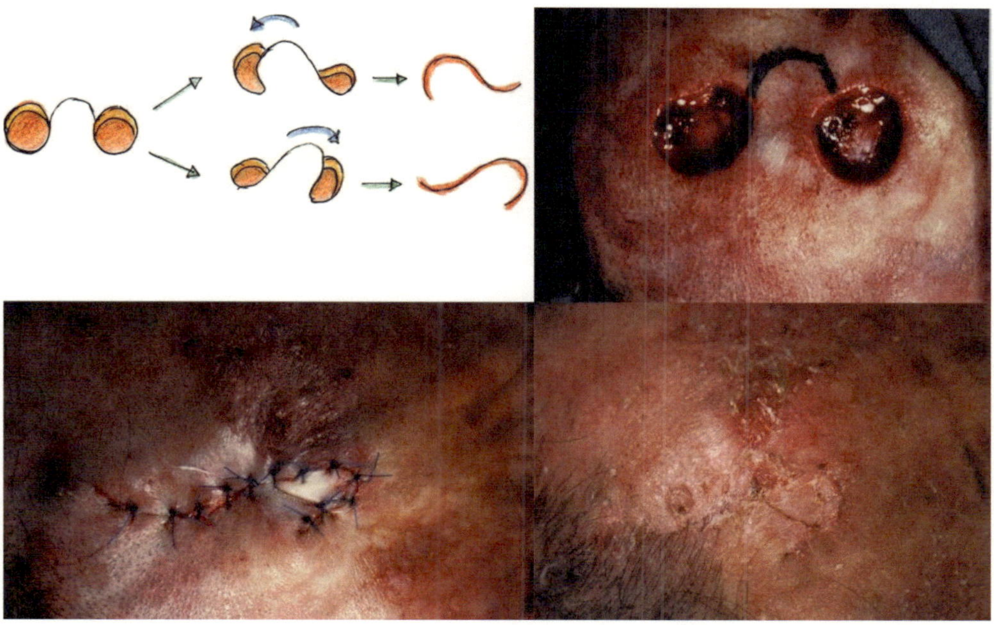

Figure 16. A clinical example of simple transposition flap and a graphic scheme of the direction of tension lines.

the first breach is closed orthogonal to the direction of rotation, while the donor area of the second flap is closed directly in the direction to the rotation, thus facilitating the movement of the flap itself (**Figure 17**).

4.1.3. Interposed bilobed flap

If the distance between the breaches is greater than 1 diameter, a bilobed flap can also be built between them, covering a gap with the first lobe and the donating area of this with the second lobe. The second breach is sutured directly, facilitating in this way the rotation of the flap. In the rotation movement, the advancement of the peduncle facilitates the direct closure of the second donor area (**Figure 18**).

4.1.4. Bilobed flap for three breach closures

It represents the extension of the concept expressed in the two previous paragraphs.

The three breaches must be spaced about a diameter and must be arranged in the shape of an arch: the most caudal of the three breaches is reduced spontaneously by the movement of the flap rotation, and the donor areas can be closed for direct suture (**Figure 19**).

4.1.5. Trilobed flaps

The concept of bilobed flap can be further expanded as trilobed flap, for multiple excisions. When the breaches are arranged along an arched line and spaced apart about 1 diameter, the flap lobes are drawn by interposing them at breaches, so that each one facilitates the rotation of the following. This can be done for three cutaneous lesions and also for four lesions (**Figure 20**).

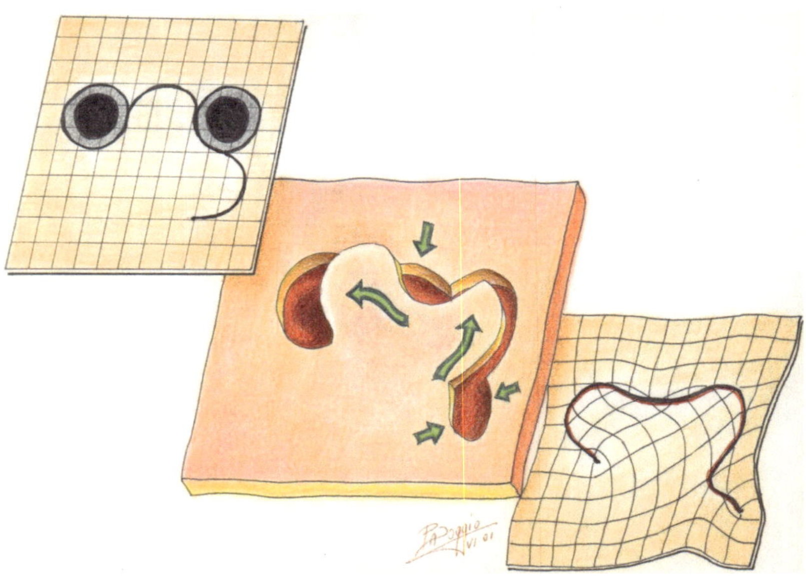

Figure 17. A graphic representation of bilobed flap.

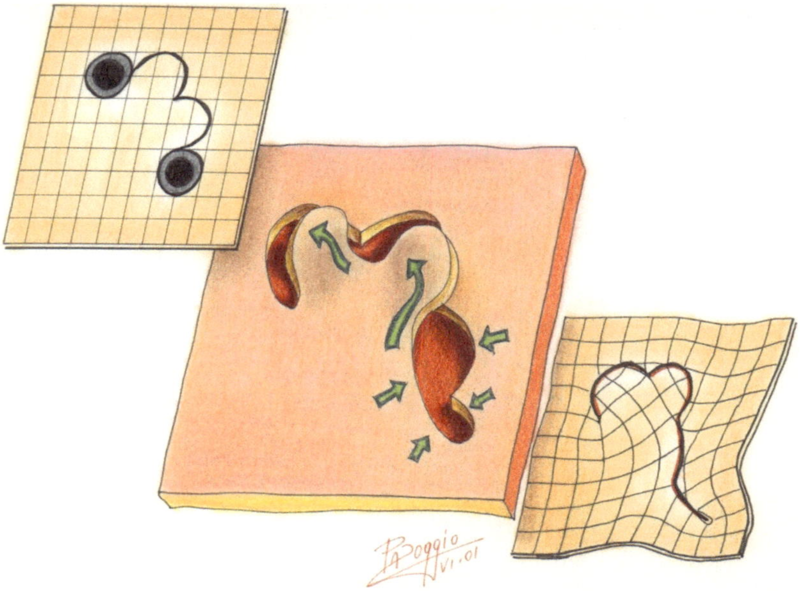

Figure 18. A graphic representation of interposed bilobed flap.

A practical application of the trilobed transposition flap is shown in **Figure 21**.

An indispensable condition for the realization of this type of plastic is that the arch along which the breach is placed should not be too tight or too large. We underline the affinity of this plastic with the multidentate flap (**Figure 13**).

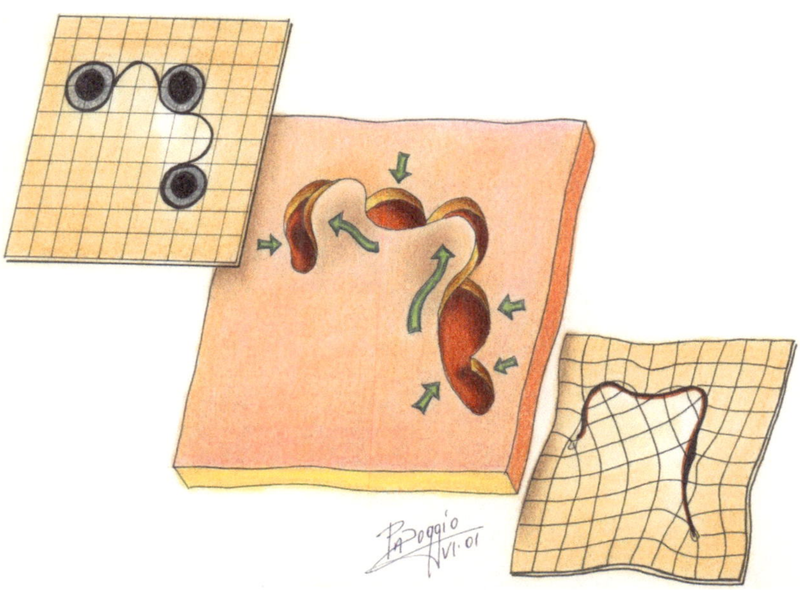

Figure 19. A graphic representation of bilobed flap for three lesions.

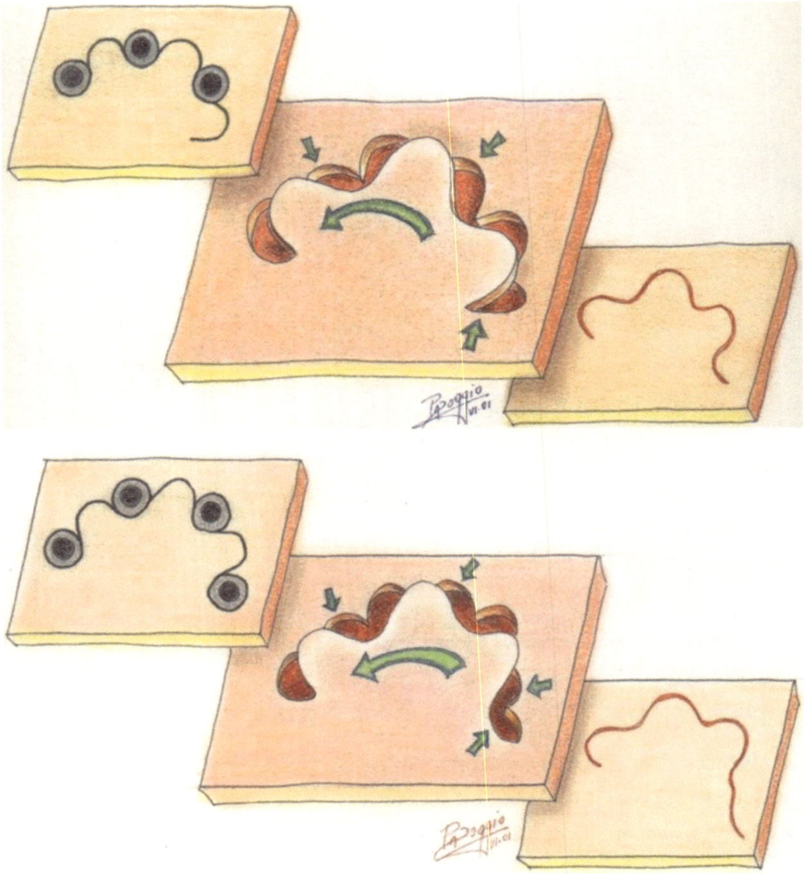

Figure 20. A graphic representation of trilobed flap and for four lesions.

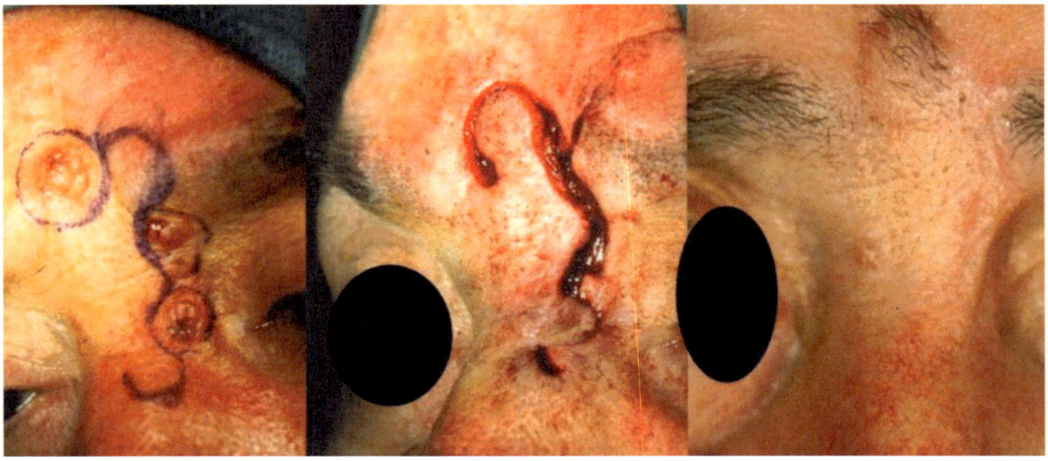

Figure 21. Clinical application of trilobed flap.

http://dx.doi.org/10.5772/intechopen.71691

4.1.6. *Centripetal and centrifugal opposite transposition flaps*

In the case of three lesions of a similar size, aligned and spaced of about a diameter, we can perform a closure with a transposition flap that can be applied bilaterally in the same way. On the basis of the skin distensibility and according to the final suture shape, two flaps can be rotated in the opposite direction, exploiting, respectively, the lateral and central breaches as areas for facilitating rotation (**Figure 22**).

4.2. Coaxial transposition flaps

In case of excisions of multiple lesions, this type of plastic repair can be used when one of the gaps is localized in a fairly resilient region. A flap is cut out with the gap localized at its apex in the more resilient area, in order to create a unique gap that is directly suturable and make the flap rotation easier to the lower-resilient area.

4.2.1. *Simple coaxial transposition flap*

In the case of two close lesions, this type of plastic repair can be used especially when one of the two gaps is localized in a fairly resilient region. The flap is drawn with the gap localized in the more resilient area, in order to create a unique gap easy to close directly (**Figure 23**). The possibility to adopt this technique depends on the distance between the lesions, which should not exceed 1.0–1.5 diameters; in fact, the length of the flap must be proportional to the receiving wound, to avoid waste of redundant skin. In this technique, two theoretical variants of the direction of the cut are possible in order to achieve the best cosmetic result. This is obtained cutting the flap to the left or to the right of the less-resilient gap (**Figure 23**).

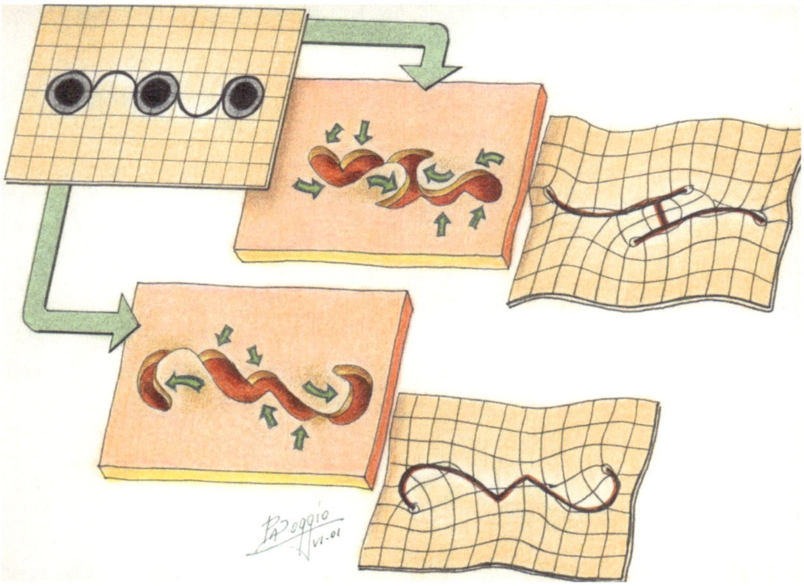

Figure 22. A graphic representation of centripetal and centrifugal opposite transposition flaps.

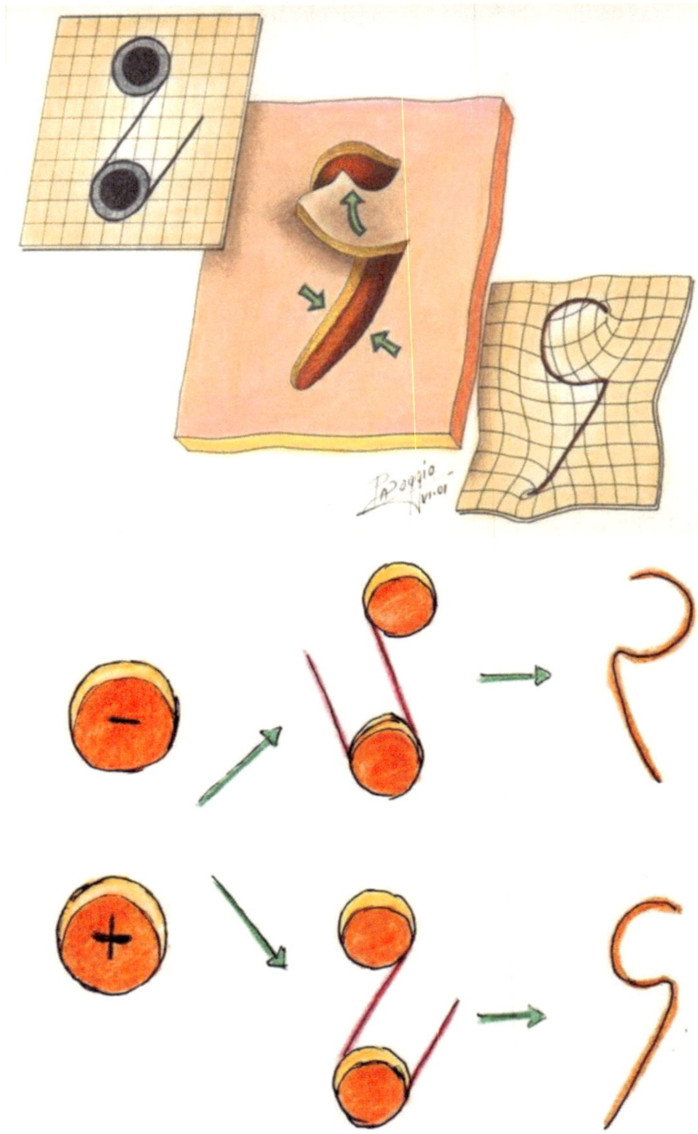

Figure 23. A graphic representation of coaxial transposition flaps.

Practical examples of the application of this technique are represented with two clinical cases; in the first one, lesions are localized in the temporal region (**Figure 24**), whereas in the second case, two lesions are localized in the retroauricular region (**Figure 25**).

4.2.2. Coaxial transposition bilobed flaps

From the type of flap described above, a variant has been developed; in this case the alignment occurs with a second accessory lobe when the lesions between them are more distant (**Figure 26**).

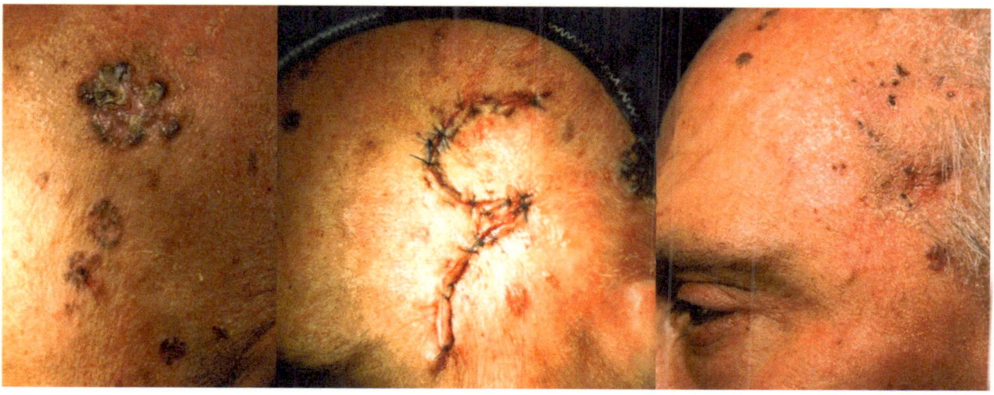

Figure 24. Clinical application of coaxial transposition flap in temporal region.

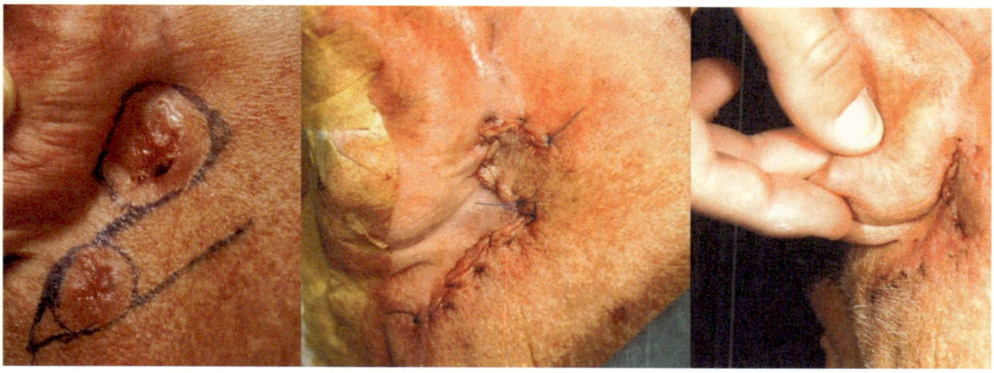

Figure 25. Clinical application of coaxial transposition flap in retroauricolar region.

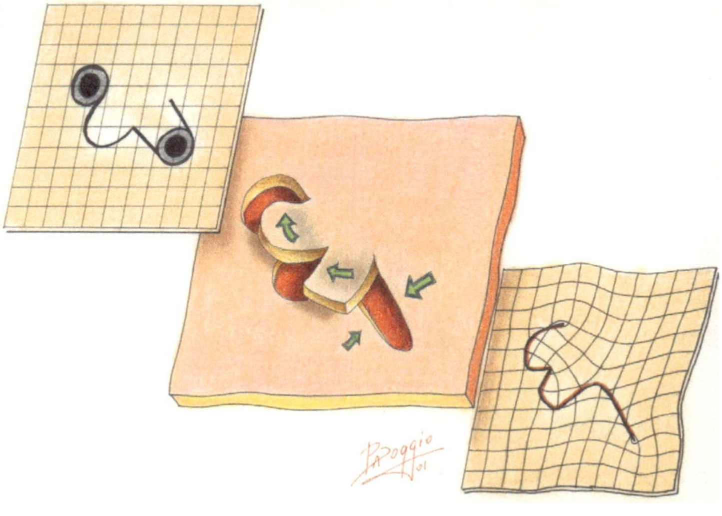

Figure 26. A graphic representation of coaxial transposition bilobed flaps.

This variant can also be applied to cases in which the second breach is in a not-sufficiently-distensible area; so, an accessory lobe is needed, to close it together with the donor area of the first lobe. **Figure 27** shows a clinical example, in which this technique is applied to the excision of two lesions on the nose.

The technique can also allow to remove three lesions: in this case, the lobes are coaxially plotted with two breaches placed in the most distensible skin areas (**Figure 28**).

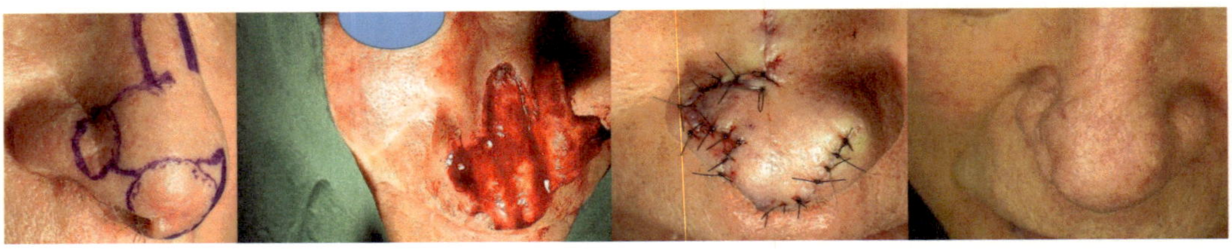

Figure 27. Clinical application of coaxial transposition bilobed flap.

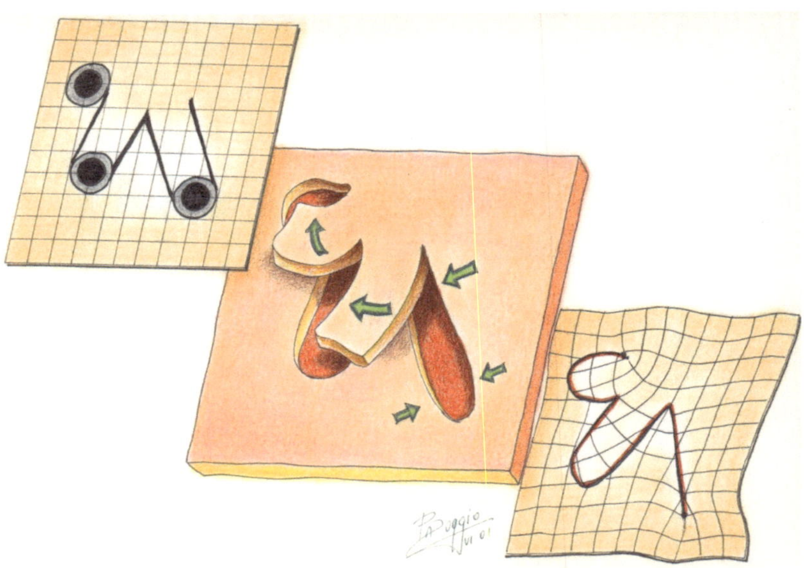

Figure 28. A scheme of a variant of coaxial bilobed flap.

5. Conclusions

We are aware of the fact that excessive schemes always have the risk of being simplistic.

The extreme variability of the cutaneous lesions areas, dimensions, and relationships between multiple lesions makes difficult to establish general rules, and at each time, the surgeon should evaluate the feasibility and the opportunity of a cutaneous plastic.

However, in this chapter we have tried to provide general guidance for the surgical treatment of multiple skin lesions, considering as many cases as possible.

In our opinion there are few general rules that you always need to keep in mind:

1. Use the minimum number of cutting lines.
2. Remove the smallest possible amount of the skin.
3. Search for the easiest plastic surgery for skin collapse.
4. Make the flaps using the cutting lines already performed for excision.
5. Search for the final suture lines respecting as much as possible the esthetic units, wrinkles, and cutaneous furrows.
6. Whenever possible, use excision areas (like Burow's triangles) to facilitate sliding of the flaps.

In conclusion, advancement, rotation, and transposition flaps should be considered as good alternatives for the simultaneous removal of close lesions, when multiple direct excisions are not feasible. However, their direction should be carefully studied in terms of distance between lesions, localization, shape, cutaneous resilience, and possible cosmetic results according to the direction of the final suture. The simultaneous ablation of multiple lesions guarantees time and cost-saving and can give better cosmetic results compared to a series of repeated rhomboid excisions. It is not possible to establish precise rules for these flaps due to the extreme variability that two close lesions can display about anatomical site, shape, and distance. For this reason, the surgeon should evaluate the advantages of a simultaneous excision with simple and conservative techniques according to each individual case. Each new case could be unique and could represent the expression of a creative, artistic, and personal intuition.

Author details

Paolo Boggio[1], Benedetta Miglino[2], Federica Veronese[2], Rossana Tiberio[1] and Paola Savoia[2]*

*Address all correspondence to: paola.savoia65@gmail.com

1 Dermatologic Department, AOU Maggiore della Carità, Novara, Italy

2 Department of Health Science, University of Eastern Piedmont, Novara, Italy

References

[1] Wheeland RG. Bilobed flap. In: Roenigk HH, editor. Dermatologic Surgery. New York: Marcel Dekker; 1989. pp. 311-313

[2] Leigheb G. Lembo bilobato di rotazione. In: Leigheb G, Tulli A, editors. Manuale di dermochirurgia. Milan: Cilag sp; 1990

[3] Kaufman R, Landes E. Simultaneous excision of two pigmented lesions. In: Kaufman R, editor. Interventi dermochirurgici. Mialno: Masson; 1994. p. 217

[4] Gormley DE. The N or reversed N closure of adjacent, parallel, ellipptical excisions. The Journal of Dermatologic Surgery and Oncology. 1985;**11**:121-123

[5] Sbano E, della Corte G. Riparazione esetetica dei difetti parziali del naso mediante lembi local. G. ital. Dermatol Chir Oncologia. 1993;**2**:80-87

[6] Salasche S. Nasal surgery. In: Roenigk RK, Roenigk HH, editors. Dermatologic Surgery. New York: Marcel Dekker; 1989. pp. 438-464

[7] Dufourmentel C, Mouly R. Chirurgie Plastique. Paris: Flammarion; 1959

Chapter 5

Mohs Micrographic Surgery

Merdan Serin

Additional information is available at the end of the chapter

http://dx.doi.org/10.5772/intechopen.70285

Abstract

Mohs micrographic surgery (MMS) is used to obtain clear margins in skin cancer treatment. MMS involves staged excisions and complete margin assessment of the specimen from fresh tissue frozen sectioning. It has been shown to achieve higher cure rates with malignancies, including basal cell carcinoma (BCC), squamous cell carcinoma (SCC), lentigo maligna, melanoma in situ and dermatofibrosarcoma protuberans. This technique is especially useful in face, feet and hand regions to avoid cosmetic deformities.

Keywords: basal cell carcinoma, squamous cell carcinoma, Mohs, skin cancer, Mohs surgery

1. Introduction

Mohs micrographic surgery (MMS) is a method used by physicians to obtain clear margins in the treatment of skin tumors. It was first described by a general surgeon, Frederick Edwards Mohs [1, 2]. Originally, this technique involved the application of zinc chloride paste to the excised tissue for overnight. The technique was later modified with the introduction of fresh tissue-frozen technique and the elimination of zinc chloride fixation [3].

MMS is characterized by complete evaluation of all tumor margins. It has been proven beneficial for various types of skin malignancies including basal cell carcinoma (BCC), squamous cell carcinoma (SCC), lentigo maligna (LM) and melanoma in situ (MIS). This technique is especially useful in face, feet and hand regions to avoid wide excision, which may not be required for tumor control [4].

2. Indications

Recurrent tumors, tumors in the "h-zone" (central face, eyelids, eyebrows, nose, lips, chin, ear, hand, genitalia, feet, nail units, ankles and nipples/areola), tumors with more than 2 cm diameter and tumors with aggressive histopathologic findings are candidates for MMS. In 2012, appropriate use criteria have been established by American Academy of Dermatology (AAD) and other collaborating organizations [5]. According to these criteria, all BCC, SCC, LM and MIS located in the "h-zone" and the "m-zone" (cheeks, forehead, scalp, neck, jawline and pretibial surface) are appropriate for MMS except focal in situ SCCs with actinic keratosis and superficial BCC with less than 0.5 cm diameter located in the "m-zone." In the "L-zone" (trunk and extremities), only aggressive, recurrent or large tumors meeting certain criteria are considered suitable for MMS.

2.1. Basal cell carcinomas (BCC)

Recurrent BCC have been shown to have subclinical extension which might not be possible to identify during conventional excision. MMS has been reported to achieve better cure rates with these cases. It has been reported by Hoorens et al. that tumor with an area more than 1 cm^2, aggressive histology and patient age more than 80 are strong indications of MMS for BCC [6]. This aggressive biological behavior is characterized by sclerodermiform, infiltrative, micronodular or basosquamous histology. MMS technique for these tumors can achieve higher cure rates when compared to standard excision [7].

2.2. Squamous cell carcinoma (SCC)

MMS can achieve better cure rates for SCC when compared to conventional surgery. Lower recurrence rates have been reported in SCC cases over 5-year follow-up periods with MMS. MMS has been shown to provide better margin control in cases with larger than 2 cm diameter, poor differentiation and perineural invasion in which tumors are frequently known to extend beyond their macroscopic margins. [8].

2.3. Melanoma in situ and lentigo maligna

The role MMS in the management of invasive melanoma is controversial since it is difficult to identify the atypical melanocytes in frozen section. On the other hand, successful treatment of melanoma in situ (MIS) has been reported with MMS. The current standard in the MIS is wide local excision (WLE) with 0.5–1 cm margin. In a recent study by Nosrati et al., 277 patients treated with MMS and 385 patients treated with WLE were compared. No significant difference between the recurrence rate and melanoma-specific survival of the patients was found. This study is especially valuable since prior studies did not involve any direct comparison of these techniques [9]. The comparison of cosmetic and functional results of MMS compared to WLE is still not clearly understood. Further studies are needed in this regard.

Lentigo maligna (LM) is considered as a type of melanoma in situ. MMS that has been reported achieves similar cure rates compared to WLE in LM cases [10].

2.4. Other tumors

Dermatofibrosarcoma protuberans (DFSP): The very high risk of recurrence associated with wide local excision has encouraged the use of MMS with DFSP. In spite of the absence of randomized controlled studies to compare MMS with WLE in DFSP, low recurrence rates associated with

http://dx.doi.org/10.5772/intechopen.70285

MMS have been reported [11]. MMS can identify the subclinical extension of the tumor much better than the conventional WLE. It has been reported in a study that DFSP requires the highest number of Mohs stages when compared to other rare cutaneous tumors treated with MMS [12].

Eccrine porocarcinoma (EPC): There are no large studies comparing WLE with MMS in EPC. Although it has been suggested by some authors that MMS outcomes could be better than WLE, many surgeons prefer to treat EPC with WLE [13–15].

Microcystic adnexal carcinoma (MAC): Recurrence rates of up to 50% have been reported with WLE. Recurrence rates with MMS have been reported from 0 to 22% [16]. One important aspect of MAC is that paraffin embedding with horizontal sectioning is usually preferred instead of frozen sectioning since it is easier to interpret. This process is also called "slow Mohs."

Merkel cell carcinoma: Kline and Coldiron have reported in a recent study that the MMS results are at least comparable to WLE. They have reported 5% recurrence rate as opposed to 32–50% recurrence rate with WLE [17].

Sebaceous carcinoma: Brady and Hurst have shown that MMS has been shown to be associated with lower recurrence and metastatic rates when compared to WLE [18].

Angiomyxoma: Despite its benign pathological features, high recurrence rates up to 40% have been reported with conventional surgery. MMS has been reported to decrease the recurrence rate significantly. But it has been argued in a paper that the pathological features of angiomyxoma might be hard to detect with a frozen section [19].

Lymphoepithelioma, trichilemmal carcinoma, spiradenocarcinoma, nerve sheath myxoma, cutaneous angiosarcoma, granular cell tumor, atypical fibroxanthoma and extramammary Paget's disease are among other skin tumors which have been treated with MMS.

3. Technique and principles

Conventional MMS begins with the removal of the tumor with a small free margin usually between 1 and 2 mm depending on the tumor location as opposed to standard excision of skin cancers, in which at least 5 mm of margin is preferred. The lateral borders are excised at a 45° angle to allow for flattening of the lateral borders of the specimen. Complete circumferential peripheral and deep margin assessment (CCPDMA) is performed following the excision. This technique provides the complete evaluation of all tumor margins as opposed to traditional margin assessment. Following mapping of the excised tissue lateral borders are delineated with a "mashing the pie pan" technique and are positioned at the same horizontal level as the deep margin (**Figures 1** and **2**). The purpose of this technique is to flatten the lateral margins at the same horizontal plane as the deep margin. Afterwards, tissue is embedded in OCT compound in cryostat to obtain horizontal–tangential sections from the deep margin, which also contains the lateral borders after the flattening, instead of conventional vertical sections. Following the staining with hematoxylin and eosin (H&E) or toluidine blue, slides are interpreted under microscopy. Consecutive re-excisions are performed until a clear surgical margin is achieved (**Figure 3**). The final step of MMS involves the reconstruction of the final defect which most frequently involves primary closure, local flaps and skin grafts [4].

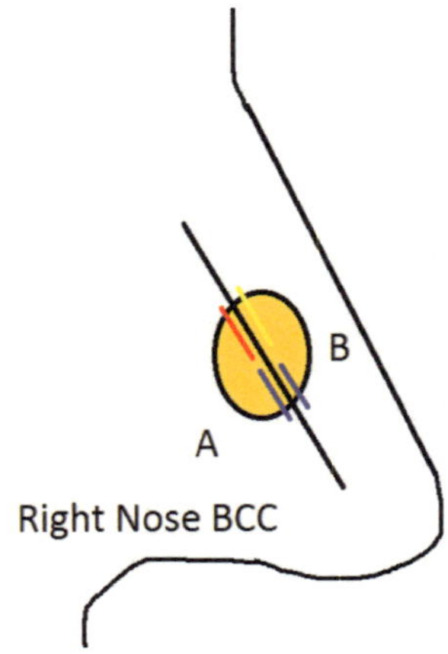

Figure 1. Mapping of the excised tissue.

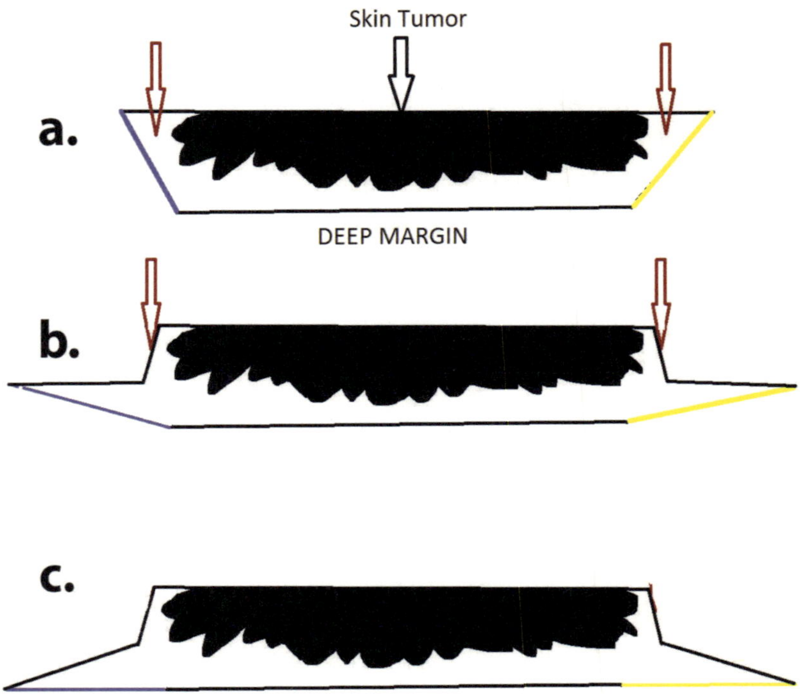

Figure 2. Flattening of the resected tissue with relaxing incisions indicated with arrows. a. b. Relaxing incisions. c. Flattening of the specimen.

4. Outcomes and complications

There is a considerable amount of variations in the reported cure rates for MMS among different surgeons. Misinterpretation of the pathological slides, misoriented tissue margins, freezing

http://dx.doi.org/10.5772/intechopen.70285

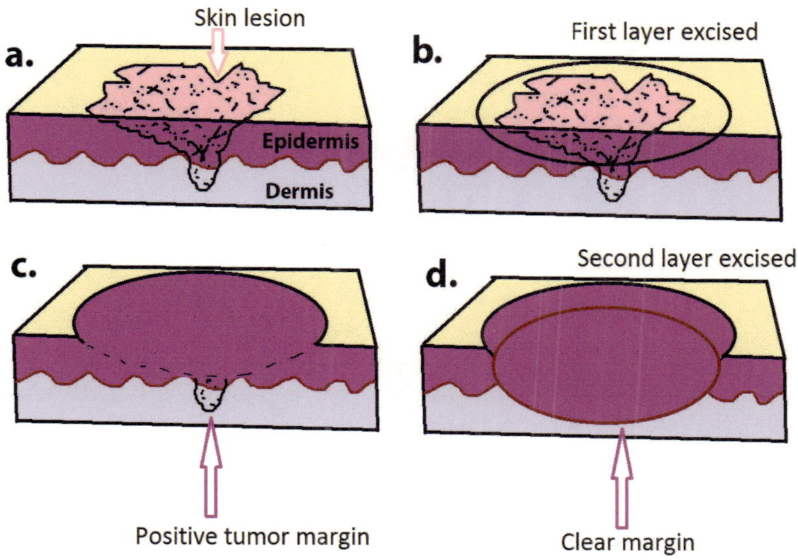

Figure 3. Illustration of staged surgical excisions. a. preoperative view b. excision of the first layer c. positive tumor margin after the excision d. clear margin after the excision of the second layer.

artifacts, poor staining, difficulty of defining atypical cells in the presence of inflammation and scar tissues, inadequate amount of sectioning and problems with flattening the resected tissues are among the reasons for less than ideal outcomes of MMS. All of these can be related to poor training of the physicians and the technicians. Certain pitfalls can be encountered during interpretation of frozen sections. These include adnexal structures which are mistaken for BCC, sun-damaged skin resembling lentigo maligna and pseudocarcinomatous hyperplasia mistaken for SCC [20, 21].

Complications such as tumor recurrence, hematoma, infection, cosmetic and functional deformities can be seen following MMS. Lips, nasal region and eyelids are among the most common sites for cosmetically poor results after MMS. Plastic surgeons should be consulted for reconstruction in cases where the primary closure of the defect with simple methods is not possible.

5. Conclusion

Mohs surgery is an important technique for the treatment of certain types of skin cancer. It is the modality of choice for high-risk basal cell carcinomas (BCC) and squamous cell carcinomas, particularly for the ones located in the facial region. This method achieves very high cure rates for both primary and recurrent BCC. Surgeons can usually avoid large deformities of the face region with application of this technique. This is an important tool that requires special training in the surgery and the pathology of the skin.

Author details

Merdan Serin

Address all correspondence to: merdanserin@gmail.com

Istanbul Training and Research Hospital, Plastic Surgery Clinic, Istanbul, Turkey

References

[1] Mohs FE. Chemosurgery: A method for the microscopically controlled excision of cancer of the skin and lips. Geriatrics. 1959;**14**(2):78-88

[2] Mohs FE. Chemosurgery: A microscopically controlled method of cancer excision. Archives of Surgery. 1941;**42**:279-295

[3] Tromovitch TA, Stegeman SJ. Microscopically controlled excision of skin tumors. Archives of Dermatology. 1974;**110**(2):231-232

[4] Kim KH, Geronemus RG. Mohs micrographic surgery. In: Thorne CH, Beasley RW, Aston SJ, Bartlett SP, Gunter GC, Spear SL, eds. Grabb and Smith's Plastic Surgery. 6th ed. Philadelphia: Lippincott Williams and Wilkins; 2007. P. 115-9

[5] American Academy of Dermatology, et al. AAD/ACMS/ASDSA/ASMS 2012 appropriate use criteria for Mohs micrographic surgery: A report of the American Academy of Dermatology, American College of Mohs Surgery, American Society for Dermatologic Surgery Association, and the American Society for Mohs Surgery. Dermatologic Surgery. 2012;**38**(10):1582-1603

[6] Hoorens I et al. Mohs micrographic surgery for basal cell carcinoma: Evaluation of the indication criteria and predictive factors for extensive subclinical spread. British Journal of Dermatology. 2016;**174**(4):847-852

[7] Cernea SS et al. Indication guidelines for Mohs micrographic surgery in skin tumors. Anais Brasileiros De Dermatolologia. 2016;**91**(5):621-627

[8] Vuyk HD, Lohuis PH. Mohs micrographic surgery for facial skin cancer. Clinical Otolaryngology and Allied Sciences. 2001;**26**(4):265-273

[9] Nosrati A et al. Outcomes of melanoma ın situ treated with Mohs micrographic surgery compared with wide local excision. JAMA Dermatology. 2017;**153**(5):436-441

[10] Hou JL et al. Five-year outcomes of wide excision and Mohs micrographic surgery for primary lentigo maligna in an academic practice cohort. Dermatologic Surgery. 2015;**41**(2):211-218

[11] Gloster HM Jr, Harris KR, Roenigk RK. A comparison between Mohs micrographic surgery and wide surgical excision for the treatment of dermatofibrosarcoma protuberans. Journal of American Academy of Dermatology. 1996;**35**(1):82-87

[12] Flohil SC et al. Mohs micrographic surgery of rare cutaneous tumours. Journal of the European Academy of Dermatology and Venereology. 2017;**31**:1285-1288

[13] Tolkachjov SN et al. Treatment of porocarcinoma with Mohs micrographic surgery: The mayo clinic experience. Dermatologic Surgery. 2016;**42**(6):745-750

[14] Tidwell WJ et al. Treatment of eccrine porocarcinoma with Mohs micrographic surgery: A cases series and literature review. International Journal of Dermatology. 2015;**54**(9):1078-1083

[15] Ghareeb ER et al. Underutilization of Mohs micrographic surgery for less common cutaneous malignancies in the United States. Dermatologic Surgery. 2016;**42**(5):653-662

[16] Diamantis SA, Marks VJ. Mohs micrographic surgery in the treatment of microcystic adnexal carcinoma. Dermatologic Clinics. 2011;**29**(2):185-190 viii

[17] Kline L, Coldiron B. Mohs micrographic surgery for the treatment of merkel cell carcinoma. Dermatologic Surgery. 2016;**42**(8):945-951

[18] Brady KL, Hurst EA. Sebaceous carcinoma treated with Mohs micrographic surgery. Dermatologic Surgery. 2017;**43**(2):281-286

[19] Aberdein G, Veitch D, Perrett C. Mohs micrographic surgery for the treatment of superficial angiomyxoma. Dermatologic Surgery. 2016;**42**(8):1014-1016

[20] Denkler K, Kivett W. Management of non-melanoma skin cancer. In: Mathes SJ, ed. Tumors of head, neck and skin. Plastic Surgery. 2nd edn. Philadelphia, Elsevier Inc: 2006;**5**:437-439

[21] Thorne C, Grabb WC, Smith JW. Grabb and Smith's Plastic Surgery. 6th ed. Vol. xix. Philadelphia: Wolters Kluwer Health/Lippincott Williams & Wilkins; 2007, 929 p

Section 3

Advanced Dermatologic Procedures

Chapter 6

CO_2 Laser-Assisted Otoplasty: A New Dermatosurgical Procedure

Hector Leal Silva

Additional information is available at the end of the chapter

http://dx.doi.org/10.5772/intechopen.71992

Abstract

Otoplasty is the surgical procedure characteristically performed to improve the appearance of unpleasant, protruding auricles. An incision in the back of the ear with or without excision of cartilage is the usual approach. A novel technique performed with CO_2 laser is presented. The objective of CO_2 laser-assisted otoplasty is to decrease the mastoid-scapha angle up to approximately 30°; also, the conchal-scapha angle should be reduced to its usual of approximately 90°. The aims of this procedure are to restructure the scapha and the antihelix fold, to diminish the size of the concha (hinge effect), and to relocate the reshaped ear closer to the head in esthetically desired angles, not only horizontally (lateral angle), but also (and of extreme importance for most patients) vertically (superior angle).

Keywords: CO_2 laser, otoplasty, cosmetic surgery, correction of the angle of the ears, reduction of the ears

1. Introduction

Protuberant ears (apostasies, Otis) are one of the most common physical aesthetical variations (grade I abnormalities according to Weerda) of the head and neck regions, occasionally called otocleisis [1]. Actually the most frequent causes of this undesired condition are a disproportionately shaped cavity of the concha and an underdeveloped antihelical fold.

A large diversity of otoplasty methods have been described and all of them have the goal of recreating the normal facade of the ear and achieving symmetry. Current developments in otoplasty methods have steadily progressed in the direction of less to noninvasive procedures, from nonsurgical newborn ear molding to cartilage-sparing surgical techniques and even incisionless, office-based procedures [2].

2. Candidates and psychological specifics

Prominent ears are present in approximately 5% of the general population and can encompass a considerable psychological effect on individuals [2]. Children with protruding ears are often exposed to significant psychological stress, such as being bullied at school. Otoplasty can in general be implemented in patients aged 5 years and older (prior to the start of schooling), from the time when no significant growth or modification of the shape of the pinna can be expected. Otoplasty in pediatric patients has no significant influence on later auricular growth [3].

Kalcioglu et al. compared the growth ratios of the auricle in 1552 subjects from birth until age 18 years, assessing the longitudinal length (upper rim of the helix-lobule), the external transverse length (lateral rim of the helix-tragus), and the internal transverse length (outer rim of the antihelix-tragus), additionally measuring the conchal depth [4]. The development of the pinna regarding the transverse growth and the growth of the conchal depth was entirely completed by the age of 6 years. The length of the auricle increases during chronologic aging process because of the skin and soft tissue expected elasticity.

Schwentner et al. interrogated subjects pre- and postotoplasty concerning their emotional state, by means of a standardized questionnaire. The results of this retrospective revision demonstrated a significant enhancement in attitude toward life, greater than before courage to face life, and healthier self-confidence [5].

3. Anatomical aspects

The auricle anatomy is complex, by means of thin skin surrounding resilient cartilage. These fundamental characteristics make the ears prone to the unconcealed flaunt of surgical correction [6]. Multiple anthropometric studies have been carried out to determine the distance or to calculate the angles between the ear and the head (cephalo-auricular angles). The angle between the mastoid and the helix of a normal shaped auricle should not exceed 30° [7]. Numerous additional criteria for a suitably formed ear have been recommended by various authors:(1) the axis of the ear should be almost parallel to the bridge of the nose; (2) the position of the auricle should be approx. One auricular length behind the lateral orbital margin (55–70 mm); (3) the width of the auricle should be 50–60% of the auricular length (width: 30–45 mm, length 55–70 mm); (4) the anterolateral angle should be 21–30°; and (5) the lobule should be positioned parallel to the antihelical fold in the same plane [8]. In protruding ears, deviations from the normal shape are especially apparent at the antihelix, the concha, the mastoid-helix angle, and the lobule [9]. The angle between the mastoid and the helical rim should be between 20° and 30° according to Vargas [10]. In protruding ears, this angle can be up to 90°, due mainly to hyperplasia of the conchal bowl (**Figure 1**).

Subsequent to a detailed medical history, a thorough physical examination is performed to leave out potential treatable causes of prominent ears, for instance, retroauricular space-occupying lesions or traumatic deformity of the cartilage [11]. A meticulous examination of the antihelix fold, helix-mastoid angle, helix-head distance, position of the lobule, and depth,

http://dx.doi.org/10.5772/intechopen.71992

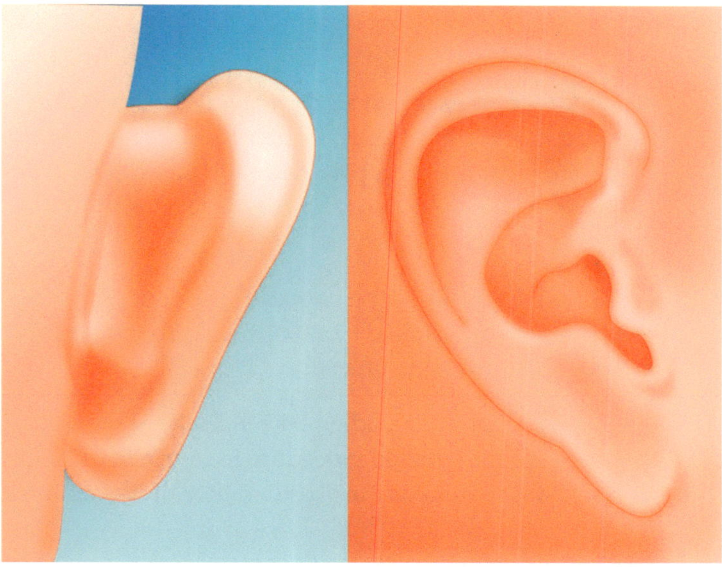

Figure 1. The aim of CO_2 laser otoplasty is to decrease the mastoid-scapha angle, and the conchal-scapha angle should be reduced.

size, and shape of the cavum conchae, is crucial (**Figure 2**). One more feature vital on procedure planning is the evaluation of the consistency of the cartilage and particularly its stiffness and thickness; the cartilage consistency is typically evaluated by palpation and careful bending. Additional abnormalities of the external ear, including auricular appendages or the existence of a Darwin tubercle, can also be discarded merely by physical inspection.

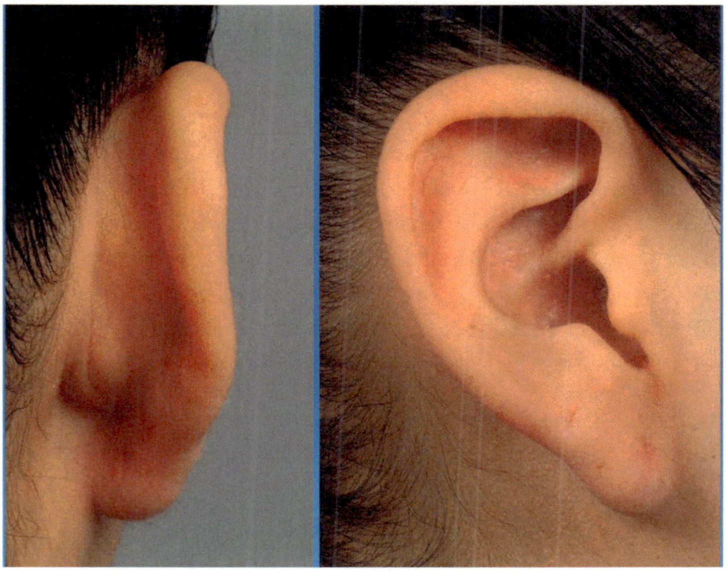

Figure 2. Cosmetically pleasing appearance of the ear.

4. History

During the nineteenth century, reports on surgical techniques described to improve prominent ears for esthetic purposes were published. Dieffenbach, in 1845, was among the first, describing a surgical technique to correct a posttraumatic prominent auricle in a patient. He excised retroauricular skin and used a concho-mastoidal suture for the fixation of the ear [12].

Following Dieffenbach, Ely published in 1881 a crescentic continuous resection of a cartilage strip in combination with a concho-mastoidal fixation suture. To correct bilateral prominent ears, Ely performed otoplasty as a two-step procedure [13].

A review article published by Weerda, including 94 publications on otoplasty techniques, makes it clear that the choice on the suitable procedure to improve protruding auricles can only be selected on an individual basis, taking in consideration all the variants associated with prominent ears [14].

In 1955, Converse published an excision surgical procedure with retroauricular access, supporting a spindle-shaped excision of a cartilage strip, sparing the anterior perichondrium, to reduce the concha [15]. Ultimately, of the numerous different surgical methods and their adaptations, three procedures, alone or combined, have demonstrated their efficacy in the amendment of protruding ears: Converse's incision-suture technique [15], Stenström's incision technique [16], and Mustardé's suture technique [17]. Beasley and Jones cut out the lower conchal bowl segment via a posterior access to diminish the height of the antitragus [18].

In 2007, during the 28th Annual Meeting of the International Society of Dermatologic Surgery in Venice, Italy, the author presented his initial experience using a proprietary surgical technique in 17 patients treated with CO_2 laser-assisted otoplasty with a follow-up of at least 6 months with very good to excellent outcomes in 15 of the 17 patients as reported by the subjects in a satisfaction questionnaire [19].

Holden et al. in 2009 published a minimally invasive ear reshaping with a 1450-nm diode laser using cryogen spray cooling in New Zealand white rabbits [20]. Next year Leclere et al. introduced a noninvasive laser-assisted cartilage reshaping (LACR) technique as an alternative to invasive surgical otoplasty using a 1540-nm laser. They concluded it was a safe and reproducible method for the treatment of protruding ears [21]. In the same year, Ragab described a new technique for prominent ears: carbon dioxide laser-assisted cartilage reshaping otoplasty in subjects with ages ranging from 4 to 7 years (mean 5.5 years), and an average follow-up of 2.4 years [22]. Leclere et al. later published a prospective long-term follow-up of 32 procedures of LACR [23].

Mehta and Gantous published a laser-assisted incisionless otoplasty, a technique for the correction of prominauris. In their article, complications were reported in 10 of 70 patients [24]. The enormous quantity of ever-evolving otoplasty surgical and nonsurgical procedures evidenced its complexity.

5. Method

Our approach to this procedure is centered on the antihelix, particularly on the antihelical fold, the concha, and the scapha of the auricle, where usually the disproportion and excessive angulations of the ear reside. In order to attain a cosmetically pleasing appearance, the proportions of the ear ought to be carefully observed as a whole in the midst of the face and head shape. Asymmetries should also be carefully considered in surgical planning. Asymmetries and individual characteristics should be discussed with the patient, documented, and considered at this point. Planning includes determination of the shape, size, and position of both auricles, from every possible angle.

Naumann [25] described a useful algorithm preotoplasty for the evaluation of the ear and the planning of the procedure, recommending that attention should be paid to the following parameters:

1. Helix-mastoid angle (>30°)
2. Helix-mastoid distance:
   a. Cranial helical rim;
   b. Helical rim at the level of the cavum conchae;
   c. Lobule (>18–20 mm)
3. Hypoplastic antihelix, antihelical folding
4. Conchal hyperplasia, cavum conchae
5. Position of the lobule
6. Isolated changes at the ear: coloboma, Darwin tubercle, auricular appendage
7. Cartilage consistency:
   a. Soft, easily pliable cartilage;
   b. Thick, stiff, poorly pliable cartilage
8. First intervention or revision
9. Tendency to develop keloids
10. Age of patient

Prior to the laser-assisted procedure, patients or parents of the child are informed about the different surgical techniques available and the potential risks and complications, including hematoma and infections or necrosis of skin or cartilage, and also regarding the possibility of an unsatisfactory cosmetic result, or latent abnormal scarring.

Pre- and postoperative photographic documentation in frontal, lateral, oblique, and dorsal views for further assessment is an absolute requirement for the procedure. The uses of photographic documentation are to document preoperative condition and can also be used to outline problematic areas or phases of the laser-assisted procedure. Postoperative photos at intervals of 6 and 12 months help assessing postoperative outcome and are also recommended for medicolegal reasons [26].

The first step of the procedure is to mark unmistakably where the incisions are going to be made. To diminish the cavum-mastoid angle is necessary to bring back the ear closer to the cranial bone. A retroauricular incision parallel to the helical rim should be performed, and usually only a single incision is required, although in some cases a secondary incision is mandatory. The marks are made in of the posterior face of the ear; the main mark should be done following the posterior auriculocranial fold starting right behind the upper insertion of the ear, up to midportion of the auricular lobule. This mark should stay as close as possible to the fold, unless the patient has some excess skin in that area, and then, the mark can be made 2 or 3 mm further back, directly on the cephalic skin; then, the line for auricular incision is calculated and marked, observing how much excess of skin would have to be removed to complete the desired correction. This can be done manually by simulating the position of the ear that is to be achieved, outlining the ideal extension of the incision and the skin fold to be removed with the laser (**Figure 3**). Marking planning usually compensates previously assessed asymmetries.

When needed, the marking of a secondary incision is made on the dorsal face of the scapha, close to the tip of the ear following the curve of the antihelix. Its dimensions should be proportional to the desired degree of correction for that particular area. The reason for a secondary incision is if the patient has a disproportion in the shape and size of the scapha and an

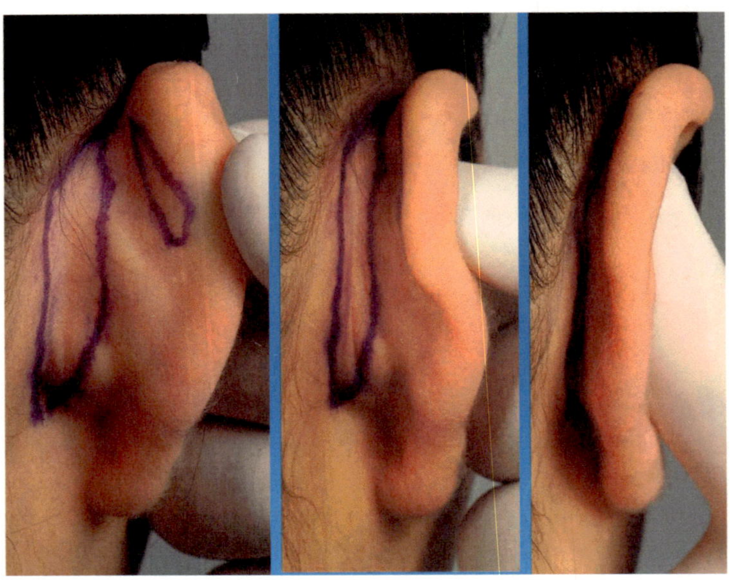

Figure 3. Manual simulation of the corrected position of the ear is used to correctly mark the incisions.

underdeveloped helix and antihelix fold (**Figure 4**), leading to a drooping and forward tilting of the tip of the ear. In some cases, this secondary incision may be unilateral.

Marking includes not only the dorsal side of the ear where the main and secondary incisions will be placed, but also the ventral side of the ear to be infiltrated in the concha and the scapha. A careful planning on the incision will lead to a full correction of the position, angles, and size of the ears, without tension and with an excellent esthetical outcome (**Figure 5**).

After marking, antisepsis is applied to the entire area and adhesive separators are placed to keep the area clear of hair. Sterile tape can be used to delimit the area around the sterile fields to later apply the local anesthetic.

The surgical correction of protruding ears in older children starting from 8 years of age, or adults with adequate compliance can be performed under local anesthesia alone; in smaller children or noncompliant adults, IV sedation is the preferred anesthetic method to complement local anesthesia. General anesthesia can also be used [27].

The local anesthesia employed usually consists of a dose of approximately 5 ml of lidocaine 2% with epinephrine 1:200,000; it is infiltrated subcutaneously in a fan-shaped pattern on the dorsal surface of each ear, directly on the retroauricular fold.

Additional infiltration in the ventral surface of the ears, always on the concha and sometimes on the scapha, is essential for this procedure (**Figures 6** and **7**). It is required that infiltration results in a precise separation of the skin and the perichondrium (hydro-dissection). Since CO_2 laser's chromophore is water, this infiltration will later serve as a natural block for the laser beam to prevent or reduce the incidence of accidental injuries on the ventral skin of the auricle.

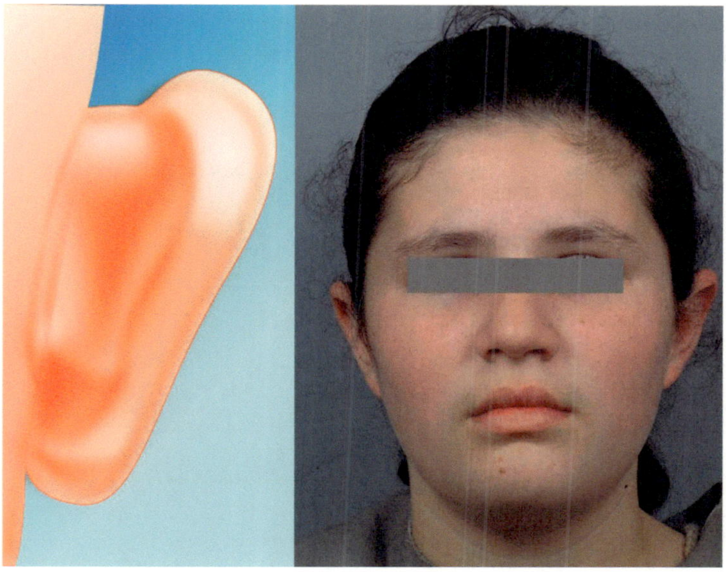

Figure 4. Drooping and protruding tip of the ear and asymmetry.

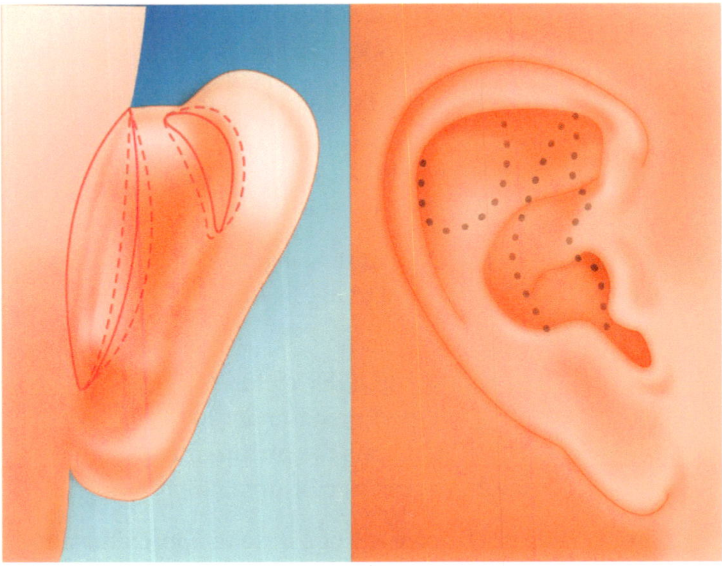

Figure 5. Examples of possible markings for the primary and secondary incisions in the dorsal face of the ear, and areas of infiltration for hydrodissection of ventral face of ear.

The retroauricular skin incisions can be extended from the upper insertion of the ear to the middle of the lobule (depending on the lobule shape), and skin excisions are then performed to the extent needed in each case [28]. The shape and extension of the incisions is directly proportional to the extent to which the auricle protrudes. The main incision is placed directly on the retroauricular fold, and it must extend superiorly as much as the superior angle needs to be fully corrected (if not carefully considered, patient's expectations may not be fulfilled; the degree the ears face downwards is usually more important to the patient than what they face forwardly). A secondary incision in the dorsal side of the scapha is sometimes required to fully correct the shape and angle of the ear.

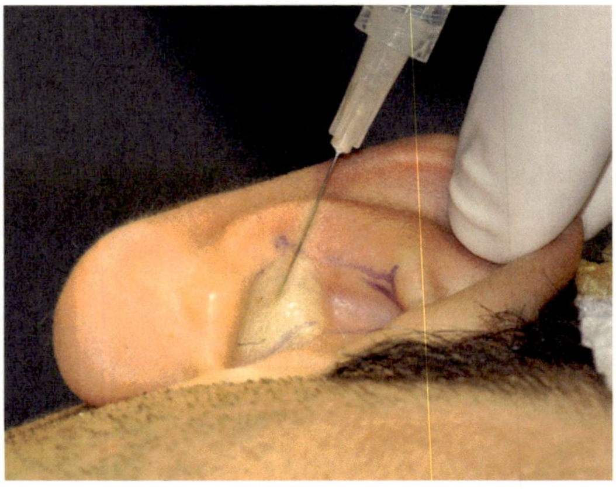

Figure 6. Infiltration of lidocaine 2% with epinephrine 1:200,000 is infiltrated subcutaneously in the concha.

http://dx.doi.org/10.5772/intechopen.71992

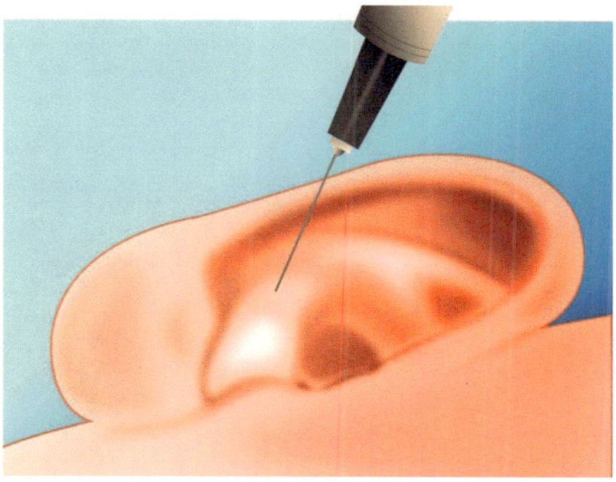

Figure 7. Schematic infiltration of the concha.

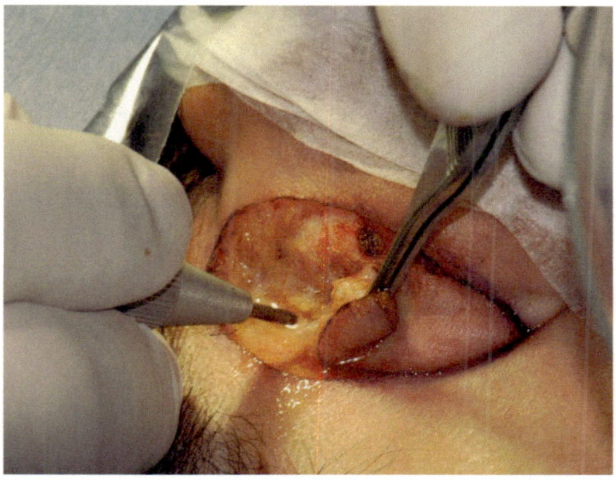

Figure 8. Incision is made directly with the CO_2 laser, layer by layer, up to a complete epiperichondral mobilization of skin and subcutaneous tissues on the dorsal side of the ear.

Incision is made directly with a high-fluence surgical narrow beam CO_2 laser (10,600 nm wavelength), layer by layer; the posterior auricular muscle is transected, and excessive retro-auricular subcutaneous fat and connective tissue is removed up to an epi-perichondral level, completely sparing the temporal fascial, and the posterior aspect of the cartilage in a caudal direction up to the mastoid plane is prepared (**Figure 8**) [29].

The amount of cartilage that is to be removed from the concha (usually 4–9 mm width), medial to the antihelix, depends on the incision that was planned, based on the amount of skin that is to be removed as well as the amount of pressure required to bend the ear properly (hinge effect). For precise marking of the perichondrium, as reference to limit the angles of the cartilage cut, two 30 G × ½ inch needles are inserted at the edges and mid-depth of the concha, transecting the auricle from the ventral side.

The marked window of cartilage is slightly incised with the laser (**Figure 9**) then blunt dissection of the cartilage is performed using tenotomy scissors with blunt tip, the cartilage

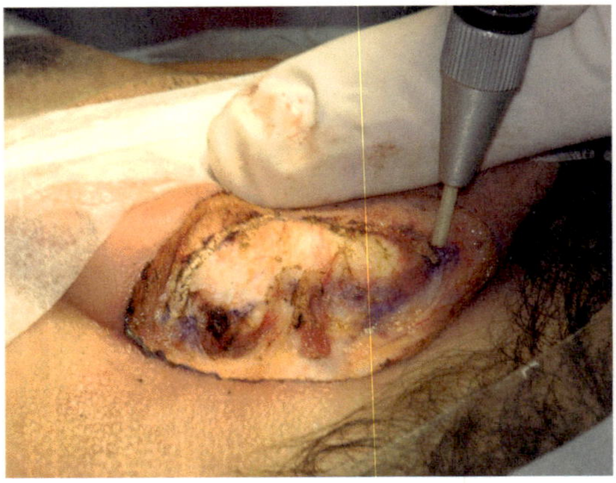

Figure 9. The cartilage is slightly incised with the laser.

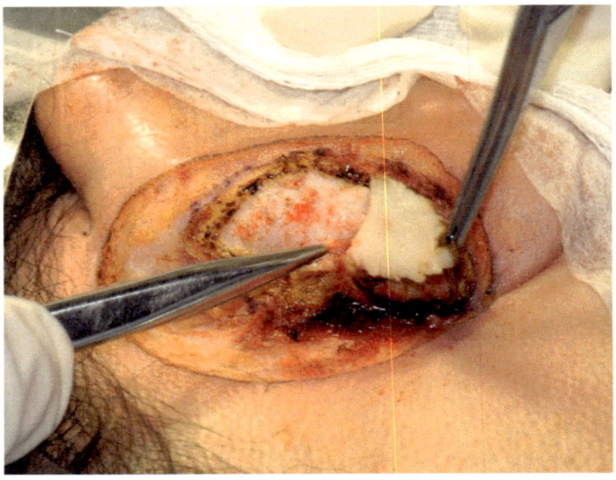

Figure 10. A window of cartilage is excised after blunt dissection.

window is then removed (**Figure 10**); adequate hemostasis of the area is key to a successful outcome; carbonized tissue should be removed (it interferes and retards wound healing process).

The same procedure is made on the dorsal side of the scapha if required. The shape of this secondary incision is determined by the degree of disproportion of the scapha and the need of correction of the conchal-scapha angle.

Then, the auricle is bent dorsally and fixed between the conchal cartilage and the dorsa mastoid periosteum, by means of mattress sutures. The wound must be closed with vicryl or monocryl, 3–0 or 4–0 sutures, depending on the strength of the cartilage and the width of the wound. The first stitch should join both edges of the posterior auricular muscle, from the perichondrium to the mastoid periosteum (**Figures 11** and **12**). After this first buried mattress suture, the desired back angle of the ear should have been achieved; if at this point the angle of the ear has not been corrected properly, then the surgeon should go to go back and

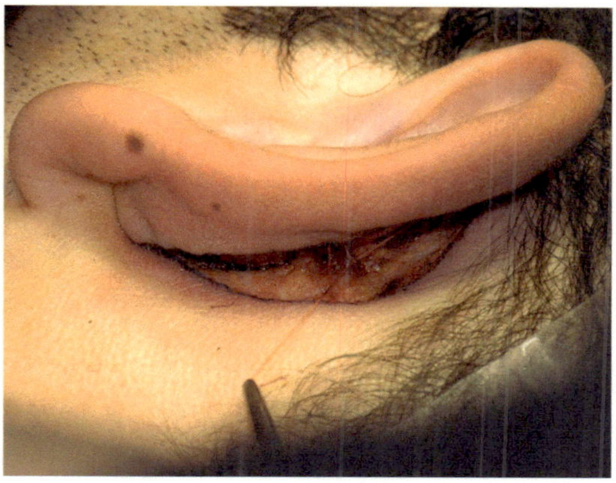

Figure 11. Surgical wound closure is made in two layers subcutaneously using a 4–0 vicryl absorbable suture starting at the posterior retroauricular muscle.

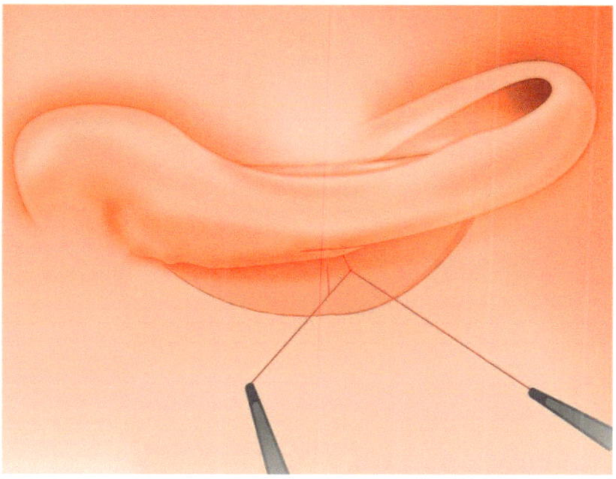

Figure 12. Buried mattress sutures are used to close the wound.

remove more skin and/or subcutaneous tissue or even cartilage as required (**Figure 13**). The same applies for the superior area of the incision, where one or two mattress sutures should correct adequately the lateral dropping of the superior portion of the ear (**Figure 14**). Once the subcutaneous suture is completed, cyanoacrylate glue is applied to the skin or a closed continuous intracutaneous suture (5–0 monocryl) is used to close the skin. No difference has been observed than our previous approach, which was to use continuous intracutaneous 5–0 prolene suture, with the inconvenience of the suture removal after 10 days.

No dressing is used after this outpatient procedure. One of the advantages of this technique is that there is no need to use any type of bandage or patches, nor does it depend on permanent sutures or bandages to force the fold of the cartilage to hold in place. A broad spectrum antibiotic can be used as prophylactic (the author usually prescribes azithromycin orally for 3 days postoperatively). Usually no postoperative analgesics are required. The patient is assessed in a week.

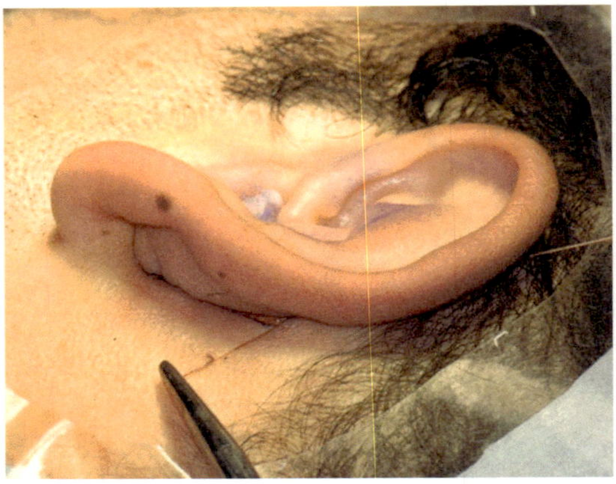

Figure 13. Complete correction of the angle with the initial suture.

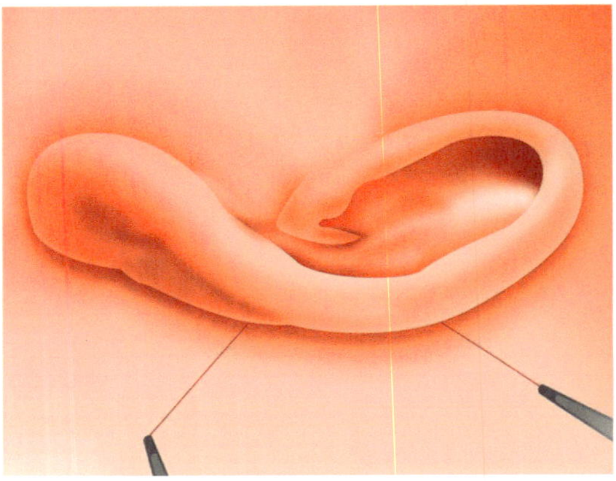

Figure 14. Additional mattress sutures are used to complete the stitching of the wound.

Early and late complications of otoplasty can be distinguished. Early complications include hematomas, and wound infection, which may be associated with perichondritis, pain, postoperative bleeding, allergic reactions, and cartilage or skin necrosis. In contrast, hypertrophic scars, keloids, suture material rejection, hypoesthesia or paresthesia, auricular deformities, or recurrence arise as late complications. Regular examination follow-up visits are strongly suggested, for early detection of complications [8, 14, 30]. With the previously described surgical CO_2 laser procedure, none of the published or any other complications has been observed nor reported by the patients. Postoperative indications include sleep in a Low Fowler's position the first 3–5 days, limit physical exercise, and the use of a travel pillow for neck support, avoiding pressure on the ears for approximately 10 days.

Swelling and bruising are expected side effects that usually last about 10 days. Moderate inflammation will usually persist for 3 weeks, and a very mild inflammation can persist up to 4 months. The final result is reached, as in most procedures, between the 5th and 6th months, although some changes may continue to develop up to 12 months postoperatively.

http://dx.doi.org/10.5772/intechopen.71992

6. Commentaries

We did re-intervene a couple of the first patients, and due to inexperience, we considered important only the lateral back angle and did not take into account the superior angle of the ear. These patients were treated afterward, and esthetic expectations were met using secondary incision

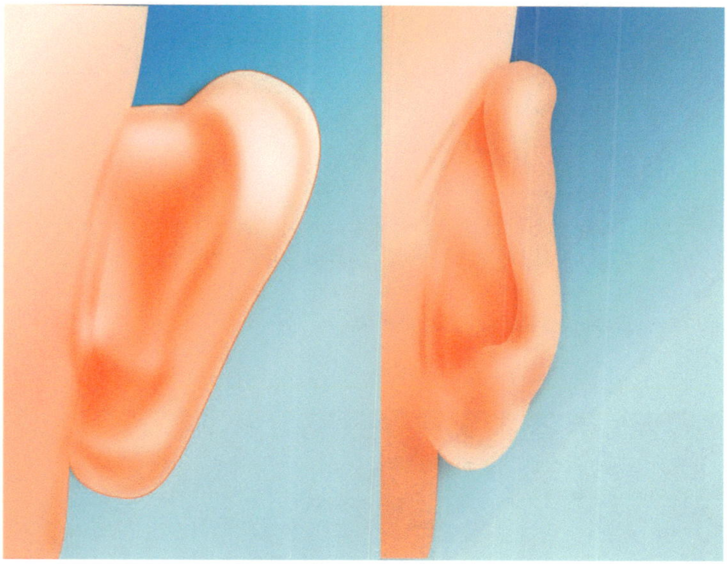

Figure 15. Schematic correction of a protruding ear from a dorsal view.

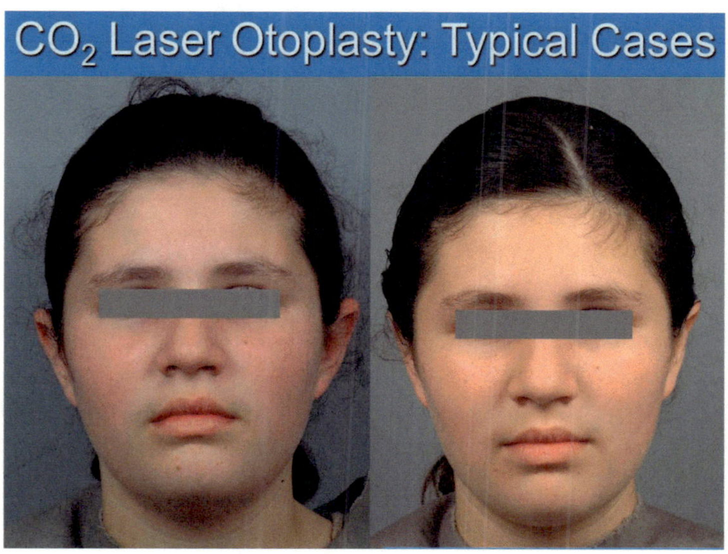

Figure 16. Before and 12 months after a CO_2 laser-assisted otoplasty.

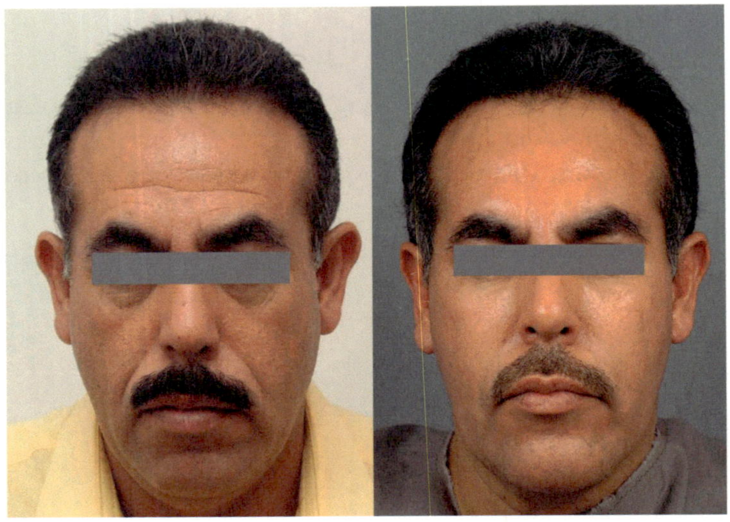

Figure 17. Before and 12 months after a CO_2 laser-assisted otoplasty.

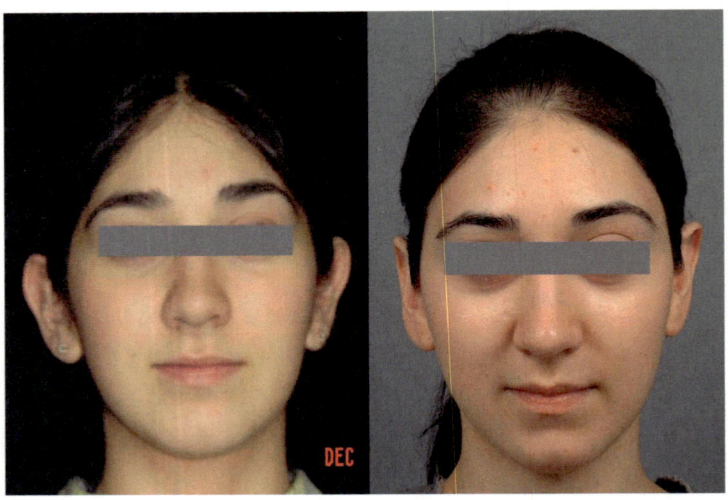

Figure 18. Before and 12 months after a CO_2 laser-assisted otoplasty.

in the back of the scapha. With time we learned that in most cases, there was no need for a secondary incision to correct a drooping ear due to the fact that more skin can be easily removed from the dorsal face of the ear in the superior area of the main incision (usually 1–1.5 cm). This can, in most cases, correct a drop or forward tilt of the superior area of the ear (**Figure 15**).

The secondary semilunar incision, parallel to the helix, is now reserved for cases where clearly there is a disproportional growth of the scapha or an almost absolute lack of the superior aspect of the antihelical fold and an underdeveloped helix. Per each case's particular needs, a second incision can be performed and a part of the cartilage removed to create a crease or fold to reduce the ear's tip size and force a posterior displacement (**Figures 16–22**).

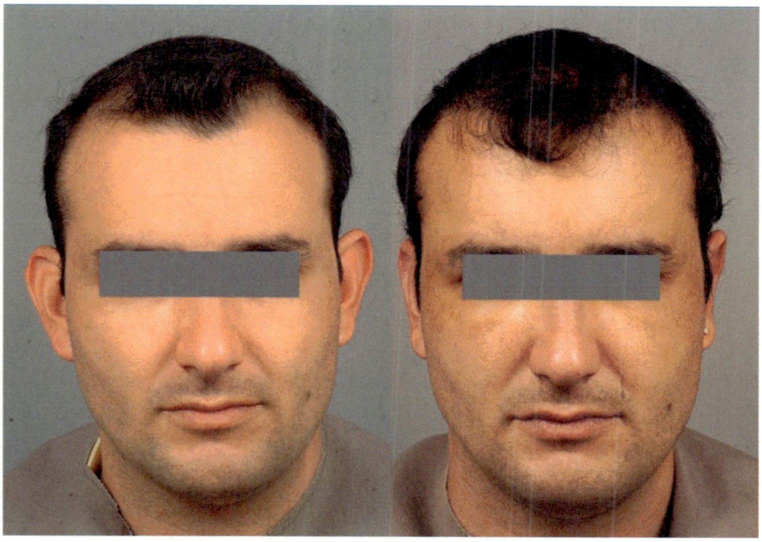

Figure 19. Before and 12 months after a CO_2 laser-assisted otoplasty.

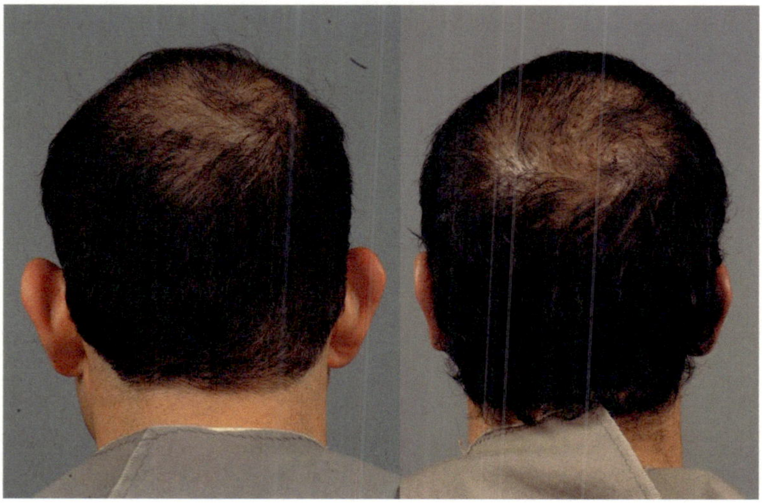

Figure 20. Before and 12 months after a CO_2 laser-assisted otoplasty.

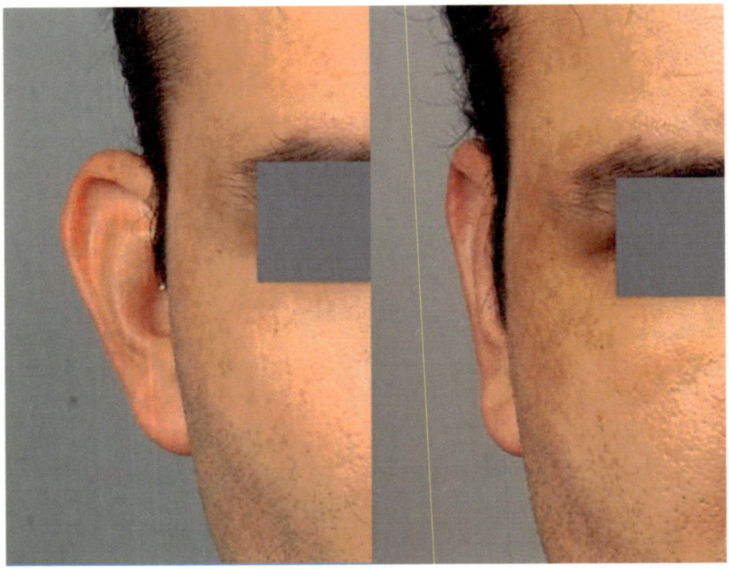

Figure 21. Before and 12 months after a CO_2 laser-assisted otoplasty.

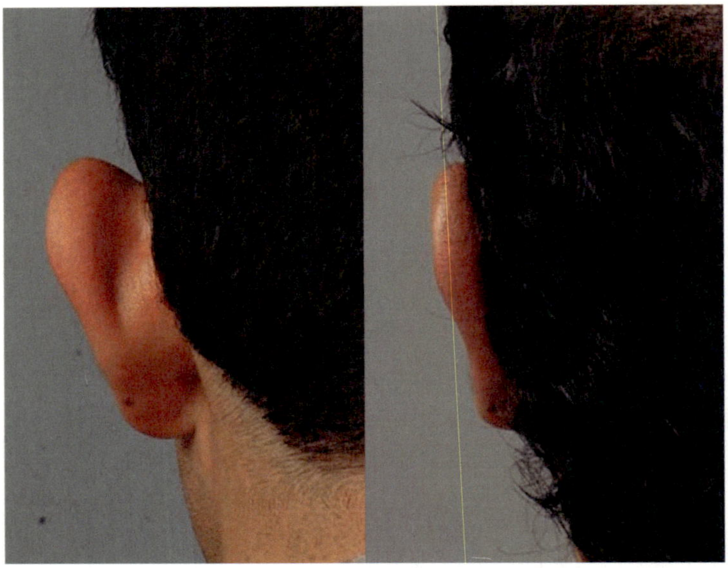

Figure 22. Before and 12 months after a CO_2 laser-assisted otoplasty.

7. Conclusion

Surgical CO_2 laser-assisted otoplasty is presented as a simple, effective, and highly safe novel approach to enhance ear cosmetics for the treatment of esthetically displeasing protruding and/or prominent ears.

Author details

Hector Leal Silva

Address all correspondence to: hleal@ultralaser.com.mx

University of Monterrey, San Pedro Garza García, Mexico

References

[1] Weerda H. Remarks about otoplasty and avulsion of the auricle. Laryngo-Rhino-Otologie. 1979;**58**(3):242-251

[2] Pawar SS, Koch CA, Murakami C. Treatment of prominent ears and otoplasty: A contemporary review. JAMA Facial Plastic Surgery. 2015;**17**(6):449-454

[3] Balogh B, Millesi H. Are growth alterations a consequence of surgery for prominent ears? Plastic and Reconstructive Surgery. 1992;**90**(2):192-199

[4] Kalcioglu MT, Toplu Y, Ozturan O, Yakinci C. Anthropometric growth study of normal human auricle. International Journal of Pediatric Otorhinolaryngology. 2003;**67**:1169-1177

[5] Schwentner I, Schmutzhard J, Deibl M, Sprinzl GM. Health-related quality of life outcome of adult patients after otoplasty. Journal of Craniofacial Surgery. 2006;**17**:629-635

[6] Handler EB, Song T, Shih C. Complications of otoplasty. Facial Plastic Surgery Clinics of North America. 2013;**21**(4):653-662

[7] Farkas LG. Anthropometry of the normal and defective ear. Clinics in Plastic Surgery. 1990;**17**:213-218

[8] Janis JE, Rohrich RJ, Gutowski KA. Otoplasty. Plastic and Reconstructive Surgery. 2005;**115**(4):60e-72e

[9] Siegert R, Krappen S, Kaesemann L, Weerda H. Computer assisted anthropometry of the auricle. Faces. 1998;**6**:1-6

[10] Wodak E. On the position and shape of the human auricle. Archiv fur Klinische und Experimentelle Ohren- Nasen- und Kehlkopfheilkunde. 1967;**188**:331-335

[11] Payasli C, Babuccu O, Kargi E, Hosnuter M, Tekerekoglu B. Traumatic prominent ear secondary to cartilage fracture without skin laceration or hematoma. Plastic and Reconstructive Surgery. 2006;**117**(3):1052-1053

[12] Dieffenbach JE. Die Operative Chirurgie. Leipzig: Brockhaus FA; 1845

[13] Ely ET. An operation for prominent auricles. Archives of Otolaryngology. 1881;**10**:97 Reprinted in Plastic and Reconstructive Surgery. 1968;**42**:582

[14] Weerda H. Chirurgie der Ohrmuschel. Vol. Bd. 1. Stuttgart: Thieme; 2004

[15] Converse JM, Nigro A, Wilson FA, Johnson N. A technique for surgical correction of lop ears. Plastic and Reconstructive Surgery. 1955;**15**:411

[16] Stenström SJ. A "natural" technique for correction of congenitally prominent ears. Plastic and Reconstructive Surgery. 1963;**32**:509

[17] Mustardé JC. The treatment of prominent ears by buried mattress sutures: A ten-year survey. Plastic and Reconstructive Surgery. 1967;**39**:382

[18] Beasley NJ, Jones NS. Otoplasty: The problem of the deep conchal bowl. Journal of Laryngology & Otology. 1996;**110**(9):864-868

[19] Leal H. 28th Annual Meeting. Venice, Italy. ISDS. 26-10-2007

[20] Holden PK, Chlebicki C, Wong BJ. Minimally invasive ear reshaping with a 1450-nm diode laser using cryogen spray cooling in New Zealand white rabbits. Archives of Facial Plastic Surgery. 2009;**11**(6):399-404

[21] Leclere FM, Petropoulos I, Mordon S. Laser-assisted cartilage reshaping (LACR) for treating ear protrusions: A clinical study in 24 patients. Aesthetic Plastic Surgery. 2010; **34**(2):141-146

[22] Ragab A. Carbon dioxide laser-assisted cartilage reshaping otoplasty: A new technique for prominent ears. The Laryngoscope. 2010;**120**(7):1312-1318

[23] Leclere FM, Trelles M, Mordon SR. Cartilage reshaping for protruding ears: A prospective long term follow-up of 32 procedures. Lasers in Surgery and Medicine. 2011;**43**(9): 875-880

[24] Mehta S, Gantous A. Incisionless otoplasty: A reliable and replicable technique for the correction of prominauris. JAMA Facial Plastic Surgery. 2014;**16**(6):414-418

[25] Naumann A. Otoplasty–techniques, characteristics and risks. GMS Current Topics in Otorhinolaryngology, Head and Neck Surgery. 2007;**6**:Doc04

[26] Spira M. Otoplasty: What I do now—A 30-year perspective. Plastic and Reconstructive Surgery. 1999;**104**(3):834-841

[27] Ganzer U. Leitlinien "Ohrplastik" online. 2003. Konsensusbericht der Deutschen Gesellschaft für Hals-Nasen-Ohren-Heilkunde, Kopf- und Hals-Chirurgie: Plastisch-rekonstruktive und ästhetische Operationen in der Hals-Nasen-Ohren-Heilkunde, Kopf-Hals-Chirurgie

[28] Kelley P, Hollier L, Stal S. Otoplasty: Evaluation, technique, and review. Journal of Craniofacial Surgery. 2003;**14**(5):643-653

[29] Furnas DW. Correction of prominent ears by conchamastoid sutures. Plastic and Reconstructive Surgery. 1968;**42**:189

[30] Elliott RA Jr. Otoplasty: A combined approach. Clinics in Plastic Surger. 1990;**17**(2):373-381

Chapter 7

Photodynamic Therapy and Skin Cancer

Eleni Papakonstantinou, Florian Löhr and
Ulrike Raap

Additional information is available at the end of the chapter

http://dx.doi.org/10.5772/intechopen.70309

Abstract

Non-melanoma skin cancer (NMSC) is the most common type of cancer among white skin individuals worldwide with an increasing incidence over the last years. NMSC is mostly treated with surgical or non-invasive methods such as cryotherapy or topical chemotherapeutics. Over the last years, there has been a rapidly growing interest in the use of photodynamic therapy (PDT) which is a well-tolerated, safe and effective alternative treatment option. PDT involves a photosensitizer, a light source and tissue oxygen and is based on a photo-oxidation reaction in the target tissue which results to a selective destruction of the cancer cells. PDT has been approved for treatment of actinic keratosis, Bowen's disease and basal cell carcinoma in Europe. Off-label uses include treatment of invasive squamous cell carcinoma, cutaneous T-cell lymphoma, Kaposi's sarcoma, Paget's disease and prevention of recurrence of squamous cell carcinoma in organ-transplant recipients. Also combination of PDT with other treatment options such as cryotherapy, surgery and topical therapies has been reported with improved efficacy, tolerability and long-term results. Development of novel photosensitizers and light sources together with targeted delivery systems will increase specificity, efficiency and treatment field of PDT in the future. This chapter aims to give the reader an overview of the important applications of PDT, including indications, approved treatments, advantages and disadvantages of this method such as future trends.

Keywords: photodynamic therapy, photosensitizer, non-melanoma skin cancer, basal cell carcinoma, squamous cell carcinoma, actinic keratosis

1. Introduction

Non-melanoma skin cancer (NMSC) is the most common type of cancer among white-skin individuals worldwide with an increasing incidence over the last years. Clinical examination, evaluation through dermoscopy and histopathology are the gold standard methods for the diagnosis of skin cancer. These diagnostic procedures together with the location and extent of the tumor will determine the choice of treatment. NMSC is mostly treated with surgical excision or non-invasive methods such as cryotherapy, application of topical chemotherapeutics or radiotherapy. However, limitations and side-effects of the conventional therapies motivate the development of other techniques.

Over the last years, there has been a rapidly growing interest in the use of photodynamic therapy (PDT) for treatment and prevention of skin cancer. PDT is a well-tolerated, safe and effective alternative in the treatment and prevention of non-melanoma skin cancer. Nowadays, it is mostly used for the treatment for actinic keratosis but also for in situ squamous cell carcinoma (Bowen's disease), superficial- and also nodular basal cell carcinoma with acceptable response rates [1].

As a non-invasive targeted therapy with a low spectrum of adverse effects, PDT has advantages concerning the patient comfort and achieves excellent cosmetic results while the response rates are comparable to that of other surgical and nonsurgical procedures [2].

The aim of this chapter is to provide an assessment of the current state of use of PDT in the treatment of skin cancer and focus on new developments and future aspects of this procedure in the treatment of non-melanoma skin cancer.

2. General principles of photodynamic therapy

The main principle of photodynamic therapy is based on photooxidation occurring in a target tissue. Key components of this technique are a photosensitizer, oxygen and light within the absorption spectrum of the photosensitizer.

The mechanism of action of photosensitizers is divided in two different types. Type I reaction involves direct oxidation by hydrogen peroxide, superoxide anion radical and hydroxyl radical of biological targets (DNA, membranes and proteins), while type II reaction includes oxidation mediated by singlet oxygen through energy transfer from triplet states to molecular oxygen [3]. The production of reactive oxygen species (ROS) depends on the uptake of a photosensitizing drug by the tumor, the subsequent irradiation of the tumor with visible light of an appropriate wavelength and the presence of an adequate concentration of molecular oxygen [3]. A photosensitizer can induce tissue damage either directly through induction of necrosis or apoptosis or indirectly by affecting its vascularization. It is important to know that in absence of any one of these components, the effectiveness of photodynamic response is disturbed. Therefore, careful selection of photosensitizer, type of tissue photosensitization and light dosimetry is essential [4, 5].

2.1. Photosensitizers

Photosensitizers (PSs) are substances capable of making an organism, a cell or a tissue photosensitive by inducing the photo-oxidation of several types of molecules through energy transfer processes. The development of an ideal photosensitizer remains a major challenge since several characteristics have to be taken into consideration. It is important for the photosensitizer to be chemically pure, to have chemical and physical stability, high selectivity and to be activated only in the presence of light, with no dark toxicity. The wavelength of the light used in PDT has to be longer than those in the UV spectrum in order to minimize the risk of UV-induced skin cancer. Its absorption peak should be a wavelength > 630 nm, where it presents an optimal tissue penetration. Furthermore, it should have a high absorption capacity being able to be rapidly and predominantly retained in the tumor tissue and eliminated from the organism in order to prevent the risk of prolonged systemic photosensitivity. The photosensitizer should also have a clearance from the tumor tissue which is slower than that of normal cells and be capable to generate reactive oxygen species [6].

For dermatological appliance, only haematoporphyrin derivatives like porfimer sodium (Photofrin H) or protoporphyrin IX (PPIX)-inducing precursors like 5-aminolevulinic acid (ALA) or methyl aminolevulinate (MAL) are of practical concern. Therefore topical photosensitizers are preferred for use in dermatology. After topical application, both ALA and MAL are mainly taken up by cells of epithelial origin and are converted into photosensitizing porphyrins [7]. After an incubation period, followed by illumination with visible light to activate the photosensitizer a type II photo-oxidation reaction takes place and produces reactive oxygen species (ROS), which destroy cell membranes and structures, ultimately leading to cell death. The appropriate wavelength of light, concentration of sensitizer and molecular oxygen level in the tissue are all critical for the efficacy of PDT [8].

2.2. Topical photosensitizing drugs

Current clinical practice utilizes the use of topical photosensitizers in PDT such as 5-aminolevulinic acid (5-ALA) or methyl-aminolevulinate (MAL), which are both precursors in the biosynthesis of protoporphyrin IX (PpIX) (**Figure 1**). PpIX is a native photosensitizing compound that accumulates in the cells and has an absorption peak at 505, 540, 580 and 630 nm.

The 5-ALA-based photosensitizers are not photoactive themselves, but show a preferential intracellular accumulation in the tissue target and particularly in the tumor cells where they are metabolized by the haem biosynthesis into photosensitizing porphyrins [7, 9].

Although these two molecules share a similar mechanism of action as prodrugs that lead to production of photoactive PpIX, they have notable differences.

ALA is a hydrophilic molecule and is used to treat more superficial lesions due to its modest tissue penetration [10]. Although the uptake of ALA is non-selective, accumulation of PpIX in tumor cells may occur selectively through alterations in enzymatic activity in the heme synthesis pathway. It is supposed, that activity of porphobilinogen deaminase (PBGD) increases in tumor tissue. PBGD synthesizes a precursor of PpIX and thus increases production of PpIX. The accumulation of PpIX in tumor tissue is further enhanced by decreased activity of ferrochelatase, which converts PpIX to heme [11]. Another postulated mechanism of selectivity for topical ALA relates to the altered stratum corneum of tumoral skin.

MAL is a more hydrophobic molecule which can better penetrate through the cell membranes and more easily reaches the deepest epidermal layers. Therefore, shows MAL a higher selectivity for tumor cells compared with ALA. However, the biosynthesis of protoporphyrin IX

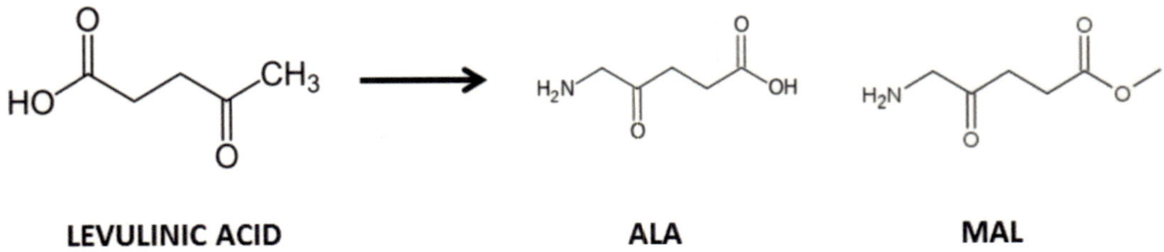

Figure 1. Molecular structures of 5-aminolevulinic acid (5-ALA) and methyl-aminolevulinate (MAL).

production from MAL is slightly slower because of the need of hydrolysis of this compound. Adjacent unaffected structures such as epidermis and mesenchymal cells show a much less pronounced production of porphyrin, thus leading to a high ratio between tumor and surrounding tissue [12]. This technique enables a selective detection (fluorescence detection) and selective destruction of the target tissue with minimal harm to the surrounding one (**Figure 2**).

Interestingly, there seems to be no significant differences in the efficacy between ALA- and MAL-PDT in the treatment of NMSC, as recently shown [13].

Standardized protocols for the application of both photosensitizing drugs have been developed. For MAL-PDT, there is a standardized protocol of two treatments 1 week apart for basal cell carcinoma (BCC) and Bowen's disease (BD), but with only one initial treatment for actinic keratosis (AK), repeated at 3 months, only if required [1]. MAL is typically applied for 3 h, but Levulan ALA although licensed for an 18–24 h application, is widely used with shorter application intervals around 1 h [14]. A shorter incubation for MAL-PDT for 1 h in AK can also be performed since no significant difference in clearance rates have been reported [15].

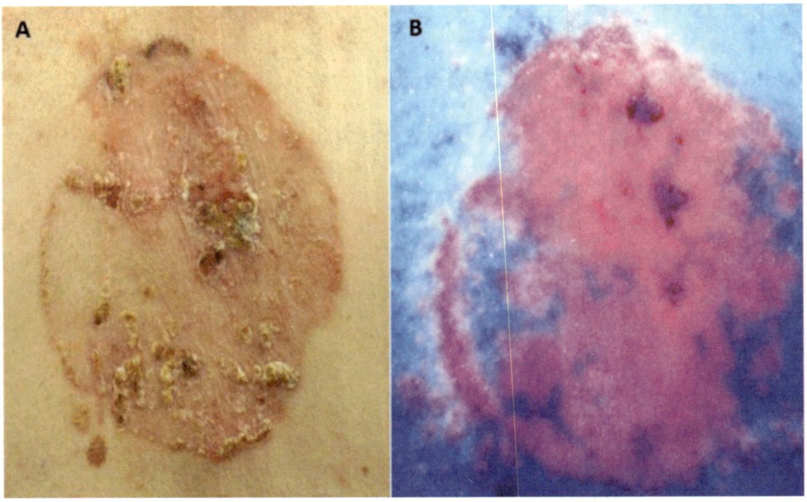

Figure 2. Selective detection of fluorescence due to prior application of ALA on a superficial BBC lesion.

Several novel topical photosensitizers such near-infrared (NIR) bacteriochlorin analogues [16], silicon phthalocyanine, alone [17] or in combination with C6-pyridinium ceramide (LCL29) [18] have promising characteristics for use in PDT but they are still in experimental level.

2.3. Light sources and action mechanism

Distinct light sources can be used for PDT. For therapy, the tissue must be irradiated with light at appropriate wavelengths (within the absorption spectrum of porphyrins) and the light source should have special characteristics for use in PDT in NMSC. Light should be perfectly absorbed by the photosensitizer, achieve a desirable penetration depth and thus reaching the target tissue, have an adequate power and duration in order to trigger the PDT reaction and cause minimal discomfort or side-effects such as erythema, crusting or dyspigmentation [19].

Porphyrins exhibit a very typical absorption spectrum with the highest peak at approximately 405 nm, called the Soret-band. Several so-called Q-bands also exist, the last having an absorption peak at 635 nm. Although the peak is much smaller than that at 405 nm, this wavelength is preferentially used for illumination since light at red spectrum results in a higher tissue penetration [20, 21].

The light sources available for PDT belong to three major groups: broad spectrum lamps, diode lamps and lasers. For a successful PDT-treatment using ALA- or MAL-PDT both laser and incoherent light sources can be used and there is no difference regarding the profile of light. Even pulsed laser light sources matching one of the Q-bands at 585 nm have comparable results to an incoherent light source in the treatment of AK [22]. Also the use of a long-pulsed dye laser at 595 nm seems to be effective for the same indication [19]. The incoherent light sources include the halogen lamps, the light-emitting diode (LED) lamps and intense pulsed light (IPL) lamps. Due to the possibility of distinct emission geometries and lower costs are an attractive option [23, 24].

Light with wavelengths of 635 nm is capable of penetrating the skin to a depth of approximately 6 mm compared to 1–2 mm with a wavelength of 400–500 nm. The effective therapeutic depth, however, appears to be close to 1–3 mm when 635 nm is used. This is due to the capacity to produce a photodynamic reaction, which depends on the dose of light and also on the quantity of photosensitizer used in the target tissue [25].

Advantages of lasers are that they provide a specific wavelength that corresponds to the peak absorption of the photosensitizer. Since lasers can emit high flux monochromatic light and have a focal precision, enable the treatment of small lesions with minimal damage to the surrounding tissue and within a short time interval. Nevertheless, for the treatment of dermatological conditions using PDT, lasers show no advantage compared to over cheaper and more practical options with non-coherent light sources. These sources emit a large radiation field, enabling larger areas of the skin surface to be treated [26]. However, the costs for purchasing and maintenance of these laser systems are extremely high. The gold standards in topical PDT are light sources with wide illumination fields which accomplish the simultaneous illumination of larger areas.

Here incoherent light sources are preferred, either lamps or light-emitting diodes (LEDs) which match the absorption maxima of the ALA- or MAL-induced porphyrins [25, 27, 28]. Using broad-spectrum red light (580–700 nm), a light dose of 100–150 J/cm^2 (100–200 mW/cm^2) is essential for tissue damage. The light intensity should not exceed 200 mW/cm^2 in order to avoid hyperthermic side effects [27]. After a photosensitizer has been activated with light of appropriate wavelength, it comes to the generation of reactive oxygen species (ROS), in particular singlet oxygen. Depending on the extend and localization of the target tissue, these ROS modify either cellular functions or induce cell death by necrosis or apoptosis [29].

MAL-PDT using daylight has been shown to be as effective as conventional red light MAL-PDT in the treatment of AK, but with minimal to no therapy-related pain [30].

There is also an option for ambulatory PDT, where portable LED light source with low irradiance can be applied for over 100 min. Satisfactory results with clearing 11 of 17 lesions and minimal pain have been reported for treatment of BD and superficial BCC [31].

2.4. Cutaneous fluorescence diagnosis

Topical photosensitizing drugs can also be applied for diagnostic purposes. Cutaneous fluorescence diagnosis (FD) is a promising dermatological procedure based on the combination of a local application of a photosensitizer such ALA or MAL and the use of a light source adapted to the absorption spectrum of these molecules. After topical application of ALA or MAL on the skin lesional and non-lesional areas, they are irradiated with blue light (408 nm). As PpIX shows red fluorescence when excited by blue light, PpIX accumulating cells can be visualized [32]. The detection of skin surface fluorescence can be made either by using simple handheld Wood's lamp (long wave UVA) or by using CCD camera systems coupled to digital imaging and helps the clinician to differentiate lesions and perform either a guided biopsy or a controlled and complete resection of tumor, or even to identify persistent or recurrent disease. By using a commercial digital CCD camera system, together with digital imaging, the contrast of the acquired fluorescence images can be significantly enhanced and allows the determination of a threshold, which can be utilized either for a directed biopsy or for preoperative planning when Moh's surgery is scheduled [33].

Furthermore, FD is probably a helpful tool to prove the efficacy of PDT. Limitations of this technique are the difficult interpretation and the low reproducibility of the obtained data. Most studies have mainly focused on BCC [34], AK and SCC [35] so far. Truchuelo et al. [36] showed that FS is a valid diagnostic tool in the diagnosis and follow up of BD with a comparable evaluation to clinical and histopathological results, a specificity of 85.7% and a 100% sensitivity (higher than clinical evaluation alone).

Although, FS cannot be used to differentiate the different stages of AK, it was shown that through differences in fluorescence ratio between AK and SCC, these entities can be differentiated [35, 37].

2.5. Practical application, tolerability and side effects

PDT with ALA or MAL conventionally begins with the topical application of the photosensitizers on the target area. In case of hyperkeratotic lesions, a keratolysis using an ointment, wet cloth or by slight non-bleeding curettage has to be performed prior to the application of photosensitizer as this may be the cause of a poor therapeutic response [38, 39].

ALA has been applied in various formulations such as creams or gels, sometimes with penetration enhancers. ALA preparations are usually applied to the target lesions with little overlap to the surrounding tissue for 4–6 h prior to illumination under occlusion and with a light protective dressing or clothing [40].

MAL is mainly applied in ointments which have a shorter incubation time of 3 h due to the preferential uptake and their higher selectivity [41, 42]. The entire area is then covered with an occlusive foil to allow a better penetration during the incubation which is then followed by illumination with blue light.

Pain is a major and serious adverse event during PDT and can lead to discomfort of the patient to incomplete treatments and need for repeat treatments [43]. The pain or a kind of burning sensation is mostly experienced during the time of illumination and a couple of hours later [9].

In a previous study it could be shown that MAL-PDT induces less pain in comparison to ALA-PDT which can be partially explained due to the differences in selectivity between the two substances [44].

Various pain-relieving approaches have been used in order to reduce pain during PDT. During extensive treatment fields administration of oral analgesia can be useful [45]. The application of local anaesthetics like lidocaine/prilocaine substances prior to illumination is generally not recommended. As previously shown also application of morphine 0.3% gel 15 min prior to illumination did not result in a significant reduction of pain as compared to a placebo gel [46]. Furthermore, due to their high pH local anaesthetics carry the risk of interaction during the incubation period of ALA/MAL and thus inactivate the photosensitizing drug. Wiegell et al. showed that application of cold water and regular pauses in illumination led to a considerable reduction of pain during PDT [47]. An alternative option with satisfactory results is a concurrent cold air analgesia which has been shown to improve the tolerability of ALA- and MAL-PDT [48]. Also analgesia by means of a nitrous oxide/oxygen mixture during PDT led to an overall reduction in pain of 55.2% and willingness of patients to continue the therapy [43].

Previous studies have also demonstrated that the type of light applied plays also a role in the development of pain. Therefore, PDT with the use of PDL coherent light, when compared to LED incoherent light led to less pain and increased willingness of patients to further perform the therapy [49].

Besides pain also burning and prickling sensations are common side effects of PDT. These sensations are usually mild to moderate in intensity and reversible [50]. In a previous study with ALA-PDT used to treat AK, it was found that about 96% of patients experienced stinging/burning sensations at 6 and 11 min during illumination. However, only 10% of them characterized pain intensity as severe [51].

Localized erythema and oedema in the treated area can also occur. Rarely a dry necrosis sharply restricted to the tumor areas can manifest over the next few days which is followed by complete re-epithelialization. Also pigmentary disorders presented as hypo- or hyper-pigmentation are also potential adverse effects of PDT treatment but are rare and of temporary duration. More often, pigmentary disorders have been noted prior to PDT-treatment and resolved at the last follow-up evaluation [51]. Allergic contact dermatitis, although extremely rare, can also occur by presence of sensitization against active ingredients of the applied sensitizers [52].

Due to the high selectivity and photosensitization preferentially to cells of epithelial origin and no fibroblasts or dermal fibers, usually no scarring or ulceration is observed clinically [9, 40]. Also irreversible alopecia could not be observed after PDT treatment series on the scalp despite the concomitant sensitization of pilosebaceous units [40, 53]. With the exception of a porphyria or previous allergic reactions to the active ingredients of the applied sensitizers in the medical history, there are no severe limitations to performance of ALA- or MAL-PDT. PDT treatment can be repeated and applied even in areas with prior exposure to ionizing irradiation [54]. During PDT treatment, both patient and clinic staff should be wearing protective goggles to avoid the risk of eye damage [38].

3. Photodynamic therapy in non-melanoma skin cancer

PDT is nowadays widely applied in the therapy of NMSC. The range of possible indications is expanding continuously, including non-malignant conditions and even premature skin aging due to chronical sun exposure. MAL is approved for use in Europe and United States in combination with red light for treating AK, superficial or nodular BCC and in-situ SCC or BD. A combination of an alcohol-containing ALA solution in a special applicator (Levulan Kerastick) and blue light is also approved in United States for the treatment of AK. For therapy of multiple lesions or by immunodeficient patients, PDT may be the treatment of first choice [23]. PDT is also indicated for patients with important comorbidities when surgery and radiotherapy are contraindicated. It may also be used for palliative care in combination with chemo- or radiotherapy for advanced tumors with skin metastases.

In the dermatological daily practice, PDT has some advantages compared to conventional treatments such as radiotherapy, chemotherapy and surgery. Some of them are the limited duration of the treatment, the efficiency and the good cosmetic outcome due to its high selectivity.

3.1. Actinic keratosis

Actinic keratoses (AKs) are premalignant disorders of keratinocytes occurring on chronically sun-damaged skin. Although a spontaneous regression may occur in up to 20% of cases [55] there is a risk of transformation to SCC within one year between 0.025 and 16% [56]. Since AK manifests in chronically sun-damaged skin and there are often multiple lesions the exact risk of malignant transformation for individual lesions cannot be estimated [57]. Various treatment options such as cryotherapy, topical immunomodulation, laser and PDT are highly effective and recommended not only for individual lesions but also for field treatment [1, 58]. Several studies have been performed analyzing the efficacy of both ALA-PDT and MAL-PDT and comparing them with other procedures in treatment of AKs. Thin AK lesions or lesions of moderate thickness on the face and scalp respond well to topical PDT with clearance rates 89–92% 3 months after therapy [59]. A phase III clinical trial of ALA-PDT for the treatment of multiple AKs of the face and scalp found that 89% of patients had a remission of 75% or more of their AKs after 3 months of treatment [60]. Tschen et al. [51] reported remission rates of 78% 12 months after a single ALA-PDT treatment, with few adverse effects.

European guidelines recommend that for AK, MAL-PDT should be performed as a single treatment and repeated if required after 3 months, reflecting equivalent efficacy in a comparable study with a double therapy 1 week apart [59].

Also compared with other treatment options such as cryotherapy PDT achieves favorable outcomes [61, 62]. A novel self-adhesive patch ALA-PDT war superior to cryotherapy and placebo after 12 weeks in a multicenter phase III trial [61]. Also MAL-PDT achieved better therapeutic results compared to single cycle cryotherapy and placebo after 3 months in another large prospective randomized study [62]. When compared to double cycle cryotherapy for AKs on the extremities in a large randomized multicenter study MAL-PDT showed superior efficacy [63].

When compared with the topical application of 5-fluouracil (5-FU) twice daily ALA-PDT showed similar outcomes in mean lesion reduction [64]. Recently Tanghetti et al. reported that patients with AK who had been treated with 5-FU prior to ALA-PDT showed a significant decrease of clinical lesions after 1 and 3 months compared to these substances alone, which indicates that 5-FU has a synergistic role to ALA-PDT [65].

No significant difference was found in treatment responses of facial AKs to topical 5% imiquimod compared to ALA-PDT in a randomized, single-blind, split-face study [66]. Tanaka et al. [67] also compared the use of topical 5% imiquimod, with ALA-PDT but also with combination therapy in a randomized study. Although the combination group showed outstanding effectiveness, it was more frequently associated with adverse events, when compared to the PDT and imiquimod alone groups. There were no differences in either efficacy or adverse events between PDT and imiquimod monotherapy, however development of pigmentation was higher in the imiquimod therapy group.

Interestingly, imiquimod 5%, showed superiority in histological and clinical outcomes over MAL-PDT for face and scalp AKs, in a further randomized study [68]. The same study found that sequential MAL-PDT and imiquimod 5% are significantly more effective than each therapy alone, indicating that combination treatment may be beneficial [68].

Compared to CO_2 laser ablation for the treatment of multiple scalp AKs in a randomized, half-side comparative study ALA-PDT showed superior efficacy [69]. By hyperkeratotic AKs, physical or chemical keratolytic pretreatment significantly improves the uptake of photosensitizer and light penetrance [70]. Topical application of 10% salicylic acid and 40% urea have similar efficacy to curettage, although chemical pre-treatment was associated with increased pain [70]. The recent introduction of ALA patch PDT reduces the need of keratolytic treatment prior to PDT [71].

Efficacy of PDT for AK on acral sites is reduced by approximately 10%, probably due to a higher proportion of thicker lesions. Compared to cryotherapy, MAL-PDT proved to be less effective for acral AK (lesion clearance 78% versus 88% after 6 months) [51].

Several novel methods of delivering PDT have been used for the treatment of AK, including the adhesive patch, daylight, ambulatory light sources and fractionated light protocols. PDT using the BF-200 ALA, has been recently licensed and proven to be superior to MAL with clearance of 90% versus 83% of thin or moderate thickness face/scalp AK (complete clearance rates of 78% versus 64%) 12 weeks after one or two PDT treatments [72].

PDT is identified as an effective therapeutic option both for lesion and field treatment for AK and by presence of multiple and/or confluent AK, at sites of poor healing, or where there has been a poor response to other topical therapies [73]. Also patient tolerance to MAL-PDT or topical imiquimod for multiple face/scalp AK and level of satisfaction were significantly higher by patients who underwent PDT treatment in a randomized comparison trial [74]. **Figures 3** and **4** present clinical outcomes of ALA-PDT in AK lesions at the head and ear of two patients.

3.2. Basal cell carcinoma

PDT is an established treatment for superficial and nodular types of BCC, but is not indicated for the more aggressive or infiltrating types [75]. Response rates of PDT in the existing

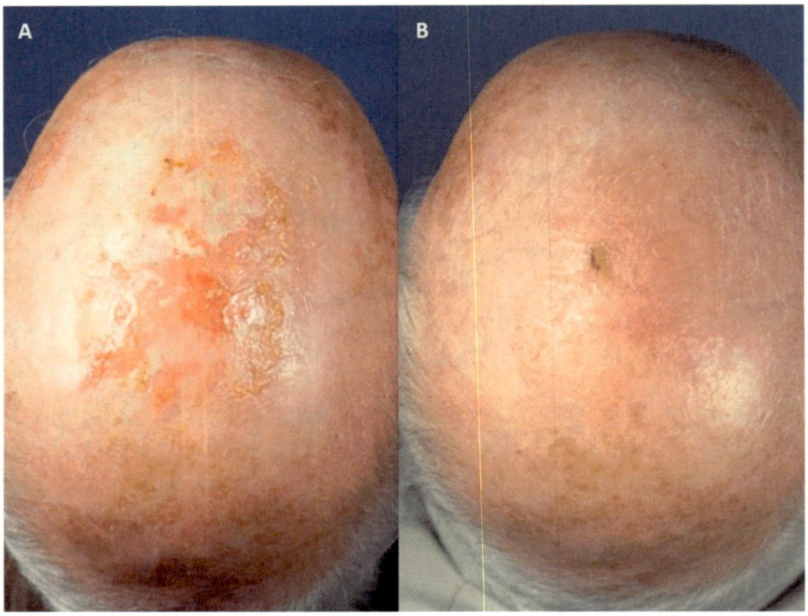

Figure 3. (A) Clinical manifestation of AKs on the head, (B) clinical outcome 4 weeks after one therapy-cycle consisting of double PDT-treatment in 1 week apart.

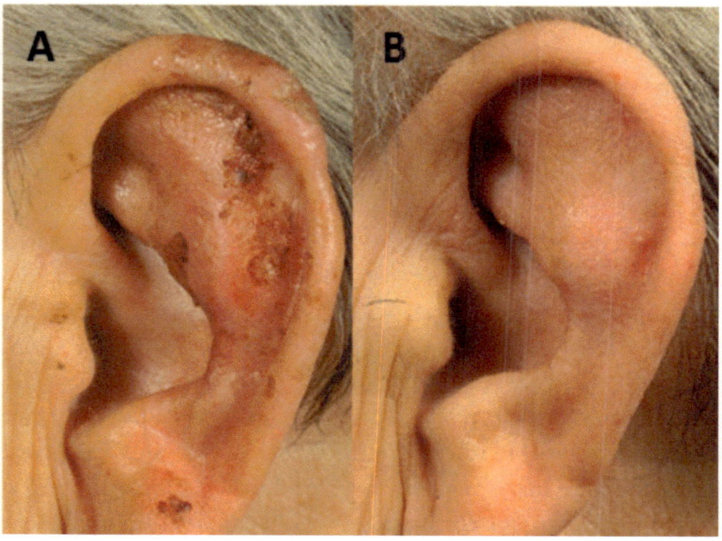

Figure 4. (A) Clinical manifestation of AKs on the helix of the left ear, (B) clinical outcome 3 years after therapy (there has been performed two therapy-cycles each consisting of double PDT-treatment in 1 week apart).

literature vary between 70 and 90%, which may depend on the kind of tumors and the exact performance of PDT [76, 77]. MAL-PDT is approved in the EU for treatment of BCC, but remains off-label in the United States. Several studies have so far assessed the efficacy, cosmetic results and recurrence rates of BCC treated with PDT [78–80].

PDT has proven to generally be more effective for superficial BCC as compared to nodular BCC and also for lesions smaller than 2 cm [65, 66, 68]. Regarding the use of PDT for the treatment of larger and nodular BCC, MAL-PDT has proven to be a more effective treatment option with lower recurrence rates as compared to ALA-PDT [66, 68].

PDT appears to have good efficacy and cosmetic outcome but results in higher BCC recurrence rates in comparison to surgical excision [77, 79, 81–83]. Szeimies et al. [77] reported a similar efficacy at 3 months for MAL-PDT and surgical excision in the management of superficial BCC in a large randomized multicenter open study (92.2% clinical lesion response versus 99.2% in the surgical group). In a recent meta-analysis Zou et al. [83] found also that PDT is comparably effective to surgical excision for treatment of BCC, but with an increased risk of recurrence. Rhodes et al. [82] showed that the recurrence rate for primary nodular BCC after treatment with PDT was 14% versus 4% with surgical excision at the 5-year follow-up point. Data from other studies support that PDT leads to better cosmetic results compared to surgical excision [81, 82]. Also PDT serves as an effective alternative treatment option in difficult cases where an extensive surgical excision should have been performed carrying the risk of a worse cosmetic outcome [84].

When compared with cryotherapy for the treatment of superficial BCC, MAL-PDT led to comparable recurrence rates after 5 years, but better cosmetic results [85]. In a recent three-year follow up randomized controlled trial Roozeboom et al. [86] compared the efficacy of

MAL-PDT, topical imiquimod and 5-FU on the treatment of superficial BCC. Topical imiquimod has shown superiority to MAL-PDT (tumor-free survival 58.0% for MAL-PDT versus 79.7% for imiquimod) but comparable results with 5-FU (68.2%).

For nodular BCC, variable response rates have been reported in several studies. Rhodes et al. [82] observed comparable response rates for primary nodular BCC treated with MAL-PDT or surgical excision at 3 months (91 and 98%, respectively), again with greater recurrence rates but better cosmetic outcomes in the PDT group. The same group showed in a later randomized study persistent complete lesion response rates at 5 years which were 76% for MAL-PDT und 96% for surgical excision of nodular BCC. PDT led consistently to better cosmetic outcomes [87]. On the contrary, Mosterd et al. [88] showed in a further randomized controlled study of 173 primary nodular BCCs that surgical excision was significantly more effective compared to a single treatment of fractionated ALA-PDT, with a failure rate of 2.3% compared to 30.3% for PDT at 3 year follow up. Performance of two ALA-PDT treatments for both nodular and superficial BCC has given comparable clinical response rates to surgery (95.83% complete response versus 95.65%). Recurrence rates were also similar (4.16% versus 4.34%) [81]. In the longest follow-up study to date lasting 10 years, Christensen et al. [89] found that the overall complete response rate for all subtypes of BCC treated with ALA-PDT was 75%, with a 60% complete response after one treatment and 87% response after two treatments.

More aggressive types of BCC, which often occur on the face, show a greater frequency of recurrence, possibly due to genetic mutations resulting to resistance to apoptosis [75]. Although long-term recurrence may limit the use of PDT for nodular BCC, PDT seems to be suitable for cases where surgical excision is not appropriate. On the other side, randomized studies with only short-term follow-up had previously reported high efficacy for facial nodular BCCs treated with MAL-PDT [90].

Since thickness of the tumor can affect the penetration capacity of the photosensitizer, various methods have been already used prior to PDT as pre-treatment in order to enhance its efficacy. Therefore, dimethylsulphoxide (DMSO), which alters the intercellular lipid structure of the stratum corneum, has been used as a pretreatment penetration enhancer [91]. Curettage and DMSO pretreatment prior to one or two sessions ALA-PDT brought favorable 10-year response rates of 75% for primary small BCC [89]. Also intralesional ALA and light source application showed promising results in a small prospective study of 20 patients with nodular BCC, with no clinical recurrence observed after 19.5 months [92].

Combination of PDT with Mohs micrographic surgery has also been performed with beneficial outcomes by reducing the tumor size and thus improving the cosmetic outcomes [93, 94].

PDT can be a useful option for patients with naevoid BCC syndrome (Gorlin syndrome) depending on the localization and thickness of the lesions [95]. In these patients can MAL-PDT significantly improve patient satisfaction and reduce the need for many surgical procedures [96].

Although topical PDT does not serve as first-line therapy for BCC, it is recommended for primary superficial and thin low-risk nodular BCC but is a relatively poor choice for high-risk lesions including nodular BCC [97]. PDT is best considered for nodular lesions where surgical excision is relatively contraindicated, or where patient preference, reflecting past therapy history, comorbidities or cosmetic considerations, although the higher risk of recurrence has to be taken into consideration. It is advised that patients receiving topical PDT for nodular BCC are reviewed for evidence of recurrence for at least 1 year. Further long-term studies are needed to better assess the effectiveness of PDT on BCC. **Figure 5** demonstrates the treatment and clinical outcome after ALA-PDT on a superficial BCC.

3.3. Squamous cell carcinoma

PDT has been also used for treatment of Bowen's disease, or squamous cell carcinoma in situ and is recommended for both extensive involvement and poor healing sites [98]. The approved MAL-PDT dosing regimen for Europe consists of two treatments 7 days apart, repeated at 3 months, if needed [99].

The clearance rates reported for BD lesions are high between 86 and 93% 3 months after one or two treatments of MAL-PDT using red light, with sustained clearance at 24 months of 68–71%, which is comparable with the conventional therapy, but with better cosmetic outcomes [100]. MAL-PDT was effective in treating lesions over 3 cm, with clearance rates of 96% in 3 months after one cycle of two treatments, with only three recurrences in a follow-up of 1 year [101]. Comparable outcomes have been reported form an observational study of 51 BD lesions which had been treated with two MAL-PDT treatments one week apart leading to clearance rates of 76.09% at 16.61 months with excellent cosmetic outcome and only mild cutaneous adverse effects [102].

Compared to cryotherapy and topical 5-FU, MAL-PDT showed similar response rates for BD at the 12 month follow-up point but superior cosmetic results [103]. Also ALA-PDT has been found to be significantly more effective for BD than topical 5-FU at 12 months (82% versus 48% complete clearance) at 12 months [104]. ALA-PDT compared to MAL-PDT, respectively, showed an 89% versus 78% response rate, at approximately 6 months after treatment [101].

Therapy guidelines recommend PDT as the treatment of choice for both large and small plaques of BD on poor-healing sites, representing the majority of lesions and a good choice

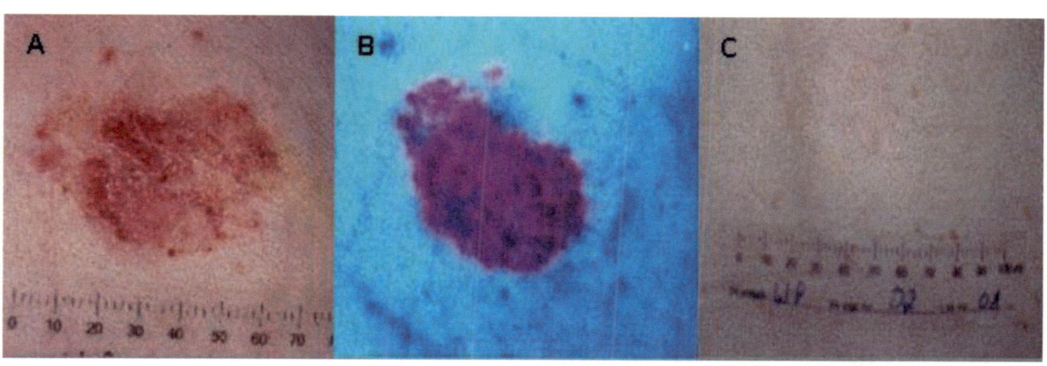

Figure 5. (A) Clinical manifestation of a superficial BCC, (B) selective detection of fluorescence after application of ALA on the lesion during PDT, (C) clinical outcome 3 years after therapy (there has been performed one therapy-cycle consisting of double PDT-treatment in 1 week apart).

for large lesions in good-healing sites [105]. However, larger studies with longer follow-up are needed to better assess response rates.

For invasive SCC there is a reduced efficacy of PDT where 24-month clearance rates of 57 and 26% have been reported. The degree of cellular atypia is a negative prognostic factor, suggesting that poorly differentiated keratinocytes are less sensitive to PDT because of reduced sensitivity to phototoxicity or decreased production of PpIX.

In some cases of invasive SCC, PDT-therapy was followed by resistance resulting in more aggressive disease. Gilaberte et al. [106] postulated that chromosomal instability is the reasonable factor through the induction of overexpression of CCND1 and aberration of the MAPK/ERK signal pathway, as previously shown in immunodeficient mice.

In view of its metastatic potential and reduced efficacy rates, PDT currently cannot be recommended for invasive SCC [100].

PDT can also be a useful treatment option by organ transplant recipients who are at an increased risk of NMSC and especially SCC due to long-term immunosuppressive therapy. Treatment with cyclic ALA-PDT at 4–8 week intervals over a 2-year period on 12 organ transplant recipients led to a significant reduction of SCC (98% mean reduction) [107]. Wennberg et al. [108] also found that repeat MAL-PDT treatments reduced the occurrence of new AKs in this special population.

4. Conclusions and future expectations

Since the incidence of NMSC is increasing over the years, available therapies should aim to deliver good cosmetic outcomes and optimize patient comfort while still achieving acceptable response rates. PDT offers an attractive alternate to surgical treatment of NMSC, as well as an alternate to non-surgical treatments such as cryotherapy, imiquimod and 5-fluorouracil. Conventional PDT is in comparison to daylight PDT a well-tolerated treatment method, with pain during and shortly after treatment being the main adverse effect.

MAL appears be associated with lower pain levels than ALA, which may be due to its greater selectivity for neoplastic lesions. New strategies, such as cooling and inhalation of a nitrous oxygen/oxygen mixture, are promising treatments to minimize pain. MAL also requires shorter incubation times compared to ALA, according to the FDA-approved treatment regimen. PDT utilizing ALA and MAL is a proven and even first line treatment for AK and superficial BCC. PDT has also demonstrated efficacy in treatment of nodular BCC and SCC in situ, although recurrence rates higher than those of standard surgical treatments preclude first-line use of PDT for these indications. Studies with MAL-PDT for superficial BCC offer acceptable response rates to consider it a reasonable therapeutic option for patients who are not eligible for surgery or do not desire surgery. PDT should be utilized with caution for nodular BCC and Bowen's disease given the risk of recurrence.

New strategies for improving the efficacy and tolerability of PDT are under continuous development. Although several classes of novel photosensitizers have been proposed, they seem to be of no advantage regarding the overall efficacy of PDT [109]. Novel delivery systems such as nanoparticles, micelles or liposomes which are promising technologies leading to a better uptake and targeting of photosensitizers may be available in the future.

New indications for PDT including cutaneous infections, inflammatory dermatoses, cutaneous T-cell lymphoma or treatment of skin photo aging are also under investigation.

Author details

Eleni Papakonstantinou[1]*, Florian Löhr[2] and Ulrike Raap[2]

*Address all correspondence to: papakonstantinou.eleni@mh-hannover.de

1 Department of Dermatology and Allergy, Hannover Medical School, Germany

2 Department of Dermatology and Allergy, Klinikum Oldenburg AöR, University of Oldenburg, Germany

References

[1] Braathen LR, Szeimies RM, Basset-Seguin N, Bissonnette R, Foley P, Pariser D, et al. Guidelines on the use of photodynamic therapy for nonmelanoma skin cancer: An international consensus. Journal of the American Academy of Dermatology. 2007 Jan;**56**(1):125-143

[2] Lehmann P. Methyl aminolaevulinate-photodynamic therapy: A review of clinical trials in the treatment of actinic keratoses and nonmelanoma skin cancer. The British Journal of Dermatology. 2007 May;**156**(5):793-801

[3] Lam M, Oleinick NL, Nieminen AL. Photodynamic therapy-induced apoptosis in epidermoid carcinoma cells—Reactive oxygen species and mitochondrial inner membrane permeabilization. The Journal of Biological Chemistry. 2001 Dec 14;**276**(50):47379-47386

[4] Henderson BW, Dougherty TJ. How does photodynamic therapy work. Photochemistry and Photobiology. 1992 Jan;**55**(1):145-157

[5] Oleinick N, Morris RL, Belichenko T. The role of apoptosis in response to photodynamic therapy: What, where, why, and how. Photochemical & Photobiological Sciences. 2002 Jan;**1**(1):1-21

[6] Dougherty TJ, Gomer GJ, Henderson BW, Jori G, Kessel D, Korbelik M, et al. Photodynamic therapy. Journal of the National Cancer Institute. 1998 Jun 17;**90**(12):889-905

[7] Fritsch C, Homey B, Stahl W, Lehmann P, Ruzicka T, Sies H. Preferential relative porphyrin enrichment in solar keratoses upon topical application of d-aminolevulinic acid methylester. Photochemistry and Photobiology. 1998 Aug;**68**(2):218-221

[8] Ericson MB, Wennberg AM, Larkö O. Review of photodynamic therapy in actinic keratosis and basal cell carcinoma. Therapeutics and Clinical Risk Management. 2008 Feb;**4**(1):1-9

[9] Morton CA, Brown SB, Collins S, Ibbotson S, Jenkinson H, Kurwa H, et al. Guidelines for topical photodynamic therapy: Report of a workshop of the British Photodermatology Group. The British Journal of Dermatology. 2002 Apr;**146**(4):552-567

[10] Wennberg AM, Larkö O, Lönnroth P, Larson G, Krogstad AL. Delta-aminolevulinic acid in superficial basal cell carcinomas and normal skin—A microdialysis and perfusion study. Clinical and Experimental Dermatology. 2000 Jun;**25**(4):317-322

[11] Kelty CJ, Brown NJ, Reed MW, Ackrovd R. The use of 5-aminolaevulinic acid as a photosensitiser in photodynamic therapy and photodiagnosis. Photochemical & Photobiological Sciences. 2002 Mar;**1**(3):158-168

[12] Ackermann G, Abels C, Bäumler W, Langer S, Landthaler M, Lang E, et al. Simulations on the selectivity of 5-aminolevulinic acid-induced fluorescence in vivo. Journal of Photochemistry and Photobiology. B. 1998 Dec;**47**(2-3):121-128

[13] Tarstedt M, Gillstedt M, Wennberg Larkö AM, Paoli J. Aminolevulinic acid and methyl aminolevulinate equally effective in topical photodynamic therapy for non-melanoma skin cancers. Journal of the European Academy of Dermatology and Venereology. 2016 Mar;**30**(3):420-423

[14] Nester MS, Gold MH, Kauvar AN, Taub AF, Geronemus AR, Ritvo EC, et al. The use of photodynamic therapy in Dermatology: Results of a consensus conference. Journal of Drugs in Dermatology. 2006 Feb;**5**(2):140-154

[15] Braathen LR, Paredes BE, Saksela O, Fritsch C, Gardlo K, Morken T et al. Short incubation with methyl aminolevulinate for photodynamic therapy of actinic keratoses. Journal of the European Academy of Dermatology and Venereology 2009 May;**23**(5):550-5

[16] Patel N, Pera P, Joshi P, Dukh M, Tabaczynski WA, Siters KE, et al. Highly effective dual-function near-infrared (NIR) photosensitizer for fluorescence imaging and photodynamic therapy (PDT) of cancer. Journal of Medicinal Chemistry. 2016 Nov 10;**59**(21):9774-9787 Epub 2016 Oct 31

[17] Baron ED, Malbasa CL, Santo-Domingo D, Fu P, Miller JD, Hanneman KK, et al. Silicon phthalocyanine (Pc 4) photodynamic therapy is a safe modality for cutaneous neoplasms: Results of a phase 1 clinical trial. Lasers in Surgery and Medicine. 2010 Dec;**42**(10): 728-735

[18] Boppana NB, Stochai U, Kodiha M, Bielawska A, Bielawski J, Pierce JS, et al. C6-pyridinium ceramide sensitizes SCC17B human head and neck squamous cell carcinoma cells to photodynamic therapy. Journal of Photochemistry and Photobiology. B. 2015 Feb;**143**:163-168

[19] Alexiades-Armenakas MR, Geronemus RG. Laser-mediated photodynamic therapy of actinic keratoses. Archives of Dermatology. 2003 Oct;**139**(10):1313-1320

[20] Szeimies RM, Abels C, Fritsch C, Karrer S, Steinbach P, Bäumler W, et al. Wavelength dependency of photodynamic effects after sensitization with 5-aminolevulinic acid in vitro and in vivo. The Journal of Investigative Dermatology. 1995 Nov;**105**(5):672-677

[21] Brown SB. The role of light in the treatment of nonmelanoma skin cancer using methyl aminolevulinate. The Journal of Dermatological Treatment. 2003;**14**(Suppl 3):11-14

[22] Karrer S, Bäumler W, Abels C, Hohlenleutner U, Landthaler M, Szeimies RM. Long-pulse dye laser for photodynamic therapy: Investigations in vitro and in vivo. Lasers in Surgery and Medicine. 1999;**25**(1):51-59

[23] Babilas P, Schreml S, Landthaler M, Szeimies RM. Photodynamic therapy in dermatology: State-of-the-art. Photodermatology, Photoimmunology & Photomedicine. 2010 Jun; **26**(3):118-132

[24] Issa MC, Manela-Azulay M. Photodynamic therapy: A review of the literature and image documentation. Anais Brasileiros de Dermatologia. 2010 Jul-Aug;**85**(4):501-511

[25] Morton CA. Photodynamic therapy for nonmelanoma skin cancer—And more? Archives of Dermatology. 2004 Jan;**140**(1):116-120

[26] Calzayara-Pinton PG, Venturini M, Sala R. Photodynamic therapy: Update 2006. Part 1: Photochemistry and photobiology. Journal of the European Academy of Dermatology and Venereology. 2007 Mar;**21**(3):293-302

[27] Clark C, Bryden A, Dawe R, Moseley H, Ferguson J, Ibbotson SH. Topical 5-aminolaevulinic acid photodynamic therapy for cutaneous lesions: Outcome and comparison of light sources. Photodermatology, Photoimmunology & Photomedicine. 2003 Jun;**19**(3):134-141

[28] Yang CH, Lee JC, Chen CH, Hui CY, Hong HS, Kuo HW. Photodynamic therapy for bowenoid papulosis using a novel incoherent light-emitting diode device. The British Journal of Dermatology. 2003 Dec;**149**(6):1297-1299

[29] Zeitouni NC, Oseroff AR, Shieh S. Photodynamic therapy for nonmelanoma skin cancers. Molecular Immunology. 2003 Jul;**39**(17-18):1133-1136

[30] Wiegell SR, Haedersal M, Philipsen PA, Eriksen P, Ed E, Wulf CH. Continuous activation of PpIX by daylight is as effective as and less painful than conventional photodynamic therapy for actinic keratoses; a randomized, controlled, single-blinded study. The British Journal of Dermatology. 2008 Apr;**158**(4):740-746

[31] Attili SK, Lesar A, McNeill A, Camacho-Lopez M, Moseley H, Ibbotson S, et al. An open pilot study of ambulatory photodynamic therapy using a wearable low-irradiance organic light-emitting diode light source in the treatment of nonmelanoma skin cancer. The British Journal of Dermatology. 2009 Jul;**161**(1):170-173

[32] Fritsch C, Neumann NJ, Ruzicka T, Lehmann P. Photodiagnostic tests. 3: Fluorescence diagnosis with delta-aminolevulinic acidinduced porphyrins (FDAP) in dermatology. Hautarzt. 2000 Jul;**51**(7):528-543 quizz 543-5

[33] Bäumler W, Abels C, Szeimies RM. Fluorescence diagnosis and photodynamic therapy in dermatology. Medical Laser Application. 2003 Jan;**18**(1):170-173

[34] Vereecken P, Da Costa SM, Steels E, Lathouwer O, Heenen M, De Mey A. Fluorescence diagnosis of face-located basal cell carcinomas: A new dermatological procedure which may help the surgeon. Acta Chirurgica Belgica. 2007 Mar–Apr;**107**(2):205-207

[35] Kleinpenning MM, Wolberink EW, Smits T, Blokx WA, van De Kerkhof PC, van Erp PE et al. Fluorescence diagnosis in actinic keratosis and squamous cell carcinoma. Photodermatology, Photoimmunology & Photomedicine 2010 Dec;**26**(6):297-302

[36] Truchuelo MT, Pérez B, Fernández-Guarino M, Moreno C, Jaén-Olaso P. Fluorescence diagnosis and photodynamic therapy for Bowen's disease treatment. Journal of the European Academy of Dermatology and Venereology. 2014 Jan;**28**(1):86-93

[37] Smits T, Kleinpenning MM, Blokx WA, van de Kerkhof PC, van Erp PE, Gerritsen MA. Fluorescence diagnosis in keratinocytic intraepidermal neoplasias. Journal of the American Academy of Dermatology 2007 Nov;**57**(5):824-831

[38] Morton CA. Methyl aminolevulinate (MetvixH) photodynamic therapy—Practical pearls. The Journal of Dermatological Treatment. 2003;**14**(Suppl 3):23-26

[39] Thissen MR, Schroeter CA, Neumann HA. Photodynamic therapy with delta-aminolaevulinic acid for nodular basal cell carcinomas using a prior debulking technique. The British Journal of Dermatology. 2000 Feb;**142**(2):338-339

[40] Nayak CS. Photodynamic therapy in dermatology. Indian Journal of Dermatology, Venereology and Leprology. 2005 May-Jun;**71**(3):155-160

[41] Szeimies RM, Karrer S, Radakovic-Fijan S, Tanew A, Calzavara-Pinton PG, Zane C, et al. Photodynamic therapy using topical methyl 5-aminolevulinate compared with cryotherapy for actinic keratosis: A prospective randomized study. Journal of the American Academy of Dermatology. 2002 Aug;**47**(2):258-262

[42] Foley P. Clinical efficacy of methyl aminolevulinate (MetvixH) photodynamic therapy. The Journal of Dermatological Treatment. 2003;**14**(Suppl 3):15-22

[43] Fink C, Uhlmann L, Enk A, Gholam P. Pain management in photodynamic therapy using a nitrous oxide/oxygen mixture: A prospective, within-patient, controlled clinical trial. Journal of the European Academy of Dermatology and Venereology. 2017 Jan;**31**(1):70-74

[44] Wiegell SR, Stender IM, Na R, Wulf HC. Pain associated with photodynamic therapy using 5-aminolevulinic acid or photodynamic therapy for non-melanoma skin cancer 5-aminolevulinic acid methylester on tape-stripped normal skin. Archives of Dermatology. 2003 Sep;**139**(9):1173-1177

[45] Touma D, Yaar M, Whitehead S, Konnikov N, Gilchrest BA. A trial of short incubation, broad-area photodynamic therapy for facial actinic keratoses and diffuse photodamage. Archives of Dermatology. 2004 Jan;**140**(1):33-40

[46] Skiveren J, Haedersdal M, Philipsen PA, Wiegell SR, Wulf HC. Morphine gel 0.3% does not relieve pain during topical photodynamic therapy: A randomized, double-blind, placebo-controlled study. Acta Dermato-Venereologica. 2006;**86**(5):409-411

[47] Wiegell SR, Haedersdal M, Wulf HC. Cold water and pauses in illumination reduces pain during photodynamic therapy: A randomized clinical study. Acta Dermato-Venereologica. 2009;**89**(2):145-149

[48] Pagliaro J, Elliott T, Bulsara M, King C, Vinciullo C. Cold air analgesia in photodynamic therapy of basal cell carcinomas and Bowen's disease: An effective addition to treatment: A pilot study. Dermatologic Surgery. 2004 Jan;**30**(1):63-66

[49] Kessels JP, Nelemans PJ, Mosterd K, Kelleners-Smeets NW, Krekels GA, Ostertag JU. Laser-mediated photodynamic therapy: An alternative treatment for actinic keratosis. Acta Dermato-Venereologica. 2016 Mar;**96**(3):351-354

[50] Lee PK, Kloser A. Current methods for photodynamic therapy in the US: Comparison of MAL/PDT and ALA/PDT. Journal of Drugs in Dermatology. 2013 Aug;**12**(8):925-930

[51] Tschen EH, Wong DH, Pariser DH, Dunlap FE, Houlihan A, Ferdon MB. Photodynamic therapy using aminolaevulinic acid for patients with nonhyperkeratotic actinic keratoses of the face and scalp: Phase IV multicentre clinical trial with 12-month follow up. The British Journal of Dermatology. 2006 Dec;**155**(6):1262-1269

[52] Wulf HC, Philipsen P. Allergic contact dermatitis to 5-aminolaevulinic acid methylester but not 5-aminolaevulinic acid after photodynamic therapy. The British Journal of Dermatology. 2004 Jan;**150**(1):143-145

[53] Morton CA, Burden AD. Treatment of multiple scalp basal cell carcinomas by photodynamic therapy. Clinical and Experimental Dermatology. 2001 Jan;**26**(1):33-36

[54] Guillen C, Sanmartin O, Escudero A, Bottela-Estrada R, Svila A, Castejon P. Photodynamic therapy for in situ squamous cell carcinoma on chronic radiation dermatitis after photosensitization with 5-aminolevulinic acid. Journal of the European Academy of Dermatology and Venereology. 2000 Jul;**14**(4):298-300

[55] Ko DY, Jeon SY, Kim KH, Song KH. Fractional erbium: YAG laser-assisted photodynamic therapy for facial actinic keratoses: A randomized, comparative, prospective study. Journal of the European Academy of Dermatology and Venereology. 2014 Nov;**28**(11): 1529-1539

[56] Glogau RG. The risk of progression to invasive disease. Journal of the American Academy of Dermatology. 2000 Jan;**42**(1 Pt 2):23-24

[57] Morton C, Campbell S, Gupta G, Keohane S, Lear J, Zaki I, et al. Intraindividual, right-left comparison of topical methyl aminolaevulinate-photodynamic therapy and cryotherapy in subjects with actinic keratoses: A multicentre, randomized controlled study. The British Journal of Dermatology. 2006 Nov;**155**(5):1029-1036

[58] Lucena RS, Salazar N, Gracia-Cazaña T, Zamarrón A, González S, Juarranz A, et al. Combined treatments with photodynamic therapy for non-melanoma skin cancer. International Journal of Molecular Sciences. 2015 Oct 28;**16**(10):25912-25933

[59] Tarstedt M, Rosdahl I, Berne B, Svanberg K, Wennberg KM. A randomized multicenter study to compare two treatment regimens of topical methyl aminolevulinate (Metvix)-PDT in actinic keratosis of the face and scalp. Acta Dermato-Venereologica. 2005;**85**(5):424-428

[60] Piacquardio DJ, Chen DM, Farber HF, Fowel JB, Glazer SD, Goodman JJ, et al. Photodynamic therapy with aminolevulinic acid topical solution and visible blue light in the treatment of multiple actinic keratoses of the face and scalp. Archives of Dermatology. 2004 Jan;**140**(1):41-46

[61] Hauschild A, Stockfleth E, Popp G, Borrosch F, Brüning H, Dominicus R, et al. Optimization of photodynamic therapy with a novel self-adhesive 5-aminolaevulinic acid patch: Results of two randomized controlled phase III studies. The British Journal of Dermatology. 2009 May;**160**(5):1066-1074

[62] Freeman M, Vinciullo C, Francis D, Spelman L, Nquyen R, Fergin P, et al. A comparison of photodynamic therapy using topical methyl aminolevulinate (Metvix) with single cycle cryotherapy in patients with actinic keratosis: A prospective, randomized study. The Journal of Dermatological Treatment. 2003 Jun;**14**(2):99-106

[63] Kaufmann R, Spelman L, Weightman W, Reifenberger J, Szeimies RM, Verhaeghe E, et al. Multicentre intraindividual randomized trial of topical methyl aminolaevulinate-photodynamic therapy vs. cryotherapy for multiple actinic keratoses on the extremities. The British Journal of Dermatology. 2008 May;**158**(5):994-999

[64] Smith S, Piacquadio D, Morhenn V, Atkin D, Fitzpatrick R. Short incubation PDT versus 5-FU in treating actinic keratoses. Journal of Drugs in Dermatology. 2003 Dec;**2**(6):629-635

[65] Tanghetti EA, Hamann C, Tanghetti MA. Controlled comparison study of topical fluorouracil 5% cream pre-treatment of aminolevulinic acid/photodynamic therapy for actinic keratosis. Journal of Drugs in Dermatology. 2015 Nov;**14**(11):1241-1244

[66] Hadley J, Tristani-Firouzi P, Hull C, Florell S, Cotter M, Hadley M. Results of an investigator-initiated single-blind split-face comparison of photodynamic therapy and 5% imiquimod cream for the treatment of actinic keratoses. Dermatologic Surgery. 2012 May;**38**(5):722-727

[67] Tanaka N, Ohata C, Ishii N, Imamura K, Ueda A, Furumura M, et al. Comparative study for the effect of photodynamic therapy, imiquimod immunotherapy and combination of both therapies on 40 lesions of actinic keratosis in Japanese patients. The Journal of Dermatology. 2013 Dec;**40**(12):962-967

[68] Serra-Guillen C, Nagore E, Hueso L, Traves V, Messequer F, Sanmartin O, et al. A randomized pilot comparative study of topical methyl aminolevulinate photodynamic therapy versus imiquimod 5% versus sequential application of both therapies in immunocompetent patients with actinic keratosis: Clinical and histologic outcomes. Journal of the American Academy of Dermatology. 2012 Apr;**66**(4):e131-e137

[69] Scola N, Terras S, Georgas D, Othlinghaus N, Matip R, Pantelaki I, et al. A randomized, half-side comparative study of aminolaevulinate photodynamic therapy vs. CO_2 laser ablation in immunocompetent patients with multiple actinic keratoses. The British Journal of Dermatology. 2012 Dec;**167**(6):1366-1373

[70] Gholam P, Fink C, Bosselmann I, Enk AH. Retrospective analysis evaluating the effect of a keratolytic and physical pretreatment with salicylic acid, urea and curettage on the

efficacy and safety of photodynamic therapy of actinic keratoses with methylaminolaevulinate. Journal of the European Academy of Dermatology and Venereology. 2016 Apr; **30**(4):619-623

[71] Szeimies RM, Hauschild A, Ortland C, Moor AC, Stocker M, Surber C. Photodynamic therapy simplified: Nonprepared, moderate-grade actinic keratosis lesions respond equally well to 5-aminolaevulinic acid patch photodynamic therapy as do mild lesions. The British Journal of Dermatology. 2015 Nov;**173**(5):1277-1279

[72] Dirschka T, Radny P, Dominicus R, Mensing H, Brüning H, Jenne L, et al. Photodynamic therapy with BF-200 ALA for the treatment of actinic keratoses: Results of a multicentre, randomized, observer-blind phase III study in comparison with registered methyl-5-aminolaevulinate cream and placebo. The British Journal of Dermatology. 2012 Jan; **166**(1):137-146

[73] De Becker D, Mc Gregor J, Hughes B. Guidelines for the management of actinic keratosis. The British Journal of Dermatology. 2007 Feb;**156**(2):222-230

[74] Serra-Guillen C, Nagore E, Hueso L, Llombart B, Reguena C, Sanmartín O, et al. A randomized comparative study of tolerance and satisfaction in the treatment of actinic keratosis of the face and scalp between 5% imiquimod cream and photodynamic therapy with methyl aminolaevulinate. The British Journal of Dermatology. 2011 Feb;**164**(2):429-433

[75] Fiechter S, Skaria A, Nievergelt H, Anex R, Borradori L, Parmentier L. Facial basal cell carcinomas recurring after photodynamic therapy: A retrospective analysis of histological subtypes. Dermatology. 2012;**224**(4):346-351

[76] Roozeboom MH, Arits AH, Nelemans PJ, Kelleners-Smeets NW. Overall treatment success after treatment of primary superficial basal cell carcinoma: A systematic review and meta-analysis of randomized and nonrandomized trials. The British Journal of Dermatology. 2012 Oct;**167**(4):733-756

[77] Szeimies RM, Ibbotson S, Murrell DF, Rubel D, Frambach Y, De Becker D, et al. A clinical study comparing methyl aminolevulinate photodynamic therapy and surgery in small superficial basal cell carcinoma (8-20 mm), with a 12-month follow-up. Journal of the European Academy of Dermatology and Venereology. 2008 Nov;**22**(11):1302-1311

[78] Lindberg-Larsen R, Sølvsten H, Kragbale K. Evaluation of recurrence after photodynamic therapy with topical methylaminolaevulinate for 157 basal cell carcinomas in 90 patients. Acta Dermato-Venereologica. 2012 Mar;**92**(2):144-147

[79] Roozeboom MH, Aardoom MA, Nelemans PJ, Thissen MR, Kelleners-Smeets NW, Kuijpers DI, et al. Fractionated 5-aminolevulinic acid photodynamic therapy after partial debulking versus surgical excision for nodular basal cell carcinoma: A randomized controlled trial with at least 5-year follow-up. Journal of the American Academy of Dermatology. 2013 Aug;**69**(2):280-287

[80] Kessels J, Hendriks J, Nelemans P, Mosterd K, Kelleners-Smeets N. Two-fold illumination in topical 5-aminolevulinic acid (ALA)-mediated photodynamic therapy (PDT) for

superficial basal cell carcinoma (sBCC): A retrospective case series and cohort study. Journal of the American Academy of Dermatology. 2016 May;**74**(5):899-906

[81] Cosgarea R, Susan M, Crisan M, Senila S. Photodynamic therapy using topical 5-aminolaevulinic acid vs. surgery for basal cell carcinoma. Journal of the European Academy of Dermatology and Venereology. 2013 Aug;**27**(8):980-984

[82] Rhodes LE, de Rie M, Enstrom Y, Groves R, Morken T, Goulden V et al. Photodynamic therapy using topical methyl aminolevulinate vs. surgery for nodular basal cell carcinoma: Results of a multicenter randomized prospective trial. Archives of Dermatology 2004 Jan;**140**(1):17-23

[83] Zou Y, Zhao Y, Yu J, Luo X, Han J, Ye Z, et al. Photodynamic therapy versus surgical excision to basal cell carcinoma: Meta-analysis. Journal of Cosmetic Dermatology. 2016 Dec;**15**(4):374-382

[84] Vinciullo C, Elliott T, Francis D, Gebauer K, Spelman L, Nguyen R, et al. Photodynamic therapy with topical methyl aminolaevulinate for "difficult-to-treat" basal cell carcinoma. The British Journal of Dermatology. 2005 Apr;**152**(4):765-772

[85] Basset-Seguin N, Ibbotson SH, Emtestam L, Tarstedt M, Morton C, Maroti M, et al. Topical methyl aminolaevulinate photodynamic therapy versus cryotherapy for superficial basal cell carcinoma: A 5 year randomized trial. European Journal of Dermatology. 2008 Sep-Oct;**18**(5):547-553

[86] Roozeboom MH, Arits AH, Mosterd K, Sommer A, Essers BA, de Rooij MJ. Three-year follow-up results of photodynamic therapy vs. imiquimod vs. fluorouracil for treatment of superficial basal cell carcinoma: A single-blind, noninferiority, randomized controlled trial. The Journal of Investigative Dermatology 2016 Aug;**136**(8):1568-1574

[87] Rhodes LE, De Rie MA, Leifsdottir R, RC Y, Bachmann I, Goulden V, et al. Five-year follow-up of a randomized, prospective trial of topical methyl aminolevulinate photodynamic therapy vs surgery for nodular basal cell carcinoma. Archives of Dermatology. 2007 Sep;**143**(9):1131-1136

[88] Mosterd K, Thissen M, Nelemans P, Kelleners-Smeets NW, Janssen R, Broekhof K, et al. Fractionated 5-aminolaevulinic acid-photodynamic therapy vs. surgical excision in the treatment of nodular basal cell carcinoma: Results of a randomized controlled trial. The British Journal of Dermatology. 2008 Sep;**159**(4):864-870

[89] Christensen E, Mørk C, Skogvoll E. High and sustained efficacy after two sessions of topical 5-aminolaevulinic acid photodynamic therapy for basal cell carcinoma: A prospective, clinical and histological 10-year follow-up study. The British Journal of Dermatology. 2012 Jun;**166**(6):1342-1348

[90] Foley P, Freeman M, Menter A, Siller G, El-Azhary RA, Gebauer K, et al. Photodynamic therapy with methyl aminolevulinate for primary nodular basal cell carcinoma: Results of two randomized studies. International Journal of Dermatology. 2009 Nov;**48**(11): 1236-1245

[91] Gerritsen MJ, Smits T, Kleinpenning MM, van de Kerkhof PC, van Erp PE. Pretreatment to enhance protoporphyrin IX accumulation in photodynamic therapy. Dermatology 2009;**218**(3):193-202

[92] Angel Rodríguez-Prieto MA, González-Sixto B, Pérez-Bustillo A, Alonso-Alonso T, Ortega-Valín L, Martínez-Valderrabano V, et al. Photodynamic therapy with intralesional photosensitizer and laser beam application: An alternative treatment for nodular basal cell carcinoma. Journal of the American Academy of Dermatology. 2012 Oct;**67**(4):e134-e136

[93] Kuijpers DI, Smeets NW, Krekels GA, Thissen MR. Photodynamic therapy as adjuvant treatment of extensive basal cell carcinoma treated with Mohs micrographic surgery. Dermatologic Surgery. 2004 May;**30**(5):794-798

[94] Al-Niajmi F, Sheth N, Kurwa HA, Mallipeddi R. Photodynamic therapy followed by mohs micrographic surgery compared to mohs micrographic surgery alone for the treatment of basal cell carcinoma: Results of a pilot single-blinded randomised controlled trial. Journal of Cutaneous and Aesthetic Surgery. 2015 Apr-Jun;**8**(2):88-91

[95] Loncaster J, Swindell R, Slevin F, Sheridan L, Allan D, Allan E. Efficacy of photodynamic therapy as a treatment for Gorlin syndrome-related basal cell carcinomas. Clinical Oncology (Royal College of Radiologists). 2009 Aug;**21**(6):502-508

[96] Pauwels C, Mazereeuw-Hautier J, Basset-Sequin N, Livideanu C, Viraben R, Paul C, et al. Topical methyl aminolevulinate photodynamic therapy for management of basal cell carcinomas in patients with basal cell nevus syndrome improves patient's satisfaction and reduces the need for surgical procedures. Journal of the European Academy of Dermatology and Venereology. 2011 Jul;**25**(7):861-864

[97] Telfer N, Colver G, Morton C. Guidelines for the management of basal cell carcinoma. The British Journal of Dermatology. 2008 Jul;**159**(1):35-48

[98] Morton CA, Szeimies RM, Sidoroff A, Braathen LR. European guidelines for topical photodynamic therapy part 1: Treatment delivery and current indications actinic keratoses, Bowen's disease, basal cell carcinoma. Journal of the European Academy of Dermatology and Venereology. 2013 May;**27**(5):536-544

[99] Morton CA. Methyl aminolevulinate: Actinic keratoses and Bowen's disease. Dermatologic Clinics. 2007 Jan;**25**(1):81-87

[100] Calzavara-Pinton P, Venturini M, Sala R, Capezzea R, Parrinello G, Specchia C. Methylaminolaevulinatebased photodynamic therapy of Bowen's disease and squamous cell carcinoma. The British Journal of Dermatology. 2008 Jul;**159**(1):137-144

[101] López N, Meyer-Gonzalez T, Herrera-Acosta E, Bosch R, Castillo R, Herrera E. Photodynamic therapy in the treatment of extensive Bowen's disease. The Journal of Dermatological Treatment. 2012 Dec;**23**(6):428-430

[102] Truchuelo M, Fernandez-Guarino M, Fleta B, Alcantara J, Jaen P. Effectiveness of photodynamic therapy in Bowen's disease: An observational and descriptive study in 51 lesions. Journal of the European Academy of Dermatology and Venereology. 2012 Jul;**26**(7):868-874

[103] Morton C, Horn M, Leman J, Tack B, Bedane C, Tjioe M, et al. Comparison of topical methyl aminolevulinate photodynamic therapy with cryotherapy or fluorouracil for treatment of squamous cell carcinoma in situ—Results of a multicenter randomized trial. Archives of Dermatology. 2006 Jun;**142**(6):729-735

[104] Salim A, Leman JA, McColl JH, Chapman R, Morton CA. Randomized comparison of photodynamic therapy with topical 5-fluorouracil in Bowen's disease. The British Journal of Dermatology. 2003 Mar;**148**(3):539-543

[105] Cox N, Eedy D, Morton C. Guidelines for management of Bowen's disease: 2006 update. The British Journal of Dermatology. 2007 Jan;**156**(1):11-21

[106] Gilaberte Y, Milla L, Salazar N, Vera-Alvarez J, Kourani O, Damian A, et al. Cellular Intrinsic factors involved in the resistance of squamous cell carcinoma to photodynamic therapy. The Journal of Investigative Dermatology. 2014 Sep;**134**(9):2428-2437

[107] Willey A, Mehta S, Lee PK. Reduction in the incidence of squamous cell carcinoma in solid organ transplant recipients treated with cyclic photodynamic therapy. Dermatologic Surgery. 2010 May;**36**(5):652-658

[108] Wennberg AM, Stenguist B, Stockfleth E, Keohane S, Lear JT, Jemec G, et al. Photodynamic therapy with methyl aminolevulinate for prevention of new skin lesions in transplant recipients: A randomized study. Transplantation. 2008 Aug 15;**86**(3):423-429

[109] Neittaanmaki-Perttu N, Gronroos M, Karppinen TT, Tani TT, Snellmann E. Hexyl-5-aminolaevulinate 0.2% vs. methyl-5-aminolaevulinate 16% daylight photodynamic therapy for treatment of actinic keratoses: Results of a randomized double-blinded pilot trial. The British Journal of Dermatology. 2016 Feb;**174**(2):427-429

Chapter 8

Advanced Technologies in Dermatology

Diana Kitala, Agnieszka Klama-Baryła,
Wojciech Łabuś, Marcelina Misiuga,
Mariusz Nowak and Marek Kawecki

Additional information is available at the end of the chapter

http://dx.doi.org/10.5772/intechopen.70288

Abstract

Cellular therapies are an attractive area of regenerative medicine. For large partial thickness wound, keratinocytes transplant is suggested. The transplantation of cell graft is achieved by obtaining large amounts of cultured cells from a skin biopsy in 3 weeks. Stem cells can be applied before that, but are also efficient in chronic wound closure. Alternative treatment methods are transplants of allogeneic, biostatic skin and amnion. Amnion can be applied as a skin substitute on shallow facialburn wounds, hand burn wounds, on donor areas and granulating wounds. For medium depth or even deep burns, allogeneic skin is recommended. Thanks to the removing of cells from human allogeneic dermis, collagen scaffolding is obtained. It can be populated *de novo* by autologous skin cells. Artificial skin substitutes are especially good for hand burns and shallow burns. Even though scarring is a part of normal wound healing, it often leads to a pathological process. When scar treatment methods prove insufficient, surgical intervention becomes necessary. Surgical scar intervention involves removal of the pathological skin tissue fragment and replacing it with healthy skin or application of expanders. Improvement of the visual features can be also achieved by laser therapy.

Keywords: skin graft, skin cell graft, amniotic membrane, acellular dermal matrix, laser therapy, skin substitutes, scars

1. Introduction

The current trend in medicine is focused on two aspects of healing: on preventive medicine, preventing disease when possible and regenerative medicine, regenerating fractured cells [1]. The methods of treating burn wounds and chronic wounds have changed over the last decades [2]. Early removal of the dead necrosis and closing the wound with an autologous skin transplant of medium thickness (STSG) is still the basis of wound treatment [3], yet new methods that could provide a better esthetic effect continue to be sought after. This change follows a growing consciousness of the patients and the resulting growing demand for new methods of wound treatment and scar healing.

2. Cellular therapies

Cellular therapies used to return the patient to the stage of skin completeness are an attractive area of translational medicine [4]. One should remember, however, that cell transplants (autologous keratinocytes or stem cells) were qualified as a healing product for advanced therapy by the Commission for Advanced Therapies of the European Medicines' Agency (EMEA). Their manufacturing is thus, with all consequences, regulated by the rules of Good Practice [5–8]. Cultivated skin cells and products obtained by bioengineering means are used in treating patients with both genetic and acquired skin diseases [4]. They are especially useful in the treatment of traumas of chronic surface or depth, such as burns [9]. One of the methods is the delivery of cultured cells to the bed of the wound [10] by, among others, applying autologous cultured cells or skin substitutes obtained by cellular bioengineering [11]. The transplantation of keratinocytes is achieved thanks for obtaining large amounts of cultured cells from a skin biopsy in 3–4 weeks [12]. One of the benefits of using stem cells is their ability to migrate and differentiate the endothelium [13], which promotes revascularization [14]. The increased optimization of microvascular activity is the result of the injection of stem cells into a protracted wound [13]. What is more, the application of cells affects local cellular response, which plays an important role in the rebuilding of skin integrity in the infected wound [15]. It has been proven that stem cells from adipose tissue rebuild skin layering [7]. In our clinic, a positive result was obtained in all the cases of injecting stem cells from adipose tissue into the wound bed [16] (20 patients). There is a thesis that the transplant of allogeneic cells of the amnion can be more effective in the treatment of chronic wounds than autologous stem cells from adipose tissue or bone marrow [17]. Skin epidermis transplants with amniocytes act in an almost physiological way, which suggests that in the stimulation of the stratification of keratinocytes, fibroblasts can be replaced [18]. Fibroblasts seeded over the amnion show good adherence and longevity [19]. This type of wound dressing is suggested for chronic wounds and burn wounds [19, 20]. Alternatively, seeding the keratinocytes over the allogeneic, acellular amnion stimulates their proliferation. The life span of seeded cells is up to 4 weeks [20]. Experience shows that stem cells of the amnion shorten the time of wound healing by twofold. The culturing of keratinocytes was implemented in the Center in 2008. Since then, about 200 cellular transplants have been effectuated in patients with burn wounds, mostly thermal wounds. About 75% of the patients where qualified for the culturing (**Figure 1**). The size of the wound was 40–79% total body surface area (TBSA) in more than half of the patients who were subject to a cellular transplant. According to Sood et al., the average life of patients subject to the cultured epidermal autografts (CEA) transplant is 91%, while we obtained 88%. It is worth remembering that when it comes to cells of the epidermis, key is the right matching of the patients as leading complications are dermal blisters, itchiness and the loss of the cellular transplant. A common and chronic after-effect is the occurrence of swollen scars [21]. One

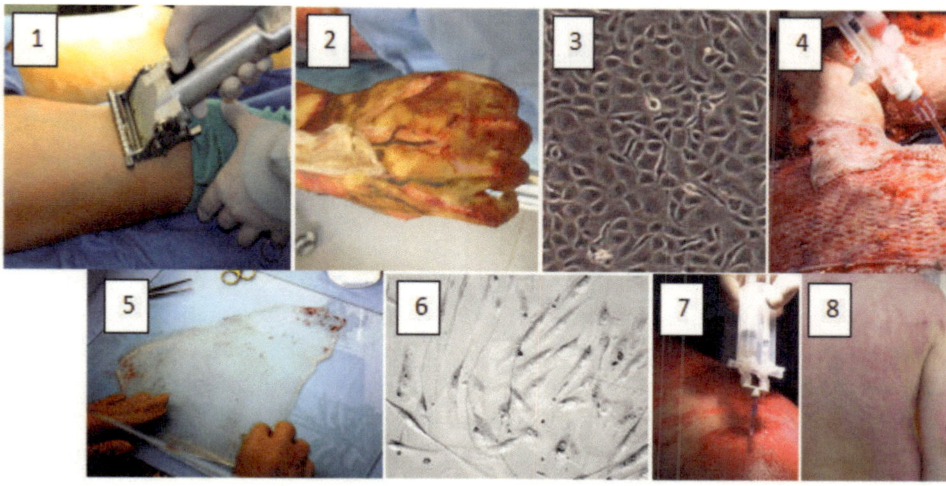

Figure 1. The right choice of the research field for the sourcing of autologous skin for culturing (1) is often problematic due to the limited amount of available research fields (2). The culturing of the epidermis for the transplant (3) and wound before the transplant (4). The source material for the isolation of stem cells (5), stem cell culture (6), the transplant (7) and the final result (8).

solution seems to be the use of stem cells [22] which help reduce the scarring [23]. The cells of the epidermis help the heeling of wounds to the maximum depth of IIb. Mansilla et al. and Rasulov et al. suggest the use of stem cells for wounds of great depth [24, 25].

RenovaCare is now performing clinical trials of the SkinGun™, which is to distribute stem cells as a suspension (fog) into the wound bed. The isolation, processing and application of the autologous cells takes only 90 min. The inventors of the gun have obtained an award for the patent and assure users that the vitality of the obtained stem cells is up to 97.3% [26]. HARVEST TERUMOBCT used the The Harvest® AdiPrep® system, allowing to obtain a suspension of cells (containing mesenchymal stem cells) in 4 minutes. The singular platform produced by this company allows to transform the platelet rich leukocyte concentrate of bone marrow and fatty tissue into stem cells with the concentration of 160,000/ml and vitality from 78 to 95% [27]. Cytori Therapeutics, Inc. also proposes a device for autologous cell therapy using fractions of cells sourced from fatty tissue (ADRCs). Adipose tissue is a good source of stem cells, but the sine qua non condition for the use of The Celution® System is the minimal amount of fatty tissue of 200 g. In our experience, the whole sourcing and transformation process takes about 2.5 h even though Fraser and associates cites 1.5 h [28], the equivalent of the transformation of the framework in our device. Our Center uses this system as liposuction is a noninvasive procedure while the amount of sourced stem cells and regenerative cells does not require a long cell culturing process. The vitality of cells obtained using the The Celution® System is 93% and is higher than that coming from the PNC's Multi Station (a manual device), the CHA Biotech Cha-Station and the Medi-Khan's Lipokit from MaxStem [29]. In our Center, this system is used for the treatment of chronic wounds as it allows for the operation to be performed on the day of admission which shortens the patient's hospitalization time and allows for the assurance of enough hospital beds to meet the needs of the other burn patients. Subjects included for this procedure contained patients who did not properly responded to CEA therapy and those with non-healing wounds. The procedure of applying ADRC cells sourced from The Celution® System was performed since 2011 in 20 patients (aged 18–80 years old). Good clinic results (final wounds closure) were obtained, which is a huge success preceded by the many months of non-responsive to healing wounds before the procedure (**Figure 2**).

The biggest limitation of the commercially available systems of sourcing stem cells for transplants is the amount of obtained cells, which is why burn patients qualify for stem cells cultured in a Stem Cell Bank. This is most effective from the point of view of a therapeutic success, yet much more complicated from the legal and financial point of view. It requires the production of stem cells in accordance with pharmaceutical law in Clean Rooms. Our Center has carried out a transplant of amniotic stem cells in a hospital exclusion which requires an extra permission from the bioethical commission and the signing of a conscious consent from the recipient. A 30-year-old patient with a thermal wound of 36% IIb/III got the cells in the fourth day after the burn. In 12 days, the wounds healed to a very good esthetic effect. It was

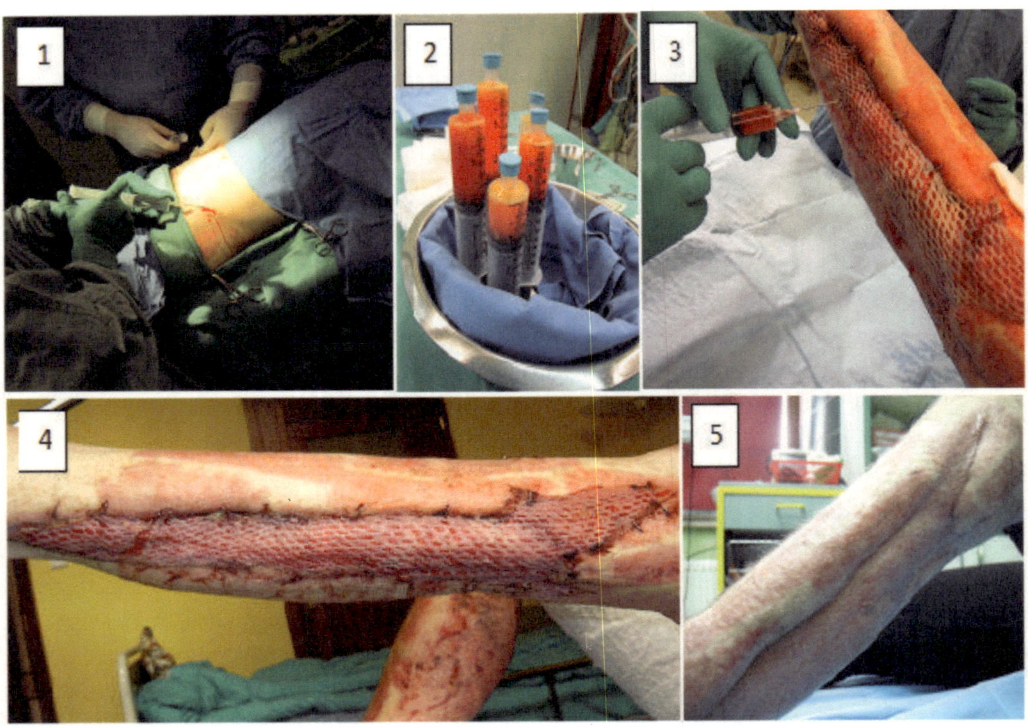

Figure 2. The isolation and application of regenerative cells from fatty tissue: liposuction (1), the sourced lipoaspirate (2), wound bed injection combined with a grated autologous skin cell transplant (3), the healing of the wound 7 days after the procedure (4), the final effect: a functioning, intact limb (5).

said that the legal regulations prevent the procedure from being routinely used. To sum, the good effects of cellular engineering in the last 30 years have been achieved in field of treatment of chronic wounds, such the diabetic foot and venous ulcers as well as deep wounds [30, 31]. It seems they will become a canonical medical practice. The only question is the right choice of therapy methods for the given patient.

3. The allogeneic amnion

The preparation which is an optimal alternative for traditional treatment methods is a transplant of allogeneic, biostatic amniotic tissue [19]. Amniotic tissue is a thin, half-permeable tissue which constitutes the most inner layer of the amnion and is obtained from seronegative donors during pre-planned Cesarean sections. Histologically, the amnion is a five-layer membrane from 0.02 to 0.5 mm thick. Amniotic membrane transplants are undertaken in sterile environments and undergo a final radiative sterilization [20]. The clinical reason for amniotic membrane transplants stems from its natural properties, such as

- it being non-immunogenic, mainly an effect of the expression of HLA-G genes in the placenta and amniotic liquid, which are responsible for the immune response during the pregnancy [34],
- reducing the risk of infection; it has been proven that the aqueous solution of the amniotic membrane promotes the apoptosis of monocells, such as lymphocytes and macrophages. [35]. This effect is proven by the latest research of Alikarami et al., which have proven the limiting effect of mesoenchymal amniotic liquid cells on the proliferation of mitogenically active T lymphocytes in the *in vitro* coculturing of T lymphocytes [36],
- its anti-inflammatory properties; the antibacterial effect observed during the application of the amniotic membrane in the process of wound healing is a common and documented phenomenon. The antibacterial effect is thought to be due to the presence of lysozyme and progesterone in the amniotic liquid as well as the very exact link between the dressing and the wound. Lysozyme is a protein with the properties of a hydrolytic enzyme which breaks down the peptidoglycan present in the cell wall of the bacteria. Progesterone is bacteriostatic against many Gram (+) bacteria [32, 33, 37, 38],
- as well as modulating the stroma of the wound; the stromal matrix amnion is rich in extracellular matrix content, such as hyaluronic acid from the embryon, glicosaminoglicanos, various types of collagen and growth factors which promote and modulate the regenerative processes occurring in the wound [39],
- stimulating proliferation processes; due to the rich ECM content. The amniotic membrane of the amnion included laminin, fibronectin, collagen IV, V and VII, as well as growth factors such as TGF, which greatly facilitates the adhesion and anchoring of the endothelial cells in the stroma and their proliferation [39, 40],

- minimizing pain; the painkiller effect is due to the very close link between the amniotic membrane and the wound, thanks to which the exposed, irritated nerve endings are protected [19, 33].

The clinical scope of the use of the amniotic membrane may include its application as a skin substitute on facial burn wounds, hand burn wounds, on donor areas and granulating wounds. An alternative is the STSG wound dressing of high gradation. Amniotic membrane transplants are useful also in the treatment of autoimmune diseases, for example, the Lyell's disease [18, 19]. The amniotic membrane can be used together with biological wound dressings, such as allogeneic skin [12, 20]. Properly aseptically prepared biovital transplants such as allogeneic transplants of the amniotic membrane are of high interest today. Good results of intravital transplants of the amniotic membrane in the treatment of wounds can result from the physiological functions of secretion of the amnion cells [41].

The Dr Stanisław Sakiel Centre for Burn Treatment in Siemianowice Śląskie, we began the undertaking of biostatic transplants of the amniotic membrane in 2011. The transplants are produced in the Clean Rooms of the Cell Bank in accordance with the Good Manufacturing Practice (GMP) (**Figure 3**). From August 2011 to March 2017, 245,229 cm^2 transplant cells have been produced. 513 patients have been served by a total of 235,317 cm^2, including 9 patients with the Lyell's Syndrome (**Figure 4**).

The obtained evidence and clinical observation suggest a conclusion that the amniotic membrane is an optimal skin substitute in the treatment of shallow burn wounds, specifically facial burn wounds.

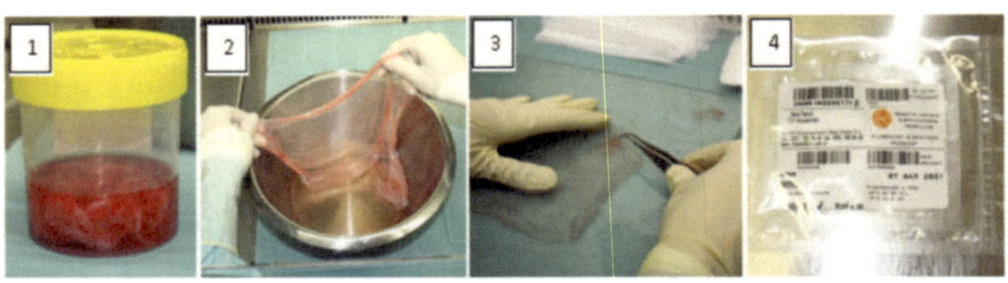

Figure 3. Select stages of production of allogeneic, biostatic transplants of human amnion: (1) the amniotic membrane in a transportation container; (2) rinsing; (3) cutting uneven fragments, measuring the surface; (4) a packaged transplant before sterilization by radiation.

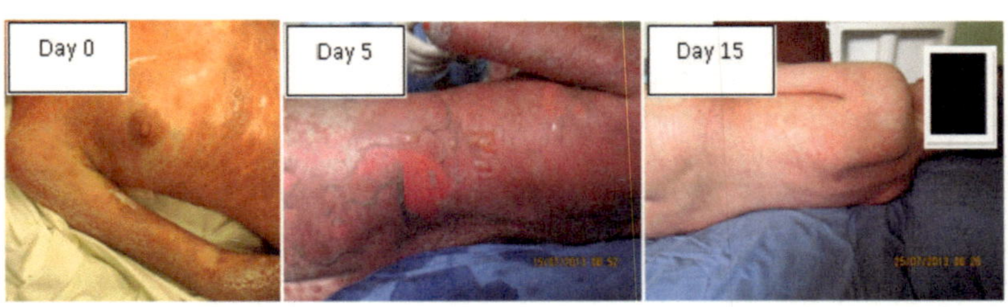

Figure 4. The clinical effect of the therapy of Lyell's effect in days: 0, 5 and 15.

http://dx.doi.org/10.5772/intechopen.70288

4. The allogeneic skin

Allogeneic skin, obtained mainly from dead, and rarely from living donors, has the properties of an ideal wound dressing: it protects the wound, stimulates healing and reduces pain. This is why is so successful in treating skin diseases such as Stevens-Johnson's disease and Lyell's disease [22]. Allogeneic skin is also used for the treatment of topical burn wounds and deep wounds alike, especially when there is not enough of the patient's skin available to dress their wound [43, 44]. One of its biggest advantages is the ease of gathering it, the possibility of gathering enough for a huge grafting surface, its low toxicity, the ease of keeping it and the relative ease of application [45]. In the case of both widespread and deep wounds, allogeneic skin used to dress a surgically cleaned wound prevents the skin from loosing water, electrolytes and proteins, while at the same time preventing the dehydration of other cells. Moreover, by being a barrier against environmental stimuli, it reduces the proliferation of microorganisms [46]. Thanks to a lowered heat loss experienced by the wound, the hypermetabolic response of the skin to the burn wound diminishes. In wounds suffered by all the layers of skin and thus lacking regenerative potential, an allogeneic skin transplant stimulates the granulation process and wound epithelization, thus creating a stroma for further surgical intervention [47]. The allogeneic skin is also a good biological dressing, which is effective in the treatment of burn wounds of medium depth, covering the epidermis and the dermis. The allogen initiates the growth of blood vessels in the wound bed and stimulates revascularization. While closely adhering to the stroma, it minimizes the level of pain and reduces the amount of necessary dressing changes, allowing for the process of the recreating of the epidermis to continue while the allogen disassociates itself from it without violating the emerging epidermis [48]. In certain cases, allogeneic skin serves as a dressing of wounds previously covered by mesh transplants of autologous skin, allowing to minimize metabolic stress and prevent infections within the wound and creating scaffolding for in vitro cultured keratinocytes [42]. In the Center of Wound Treatment in Siemianowice Slaskie, allogeneic skin is the standard operating procedure for patients with severe wounds, allowing for the temporary dressing and protection of wounds [49]. Moreover, it is also used when the exact depth of the wound cannot be determined while a risk of the wound deepening and the loss of the entire autologous transplant exists [50]. In our clinic, allogeneic skin is used also for the treatment of wounds of medium depth as a dressing meant for the stimulation of granulation tissue and the final closing of the wound thanks to its initiation of the epithelization process [51]. Allogeneic skin was first included in preparations in 2009 while the first transplant was executed in early 2010. At first, it was sourced from multiple organs. Due to clinical demand, from 2014 skin from Departments of Forensic Medicine is being used. Skin sourced in the latter way carries the risk of infected material increased by 58%, with the most common pathogen being *Klebsiella pneumoniae* [52]. In 2016, allogeneic skin was transplanted 235 times. The skin was sourced from about 50 donors. Until the end of 2016, the total amount of donors grew to 163. Allogeneic skin transplants sourced from dead people fulfilling the criteria of donors in accordance with the Bill of Law from July 1, 2005 on the sourcing, storage and transplantation of cells, tissue and organs is being prepared in the Cell Bank and *in vitro* Cell Culture Center in the Center for Burn Treatment. The transplants are then sterilized by radiation to eliminate dangerous pathogens, microbiologically tested and checked for viruses to conclude the sterilization process. If the results of the tests are negative, skin substitutes are stored in −80°C until application. The next stage, performed under anesthetics at the Surgical Ward, the burn wounds are surgically cleaned from dead tissue. Then the allogeneic skin is grated and applied to the wound. After the application of the transplant, the wound is dressed in an external wound dressing. The next stages of the dressing of burn wounds by allogeneic skin transplants are pictured in **Figure 5**.

Patients of our Center with IIB wounds and some patients with IIB/III wounds had the allogeneic skin transplant lead to a definitive closing of the wound, despite a previous nephrectomy, resulted in the stimulation of the growth of cells in the wound bed and the revascularization of the wound, as well the initiating of the epithelization process (**Figure 6**). This eliminated the need for an own skin transplant to be performed on the patient [49, 51]. Similar results have been observed by Oliver and associates, who have proven that allogeneic skin modulates the proliferation process, as well as differentiation of granulation tissue [53].

Other patients with deep skin burn wounds had allogeneic skin used as a dressing preventing the loss of water, microelements and proteins, as well protecting them from bacteria and viruses. The dressing was a source of cytokines and growth factors stimulating chemotaxation and the proliferation of cells, stimulated the grantulation of tissue and prepared the stroma for a surgical intervention and provided grounds for the definitive closing of the wound thanks to an autologous skin transplant. Moreover, allogeneic skin is used in the Center when it is impossible to assess the depth of the wound and when there is a clear risk that it can deepen and the transplant can be rejected, as well as when the patient has a limited amount of source beds for own skin transplants [50]. Allogeneic skin is also applied on wounds coming from as escharotomy. To conclude, allogeneic skin is a good alternative to autologous skin transplants. An allogeneic skin transplant results in the complete healing of the wound,

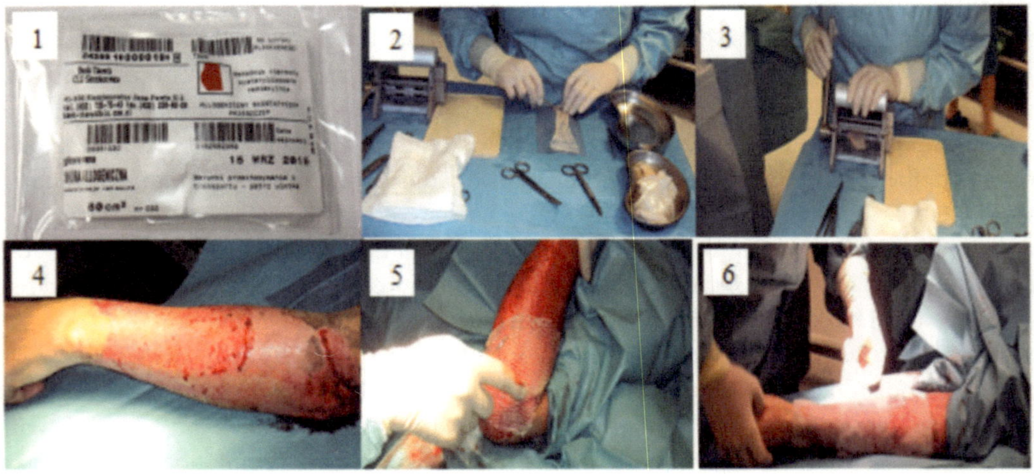

Figure 5. The allogeneic, biostatic transplant (1 and 2), the grating of allogeneic skin (3), a IIB burn wound cleaned from dead tissue (4), the application of an allogeneic skin transplant (5) and the application of an external wound dressing (6).

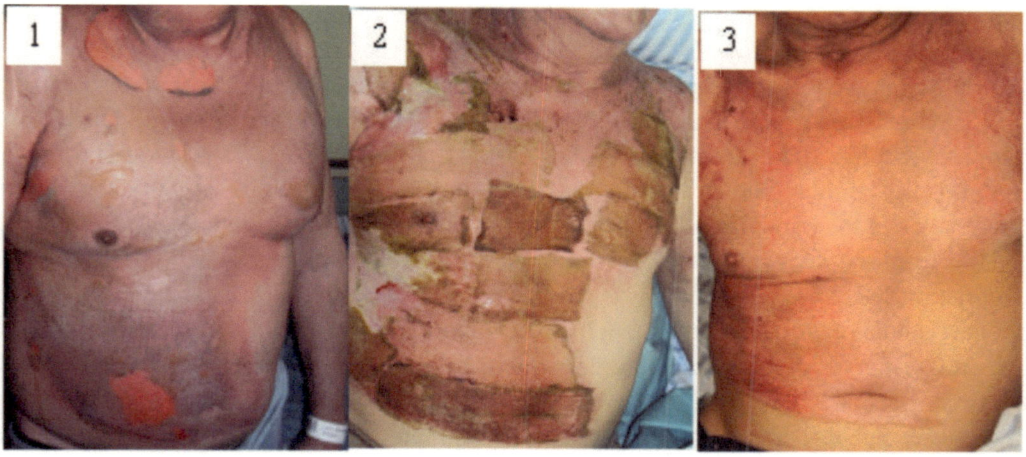

Figure 6. The patient on the day of admission to the Center (1), on the third day after the allogeneic skin transplant (2), on the 16th day from the hospital admission (the day of leaving the Center) (3).

eliminating the necessity for own skin sourcing for the transplant, which could result in further complications, pain and scarring. It is worth noting, however, than allogeneic skin can only be a temporary wound dressing, allowing for and facilitating the autologous skin transplant, which remains one of the best methods of closing a burn wound [54].

5. Acellular collagen human skin matrix (Acellular dermal matrix, ADM)

In order to improve the properties and the longevity of the transplants, tissue engineering methods such as cell removal are used. The reason for the removal of cells from tissues/organs is the obtaining of a non-immunogeneic transplant, which could be populated *in vivo* by the patients' own cells after the transplantation is completed [21]. A transplant devoid of cells is thus composed of the elements of an extracellular matrix, the ECM. The influence of the ECM on the mitogenesis and chemotaxis of cells and their targeted differentiation has been proven. It has also been proven that the ECM induces the creation and promotes the constructive remodeling of the host's tissue. Correctly used materials can modulate certain stages of healing by helping and inducing the transition from the inflammatory period to the constructive restructuring of the fractured cells. Effects observed during the interaction between the used biomaterial and the body of the recipient are complex and include immune system reactions, the proliferation of stem cells and their differentiation [55]. Moreover, ECM has many elements that are produced and populated by its colonizing cells. Between the extracellular matrix and the cells, a dynamic mutual relationship occurs. It affects their microenvironment and the proliferation and differentiation of cells. The described phenomena occur in natural body homeostasis, but are key for the healing of the wound [56]. The ECM cells regulated the biosynthesis of collagen and the processed of production of other elements of the extracellular synthesis. The role of these cells is the regulation of all the processes of biosynthesis, transformation and degradation of connective tissue [57]. Cellular residue, however, coming from the aftermath of the process of restructuring of allogeneic cells can provoke an unwanted immune response, which can in turn destroy the transplant [58, 59]. As the autoimmunological response is mostly targeted against proteins and fatty cells of the cellular tissue, the removal of cells from the tissue is a promising method that may lead to the sustaining of the induction of the immune response in the patient's body after the transplant [58, 60, 61]. The removal of cellular components should minimize the immune induced inflammation, which may weaken the biodegradation of the transplanted bioprosthesis. It is worth noting that the process of removing cells from tissue does not completely eliminate the immune response [62]. The process of eliminating cells from tissue/organs is chemical, enzymatic and mechanical in the genesis of how the cellular material is eliminated. In order to the removal of cells from human allogeneic skin, a collagen scaffolding is obtained, which can be *de novo* peopled by autologous skin cells and transplanted into the are that lacks [33]. The process of removing cells from tissues/organs is comprised of chemical, enzymatic and mechanical techniques of elimination of cellular matter. Thanks to the removing of cells from human allogeneic dermis, collagen scaffolding is obtained. It can be *de novo* populated by autologous skin cells and transplanted into the skin damage area. The method of treating burn wounds based on the use of human allogeneic, acellular extracellular matrix of the dermis (acellular dermal matrix, ADM) as a matrix for *in vitro* cultivated autologous fibroblasts and keratinocytes can be an effective method in the treatment of burn wounds [22]. The clinical need of using this method arises in patients with deep burn wounds of at least 50% TBSA and when the sites from which the skin was obtained for autologous skin grafting heal badly [12, 15]. In the Dr Stanisław Sakiela Burn Centre in Siemianowice Śląskie, the application of acellular human skin matrix (ADM) began in 2015. Until March 2017, an ADM transplant was executed on six patients. Those qualified for the procedure had deep burn wounds which healed badly. Based on the obtained results and clinical observation, we concluded that the use of ADM with *in vitro* cultured skin cells can be an optimal treatment method for burn wounds. To obtain a definitive scientific result, however, the number of the analyzed cases has to be increased [63–66].

6. Skin substitutes

The use of skin substitutes is an alternative to auto-and allogeneic transplants in the treatment of wounds of various provenance, including burn wounds and chronic wounds. Skin substitutes have to meet certain criteria to fulfill their function as actual "substitutes". They should not be immunogenic for the patient. They should modulate the proteolytic activity of the wound. The main role of synthetic skin substitutes is the provision of a bioresorptive scaffolding which facilitates cellular migration and deposition of the extracellular matrix [23]. This scaffolding should also stimulate angiogenesis and promote the migration of skin cells (fibroblasts), stimulate the synthesis of granulation and absorb and neutralize free radicals. The ideal skin substitutes should be commonly available and able to recreate various functions and layers of the skin in a short time. Skin substitutes have to undergo vascularization quickly and integrate fast into the wound bed of the patient. The majority of the currently available materials are based on scaffoldings of cattle collagen (e.g. Integra) or beef collagen as well as allogeneic keratinocytes and fibroblasts (Apligraf) [24]. Other substitutes are human-based skin equivalents, such as Apligraf®, Dermagraft® or TheraSkin® [25]. Other substitutes are acellular, natural biopolymer scaffoldings, such as Kolagen, Oasis®, GraftJacket®, DermACELL®, EpiFix®, Integra™, Promogran™, alginians and chitozans.

In the case of burn wounds, the first stage of treatment is the removal of dead tissue and a temporary wound closing, which at best may be definitive [30, 67]. A necrotomy procedure, removing the source of the infection, which is dead cells, affects the humoral reaction of the system and the amount of endotoxins in the patient's blood [30, 68]. There are many substitutes that can be used for wound dressing. In our Center, we use human biostatic transplants skin, allogeneic amnion, cellular transplants (of keratinocytes and fibroblasts) as well as commercially available synthetic substitutes. Based on years of clinical research, we developed recommendations for the use of particular skin substitutes. We have experience in the use of three commercially available skin substitutes: Suprathel, Oasis and Biobrane. Shallow wounds, usually of the IIA type, benefit from Suprathel as an epidermis substitute. The decision on using a certain skin substitute is made every time by the lead doctor for every given patient. The final decision on the use of a synthetic substitute instead of an own skin transplant of an allogeneic transplant is often made in the operations room after the cleansing of the wound.

Suprathel is a resorbed epidermis substitute characterized by a high permeability of oxygen and steam and matching the physiological qualities of human skin. The pH of the dressing is initially 5.5 and a later 4.0 (in *in vitro* conditions). The risk of infection when using this dressing is minimal. Suprathel is made of lakto-kapromer, its main ingredient being *polylactic acid*. It is fully synthetic and does not include collagen, so the biological risk is fully eliminated here. The time of hydraulic degradation of the dressing is 4 weeks.

We use Suprathel in our Center since 2011. That year, we used this substitute on burn wounds of 5 × 5 cm area in five patients and on the 9 × 10 cm in five patients. Starting in 2012 and upon the observation of the first clinically positive effects of the dressing, Suprathel became more and more popular in our Center. Below is a diagram detailing the use of Suprathel in 18 × 23 cm increments in 2012–2016 (**Figure 7**).

During these years, Suprathel was mainly used in the Surgical Ward in artificial skin transplants. However, it was used twice in the Anesthesiology and Intensive Therapy Ward (**Figure 8**).

Deeper, IIB wounds are treated by Biobrane and Oasis in our Center. Biobrane is a dressing made of ultrathin, half-permeable membrane kept together by an elastic nylon band. It is made of a nontoxin mix of highly purified peptides made from collagen isolated from porcine skin and kept together by a nylon/silicone membrane. This structure ensures high elasticity and a fitting of the dressing to the wound. This substitute is highly adjoined and very hydrophilic and biocompatible. It is a 3D structure, containing a natural extracellular matrix facilitating the migration of cells, the filling of the wound and the stimulation of healing [45, 69]. In our Center, Biobrane was used as the first commercially available skin substitute. In 2008–2012, it was used in the burn wound ward: once in the 13 × 13 cm size and nine times

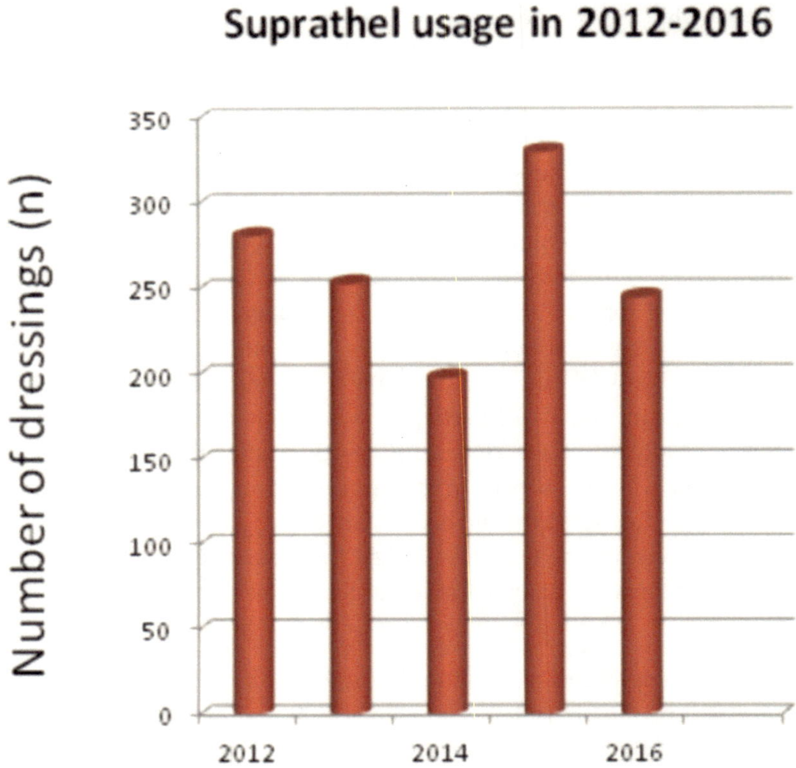

Figure 7. The amount of Suprathel used in 2012–2016.

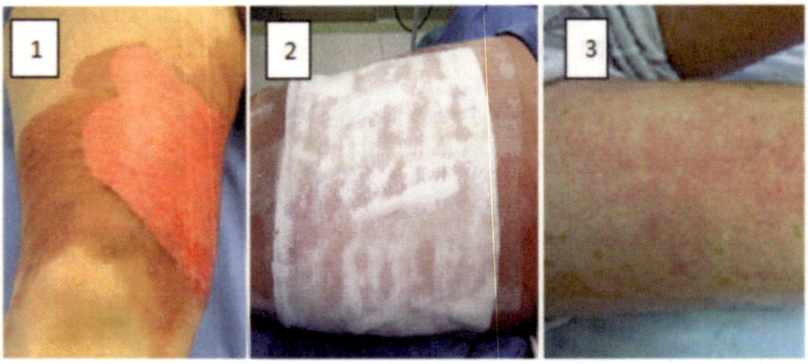

Figure 8. The wound (1) before the application of Suprathel (2) after the application of a substitute (3) upon heeling with Suprathel.

in the 13 × 38 cm size. In the first stage, Biobrane was used in the cosmetic treatment of burn and chronic wounds and used with anesthetics. Later on, Biobrane was also used during surgery. Biobrane is a mutlipurpose biosynthetic dressing [70]. It is a relatively inexpensive, easy to store and reliable dressing when used according to recommendations [71]. Despite its several pros, Lal et al. suggest that it should only be used on wound not deeper than 25%

TBSA to exclude the risk of infection [72]. Hubik et al. confirm that Biobrane carries a 37.8% risk infection [73]. Our experience confirms this data: in rare cases, an infection of the substitute occurred after it was transplanted on the cleansed burn wounds. Oasis is another skin substitute good for deeper wounds and chronic, seeding wound of the IIB type. This substitute is a natural matrix (Healthpoint) made of submucosal porcine lower intestine containing ECM (>90% collagen). It is thin (ca. 0.15 mm), half transparent and contains mainly type I collagen. The porcine component has a porous structure with pores of 20–30 μm that allow for the diffusion of oxygen and facilitates the survival of cells [74]. It maintains the biological activity of other skin elements that allow for binding of the cell growth factor and enzymes degrading the matrix, which allows an increased permeability of the cells and their accessing the fractured tissue. The matrix is the place of settling of glycosaminoglycans, proteoglycans, fibronectin and other growth factors, which gives is responsible for the substantial biological activity of this substitute [75–77]. This way, it gives not only the structural matrix, but provides growth factors as well, stimulating the angiogenesis and cellular migration, regulating the proteolytic activity and halting the extracellular matrix metalloproteinase: MMP-1, MMP-2 and MMP-9, affecting the migration of keratinocytes [78]. In our Center, we demarcated the matrix and applied the Oasis dressing during one procedure in the case of six patients between 2009 and 2015. In the case of each of these substitutes, the proper preparation of the wound bed is key. The wound has to be chemically or surgically cleansed. A very good method is VersaJet—a water knife removing dead cells. A wound cleansed of dead tissue has to be dressed with the substitute as recommended by the producer in terms of direction. The protection of the substitute is achieved by covering it with gauze soaked in vaseline (e.g. Jelonet), which is further covered by gauze dressings ready to injected with water and covered with bandage. The change of the dressing should happen no earlier than in the second day after the surgical procedure. Due to Suprathel being biodegradable, there is no need to remove it after the changing of the dressing unless and infection occurs. In this case, the infected substitute has to be removed immediately, cleanse the wound again and introduce antibacterial or antifungal procedures. To conclude, the use of commercially available skin substitutes in the treatment of burn and chronic wounds is a common practice in most Centers dealing with these kinds of wounds. Due to the high differentiation of the available products, each Center should develop its own procedure governing their good use. The procedures we described are ready recommendations for the use of commercially available skin substitutes which can be implemented in the treatment of patients with burn and chronic wounds. Due to their structure, epidermis substitutes are good for shallow wounds no deeper than IIA. Synthetic epidermis substitutes and natural skin substitutes may be equivalent to free skin transplants of medium depth and can be used on cleansed wounds no deeper than IIB [79, 80].

7. Scars treatment

Another group of skin substitutes is made of acellular synthetic polymer matrix. While they are available on the market of skin substitutes, they have various limitations, such as limiting vascularization, heightening scarring, low mechanical resistance and the danger of being rejected by the patients' immunological system. Synthetic skin substitutes often do not vascularize, which leads to the necrosis of cells and the final separation of the transplant from the wound [26]. An important limitation for the use of commercially available skin substitutes is the creation of scars, which lead to functional, mechanical and esthetic problems [27]. Even though scarring is a part of normal wound healing, it often leads to a pathological process. When the connective tissue fills the fractured skin part, it does not lead to the creation of a regular skin tone as the fibrous tissue lacks natural skin pigment. The connective tissue lacks hair follicles as well, which is why scars in hairy places can pose serious esthetic challenges. The uncovering and mechanisms of scarring would allow to determine the exact prophylaxis and therapeutic measures to undertake. A series of methods for the treatment of scars exist, yet neither one of them is fully effective. Since the use of one single method provokes a rapid relapse of the illness, a combined therapeutic approach is usually administered, allowing for a good cosmetic effect [28]. The combined therapeutic approach employing cryotherapy alone or combined with the use of steroids is one of the leading ways of scar treatment. Another method of improvement of the visual features of wounds is laser therapy. Its effectiveness is judged in various ways because of the type of wounds that can undertake this therapy. Its effects are usually augmented by corticosteroids. Another method, pressotherapy is based on treating scars by administering controlled pressure. Different compression models, compression clothes and clips' are used to this effect [29]. When scar treatment methods prove insufficient, surgical intervention becomes necessary. It involves the removal of the pathological skin tissue fragment and replacing it with new and healthy skin, usually sourced from other parts of the patients' body. Another surgical method for burn removal is the application of tissue stretchers (expanders). The use methods of burn treatment should result in the improvement of esthetic qualities of the patient, which further affect their self-confidence and quality of life [81]. More importantly, however, the aim of the therapy is to minimize clinical symptoms by minimizing or eliminating pain and burning and obtaining the full functionality of the joints affected by scarring. Wound treatment is a process of many stages, including various therapeutic methods depending on the level of maturity of the wound. The surgical procedure itself must be planned in a way that has in mind the caring for the scars. The removal of the necrosis should lead to retention of a reticular layer of the dermis, which allows for the faster healing of a wound thanks to less closely adhering scar. The use of VersaJet in the early resection of the necrosis positively impacts the look of the cleansed wounds. Depending on the type of transplant, the look of the wound at various stages of healing can be very different. The best esthetic effects are obtained by closing the wound with an autologous transplant of medium depth. A good cosmetic effect is also obtained by an *in vitro* transplant of autologous keratinocytes and fibroblasts in the grafted transplant of medium density. We have observed a good cosmetic effect of commercially available skin substitutes (Oasis, Biobrane). Besides prophylaxis, the treatment of wounds should lead to the creation of a soft, regular, non-discolorated surface. During the treatment, the creation of pathological wounds has to be avoided thanks to the provision of quick wound healing, the prevention of infections or and scar contractures (thanks to railing and rehab). At the first stage, a mild finger massage of the wound and the use of silicone gels and ointments are recommended. The silicone prevents the loss of water, the drying and chapping of the wound and alleviates the burning sensation. A layer of ointment or gel protects the wound from external dangers and mechanical damage, as well as creating slight pressure, which is why a finger massage is recommended before its application. The use of silicone band aids is recommended at the night-time, as they delicately pressurize the wound, preventing its drying. The most common silicone gels are Dermatix, Veraderm, Medigel and Cicacare and band aids are used [82]. Constant wound pressuring is obtained by pressotherapy using flexible fabrics. The effectiveness of the therapy depends on the choice of the correct pressure: too little may not be effective, too much may lead to side effects such as chafes, abrasions, maceration of the skin, sores or blisters. In the treatment of severe burn wounds, pressure clothing is used, employing slight pressure, classified by the European Standardization Commission as class I (18–21 mmHg). These clothes should be used for 6–24 months from the end of the wound healing until cosmetic effects such as the flattening, whitening and reduction of the size of the scar are achieved. The effectiveness of pressure clothing depends on their size, which is why they have to be fitted exactly and exchanged in the case of a change in body size (specifically in children) [82]. Scars can be treated by various methods. In our Center, we most commonly employ surgical treatment and laser therapy. Wound correction may comprise of their cutting out and sewing together, thus changing their direction and alleviating skin pressure. The cutting of skin must be undertaken with respect to the Langer lines. Surgical methods of wound healing used in our Center are topical, such as the "Z" method, based on making a cut of the "Z" shape. The middle part of this cut is perpendicular to the long axis of the closed wound and situated at least 3 cm from the wounds' brim. The angles between this section and the rest should be 30–90°. During the coming together of the wound brims, the resulting triangular areas change places and the "Z" shape changes from perpendicular to parallel to the long axis of the wound. This method was used six times a year. Another method of surgical wound treatment is using neighboring skin. It is thicker and stronger than the transplanted skin, which is why it can be used on areas devoid of veins. These methods are used in the treatment of contracted wound of the limbs, corpus and eyelids [83–85]. Laser therapy may, depending on the type of the laser, be used in the treatment of wounds at various stages of their maturity. At the level of wound healing, biostimulating lasers can be used. Biostimulation used low energy lasers (stimulants). These lasers emit rays up to 5 mW [83], and the wavelengths emitted by the lasers used in the biostimulation fall in the middle of the electromagnetic spectrum [84]. Biostimulation uses mainly lasers such as the He-Ne laser helium-neon and the arsen-gala semiconductor diode. The biostimulation process itself is effective in providing a predetermined amount of energy, expressed in Joules (J) to an appropriate depth. The degree of absorption and the penetration of the radiation are dependent on both the structure of the irradiated tissue, its blood flow, pH, water content, pigment, melanin and hemoglobin, as well as the wavelength, the color of light, its strength and the duration of treatment [84]. Upon the formation of the scar, our Center uses CO_2 laser ablation. The CO_2 laser emits radiation at a wavelength of 10,600 nm, which is continuous at the power of 30–100 W [83]. The radiation emitted by a CO_2 laser is invisible to the eye and absorbed by the intra- and extracellular fluid [85]. The absorption of the laser light is not selective and results in tissue damage to a depth of 0.6 mm. This causes thrombotic necrosis reaching 0.4–0.5 mm deep. A reticular layer of the skin is then formed due to thermal damage to the surrounding area of evaporation, which can sadly cause significant scarring at the site around the lesion [85]. The beneficial effect of the CO_2 laser radiation on tissue involves the evaporation of the affected tissue. This impact can, however, be complicated by adverse changes in the skin [85, 86]. This laser is used in the treatment of scars due to the very good absorption of water and shallow penetration of the tissue. Since water is the major component of tissues, it allows the beam of the laser to cut both soft tissue and even

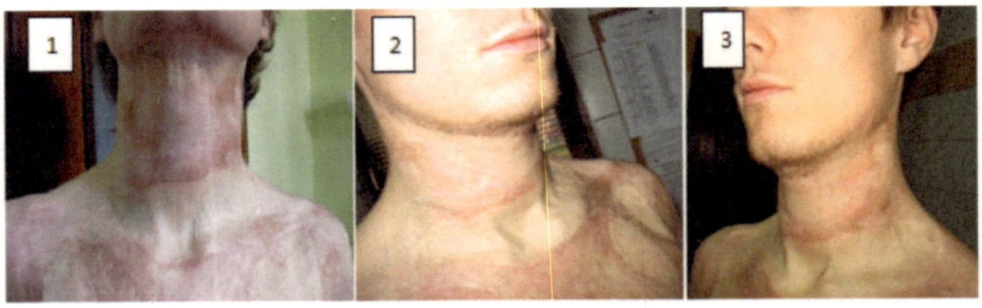

Figure 9. The wound before (1) laser therapy, after the first session (2) after the second session (3).

bone. This is why the laser is use in other medical fields such as gynecology, dermatology, ENT, where surgical intervention is necessary [83, 87]. CO_2 laser ablation procedures must be repeated three to five times to make their effects lasting and sufficient. Long intervals between treatments must be kept, allowing from 4 to 5 weeks to regenerate the patient's tissue. It is important to maintain sufficient extent of treatment, as during each session of laser therapy, it is only performed in about 15–25% of the scars (**Figure 9**). These treatments are performed in our Center's department of cosmetic surgery on an average of 96 times a year, with 93 times being laser therapy aiding in condition of scarring and fibrosis of the skin [88].

To conclude, the process of healing scars comes in stages and begins with the resection of the necrosis, which has to be carried out in such a way as to leave a layer of reticularis dermis and to perform the cuts Langer lines. This is the first stage of prophylaxis to prevent the formation of ugly scars. The type of transplant has a decisive influence on the appearance of scars, with the most cosmetically sound scars created by an medium depth solid transplant or an autologous keratinocytes and fibroblasts transplant in the scaffolding of a reticulated transplant. The very process of scar treatment should begin as soon as possible. Already the wound healing process can be aided by biostimulating lasers. The prophylaxis of scars includes the prevention of wound infection and contracted scars. Upon healing of the wound, the first step of scar treatment is a finger massage and the use of silicone gels and ointments, then pressure therapy using pressure clothing. Upon the forming a pathological scars, surgical methods such as the "Z" cut method and neighboring skin method, as well as laser therapy using the ablative CO_2 laser.

Author details

Diana Kitala[1]*, Agnieszka Klama-Baryła[1,2], Wojciech Łabuś[1], Marcelina Misiuga[1], Mariusz Nowak[1] and Marek Kawecki[1,3]

*Address all correspondence to: dp.kitala@gmail.com

1 Dr Stanislaw Sakiel's Burn Treatment Centre, Siemianowice Śląskie, Poland

2 Silesian Higher Medical School in Katowice, Katowice, Poland

3 Department of Health Sciences, Technical-Humanistic Academy, Bielsko-Biała, Poland

References

[1] Ogliari KS, Marinowic D, Brum DE, Loth F. Stem cells in dermatology. Anais Brasileiros de Dermatologia. 2014;**89**(2):286-292. DOI: 10.1590/abd1806-4841.20142530

[2] Sorg H, Betzler C, Rennekampff HO, Vogt PM. Burns. Unfallchirurg. 2012;**115**(7):635-648. DOI: 10.1007/s00113-012-2239-3

[3] Shen YM, Hu XH, Mi HR, Yu DN, Qin FJ, Chen H, Wang H, Zhang GA. Early treatment of high-voltage electric burn wound in the limbs. Zhonghua Shao Shang Za Zhi. 2011;**27**(3):173-177

[4] Petrof G, Abdul-Wahab A, McGrath JA. Cell therapy in dermatology. Cold Spring Harb Perspect Med. 2014;**4**(6):pii: a015156. DOI: 10.1101/cshperspect.a015156

[5] Official Journal of the European Union. Commission Directive 2009/120/EC of 14 September 2009 amending Directive 2001/83/EC of the European Parliament and of the Council on the Community code relating to medicinal products for human use as regards advanced therapy med [Internet]. 2009. Available from: http://ec.europa.eu/health//sites/health/files/files/eudralex/vol-1/dir_2009_120/dir_2009_120_en.pdf [Accessed: 14-02-2017]

[6] Official Journal of the European Union 10.12.2007. European Parliament and Council (2007). Regulation (EC) No 1394/2007 of the European Parliament and of the Council of 13 November 2007 on advanced therapy medicinal products and amending Directive 2001/83/EC and Regulation (EC) No 726/2004 [Internet]. 2007. Available from: http://www.biosafety.be/PDF/1394_2007_EN.pdf

[7] European Medicines Agency. Scientific advice and protocol assistance [Internet]. [Updated: 2012]. Available from: http://www.ema.europa.eu/ema/index.jsp?curl=pages/regulation/general/general_content_000300.jsp&mid=WC0b01ac058007f4bd [Accessed: 14-02-2017]

[8] Celis P. CAT—the new committee for advanced therapies at the European Medicines Agency. Bundesgesundheitsblatt, Gesundheitsforschung, Gesundheitsschutz. 2010;**53**(1): 9-13. DOI: 10.1007/s00103-009-0998-y

[9] Blais M, Parenteau-Bareil R, Cadau S, Berthod F. Concise review: Tissue-engineered skin and nerve regeneration in burn treatment. Stem Cells Translational Medicine. 2013;**2**(7): 545-551. DOI: 10.5966/sctm.2012-0181

[10] Klama-Baryła A, Kraut M, Łabuś W, Maj M, Kawecki M, Nowak M, Glik J, Cichowski A, Szydło A, Lesiak M, Anioł J, Sieroń AL. Application of platelet leukocyte gel in in vitro cultured autologous keratinocite grafts. Journal of Orthopaedics Trauma Surgery and Related Research. 2011;**2**(22):77-86

[11] Sumide T, Nishida K, Yamato M, Ide T, Hayashida Y, Watanabe K, Yang J, Kohno C, Kikuchi A, Maeda N, Watanabe H, Okano T, Tano Y. Functional human corneal endothelial cell sheets harvested from temperature-responsive culture surfaces. The FASEB Journal. 2006;**20**(2):392-394. DOI: 10.1096/fj.04-3035fje

[12] Bargues L, Prat M, Leclerc T, Bey E, Lataillade JJ. Present and future of cell therapy in burns. Pathologie-Biologie. 2011;**59**(3):e49-e56. DOI: 10.1016/j.patbio.2009.12.006

[13] Jeong JH. Adipose stem cells and skin repair. Current Stem Cell Research & Therapy. 2010;**5**(2):137-140

[14] Danner S, Kremer M, Petschnik AE, Nagel S, Zhang Z, Hopfner U, Reckhenrich AK, Weber C, Schenck TL, Becker T, Kruse C, Machens HG, Egaña JT. The use of human sweat gland-derived stem cells for enhancing vascularization during dermal regeneration. The Journal of Investigative Dermatology. 2012;**132**(6):1707-1716. DOI: 10.1038/jid.2012.31

[15] Kawecki M, Hoff-Lenczewska D, Klama-Baryła A, Glik J. Oparzenia. In: Dziki, editor. Przegląd Piśmiennictwa Chirurgicznego. Fundacja Polski Przegląd Chirurgiczny: Warsaw; 2013

[16] Hoff-Lenczewska D, Klama-Baryła A, Kawecki M, Łabuś W, Glik J, Maj M, Gola J, Mazurek U, Sieroń AL. The use of modern Technologies of cell and tissue engineering in burn treatment. Acta Biochimica Polonica. 2012;(supplement 1):17-22

[17] Kim SW, Zhang HZ, Guo L, Kim JM, Kim MH. Amniotic Mesenchymal stem cells enhance wound healing in diabetic NOD/SCID mice through high angiogenic and engraftment capabilities. PLoS One. 2012;**7**(7):e41105. DOI: 10.1371/journal.pone.0041105

[18] Hartmann-Fritsch F, Hosper N, Luginbühl J, Biedermann T, Reichmann E, Meuli M. Human amniotic fluid derived cells can competently substitute dermal fibroblasts in a tissue-engineered dermo-epidermal skin analog. Pediatric Surgery International. 2013; **29**(1):61-69. DOI: 10.1371/journal.pone.0041105

[19] Mahmoudi-Rad M, Abolhasani E, Moravvej H, Mahmoudi-Rad N, Mirdamadi Y. Acellular amniotic membrane: An appropriate scaffold for fibroblast proliferation. Clinical and Experimental Dermatology. 2013;**38**(6):646-651. DOI: 10.1111/ced.12087

[20] Wilshaw SP, Kearney J, Fisher J, Ingham E. Biocompatibility and potential of acellular human amniotic membrane to support the attachment and proliferation of allogeneic cells. Tissue Engineering. Part A. 2008;**14**(4):463-472. DOI: 10.1089/tea.2007.0145

[21] Sood R, Roggy D, Zieger M, Balledux J, Chaudhari S, Koumanis DJ, Mir HS, Cohen A, Knipe C, Gabehart K, Coleman JJ. Cultured epithelial autografts for coverage of large burn wounds in eighty-eight patients: The Indiana University experience. Journal of Burn Care & Research. 2010;**31**(4):559-568. DOI: 10.1097/BCR.0b013e3181e4ca29

[22] Pellegrini G, Ranno R, Stracuzzi G, Bondanza S, Guerra L, Zambruno G. The control of epidermal stem cells (holoclones) in the treatment of massive full-thickness burns with autologous keratinocytes cultured on fibrin. Transplantation. 1999;**68**:868-879

[23] MS H, Rennert RC, McArdle A, Chung MT, Walmsley GG, Longaker MT, Lorenz HP. The role of stem cells during Scarless skin wound healing. Advances in Wound Care. 2014;**3**(4):304-314. DOI: 10.1089/wound.2013.0471

[24] Mansilla E, Marín GH, Berges M, Scafatti S, Rivas J, Núñez A, Menvielle M, Lamonega R, Gardiner C, Drago H, Sturla F, Portas M, Bossi S, Castuma MV, Luengas SP, Roque G, Martire K, Tau JM, Orlandi G, Tarditti A. Cadaveric bone marrow mesenchymal stem cells: First experience treating a patient with large severe burns. Burns & Trauma. 2015;**3**(1):1-9. DOI: 10.1186/s41038-015-0018-4

[25] Rasulov MF, Vasilchenkov AV, Onishchenko NA, Krasheninnikov ME, Kravchenko VI, Gorshenin TL, Pidtsan RE, Potapov IV. First experience of the use bone marrow mesenchymal stem cells for the treatment of a patient with deep skin burns. Bulletin of Experimental Biology and Medicine. 2005;**139**(1):141-144

[26] Cell Renewal, Naturally™. SkinGun™ and CellMist™ Technology Overview [Internet]. Available from: http://renovacareinc.com/ [Accessed: 20-02-2017]

[27] TERUMO BCT, INC. AdiPrep® Adipose Concentration System [Internet]. Available from: https://www.harvesttech.com [Accessed: 02-02-2017]

[28] Fraser JK, Hicok KC, Shanahan R, Zhu M, Miller S, Arm DM. The Celution® system: Automated processing of adipose-derived regenerative cells in a functionally closed system. Advances in Wound Care. 2014;**3**(1):38-45

[29] Aronowitz JA, Ellenhorn JD. Adipose stromal vascular fraction isolation: A head-to-head comparison of four commercial cell separation systems. Plastic and Reconstructive Surgery. 2013;**132**(6):932e-939e. DOI: 10.1097/PRS.0b013e3182a80652

[30] Kawecki M, Glik J, Kitala D, Misiuga M. Oparzenia [Burns]. In: Dziki A, editor. Przegląd Piśmiennictwa Chirurgicznego. 1st ed. Łódź: Stowarzyszenie Popierania Rozwoju Proktologii; 2017. p. 192-196

[31] Halim AS, Khoo TL, Mohd SJ. Biologic and synthetic skin substitutes: An overview. Indian Journal of Plastic Surgery. 2010;**43**(Suppl):S23-S28. DOI: 10.4103/0970-0358.70712

[32] Gierek M, Kawecki M, Mikuś K, Glik J, Klama-Baryła A, Hoff-Lenczewska D, Nowak M. The treatment of burns wounds with human amniotic membrane dressins in the Centre for Burns in Siemianowice Śląskie—Own experience. Journal of Orthopaedics Trauma Surgery and Related Research. 2012;**3**(29):75-83

[33] Gierek M, Kawecki M, Mikuś K, Glik J, Klama-Baryła A, Hoff-Lenczewska D, Nowak M. Use of amniotic membrane in treatment of burns. Journal of Orthopaedics Trauma Surgery and Related Research. 2012;**3**(29):70-75

[34] Strom SC, Gramignoli R. Human amnion epithelial cells expressing HLA-G as novel cell-based treatment for liver disease. Human Immunology. 2016;**77**(9):734-739. DOI: 10.1016/j.humimm.2016.07.002

[35] He H, Li W, Chen SY, Zhang S, Chen YT, Hayashida Y, Zhu YT, Tseng SC. Suppression of activation and induction of apoptosis in RAW264.7 cells by amniotic membrane extract. Investigative Ophthalmology & Visual Science. 2008;**49**(10):4468-4475. DOI: 10.1167/iovs.08-1781

[36] Alikarami F, Yari F, Amirizadeh N, Nikougoftar M, Jalili MA. The immunosuppressive activity of amniotic membrane mesenchymal stem cells on T lymphocytes. Avicenna Journal of Medical Biotechnology. 2015;**7**(3):90-96. DOI: PMC4508338

[37] Barling PM, John MJ, Walsh JR, Niall HD. The isolation and characterization of lysozyme from human foetal membranes: A comparison with the enzyme from other sources. Comparative Biochemistry and Physiology Part B. 1985;**81**(2):509-513 PMID: 4017555

[38] Flores-Espinosa P, Pineda-Torres M, Vega-Sánchez R, Estrada-Gutiérrez G, Espejel-Nuñez A, Flores-Pliego A, Maida-Claros R, Paredes-Vivas Y, Morales-Méndez I, Sosa-González I, Chávez-Mendoza A, Zaga-Clavellina V. Progesterone elicits an inhibitory effect upon LPS-induced innate immune response in pre-labor human amniotic epithelium. American Journal of Reproductive Immunology. 2014;**71**(1):61-72. DOI: 10.1111/aji.12163

[39] Taghiabadi E, Nasri S, Shafieyan S, Jalili Firoozinezhad S, Aghdami N. Fabrication and characterization of spongy denuded amniotic membrane based scaffold for tissue engineering. Cell Journal. 2015;**16**(4):476-487. DOI: 10.22074/cellj.2015.493

[40] Zhang T, Yam GH, Riau AK, Poh R, Allen JC, Peh GS, Beuerman RW, Tan DT, Mehta JS. The effect of amniotic membrane de-epithelialization method on its biological properties and ability to promote limbal epithelial cell culture. Investigative Ophthalmology & Visual Science. 2013;**54**(4):3072-3081. DOI: 10.1167/iovs.12-10805

[41] DiDomenico LA, Orgill DP, Galiano RD, Serena TE, Carter MJ, Kaufman JP, Young NJ, Zelen CM. Aseptically processed placental membrane improves healing of diabetic foot ulcerations: Prospective, randomized clinical trial. Plastic and Reconstructive Surgery-Global Open. 2016;**4**(10):e1095. DOI: 10.1097/GOX.0000000000001095

[42] Rogers AD. Indications for cadaver skin in burns and complex wound care. Wound Healing Southern Africa. 2013;**6**(2):54-55

[43] Fletcher JL, Caterson EJ, Hale RG, Cancio LC, Renz EM, Chan RK. Characterization of skin allograft use in thermal injury. Journal of Burn Care & Research. 2013;**34**(1):168-175. DOI: 10.1097/BCR.0b013e318270000f

[44] Kagan RJ, Peck MD, Ahrenholz DH, Hickerson WL, Holmes J 4th, Korentager R, Kraatz J, Pollock K, Kotoski G. Surgical management of the burn wound and use of skin substitutes: An expert panel white paper. Journal of Burn Care & Research. 2013;**34**(2):e60-e79. DOI: 10.1097/BCR.0b013e31827039a6

[45] Selig HF, Lumenta DB, Giretzlehner M, Jeschke MG, Upton D, Kamolz LP. The properties of an "ideal" burn wound dressing—What do we need in daily clinical practice? Results of a worldwide online survey among burn care specialists. Burns. 2012;**38**(7):960-966. DOI: 10.1016/j.burns.2012.04.007

[46] Cleland H, Wasiak J, Dobson H, Paul M, Pratt G, Paul E, Herson M, Akbarzadeh S. Clinical application and viability of cryopreserved cadaveric skin allografts in severe burn: A retrospective analysis. Burns. 2014;**40**(1):61-66. DOI: 10.1016/j.burns.2013.05.006

[47] Zidan SM, Eleowa SA. Banking and use of glycerol preserved full-thickness skin allograft harvested from body contouring procedures. Burns. 2014;**40**(4):641-647. DOI: 10.1016/j.burns.2013.08.039

[48] Horner CWM, Atkins J, Simpson L, Philp B, Shelley O, Dziewulski P. Estimating the usage of allograft in the treatment of major burns. Burns. 2011;**37**(4):590-593. DOI: 10.1016/j.burns.2010.12.006

[49] Kitala D, Kawecki M, Klama-Baryła A, Łabuś W, Kraut M, Glik J, Ryszkiel I, Kawecki MP, Nowak M. Allogeneic vs. autologous skin grafts in the therapy of patients with burn injuries: A restrospective, open-label clinical study with pair matching. Advances in Clinical and Experimental Medicine. 2016;**25**(5):923-929. DOI: 10.17219/acem/61961

[50] Singh V, Devgan L, Bhat S, Miler SM. The pathogenesis of burn wound conversion. Annals of Plastic Surgery. 2007;**59**(1):109-115. DOI: 10.1097/01.sap.0000252065.90759.e6

[51] Misiuga M, Glik J, Kawecki M, et al. The effect of hyperbaric oxygen therapy on burn wounds covered with skin allografts. Journal of Orthopaedics Trauma Surgery and Related Research. 2016;**1**(38):17-27

[52] Kitala D, Klama-Baryła A, Kawecki M, Kraut M, Łabuś W, Glik J, Ples M, Tomanek E, Nowak M. Infections in the tissue material and their impact on the loss of transplants in the laboratory of in vitro cell and tissue culture with tissue Bank in the years 2011-2015. Cell and Tissue Banking. 2016;**17**(66):1-8. DOI: 10.1007/s10561-016-9597-y

[53] Oliver AM, Kaawach W, Mithoff EW, Watt A, Abramovich DR, Rayner CR. The differentiation and proliferation of newly formed epidermis on wounds treated with cultured epithelial allografts. British Journal of Dermatology. 1991;**125**(2):147-154

[54] Debels H, Hamdi M, Abberton K, Morrison W. Dermal matrices and bioengineered skin substitutes: A critical review of current options. Plastic and Reconstructive Surgery Global Open. 2015;**3**(1):e284. DOI: 10.1097/GOX.0000000000000219

[55] Londono R, Badylak SF. Biologic scaffolds for regenerative medicine: Mechanisms of in vivo remodeling. Annals of Biomedical Engineering. 2015;**43**(3):577-592. DOI: 10.1007/s10439-014-1103-8

[56] Kawecki M, Łabuś W, Klama-Baryla A, Kitala D, Kraut M, Glik J, Misiuga M, Nowak M, Bielecki T, Kasperczyk A. A review of decellurization methods caused by an urgent need for quality control of cell-free extracellular matrix' scaffolds and their role in regenerative medicine. Journal of Biomedical Materials Research—Part B: Applied Biomaterials, Forthcoming. DOI: 10.1002/jbm.b.33865

[57] Schmidt C, Baier JM. Acellular vascular tissues: Natural biomaterials for tissue engineering. Biomaterials. 2000;**21**(22):2215-2231

[58] Atiyeh BS, Costagliola M. Cultured epithelial autograft (CEA) in burn treatment: Three decades later. Burns. 2007;**33**(4):405-413. DOI: 10.1016/j.burns.2006.11.002

[59] Grauss RW, Hazekamp MG, van Vliet S, Gittenberger-de Groot AC, DeRuiter MC. Decellulrization of rat aortic valve allografts reduces leaflet destruction and extracellular matrix remodeling. The Journal of Thoracic and Cardiovascular Surgery. 2003;**126**(6):2003-2010. DOI: 10.1016/S0022

[60] Sullivan DC, Mirmalek-Sani SH, Deegan DB, Baptista PM, Aboushwareb T, Atala A, Yoo JJ. Decellularization methods of porcine kidneys for whole organ engineering using a high-throughput system. Biomaterials. 2012;**33**(31):7756-7764. DOI: 10.1016/j.biomaterials.2012.07.023

[61] Ott HC, Matthiesen TS, Goh SK, Black LD, Kren SM, Netoff TI, Taylor DA. Perfusion-decellularized matrix: Using nature's platform to engineer a bioartificial heart. Nature Medicine. 2008;**14**(2):213-221. DOI: 10.1038/nm1684

[62] Atiyeh B, Masellis A, Conte C. Optimizing burn treatment in developing low- and middle-income countries with limited health care resources (part 1). Annals of Burns and Fire Disasters. 2009;**22**(3):121-125

[63] Troy J, Karlnoski R, Downes K, Brown KS, Cruse CW, Smith DJ, Payne WG. The use of EZ Derm® in Partial-Thickness Burns: An Institutional Review of 157 Patients. Eplasty. 2013;**13**:e14

[64] Gould LJ. Topical collagen-based biomateriale for chronic wounds: Rationale and clinical application. Advances in Wound Care. 2016;**1**(5):19-31. DOI: 10.1089/wound.2014.0595

[65] Zaulyanov L, Kirsner RS. A review of a bi-layered living cell treatment (Apligraf (R®)) in the treatment of venous leg ulcers and diabetic foot ulcers. Clinical Interventions in Aging. 2007;**2**(1):93-98

[66] Di Domenico L, Landsman AR, Emch KJ, Landsman A. A prospective comparison of diabetic foot ulcers treated with either cryopreserved skin allograft or bioengineered skin substitute. Wounds. 2011;**23**(7):184-189

[67] Zhao JH, Diao JS, Xia WS, Pan Y, Han Y. Clinical application of full-face, whole, full-thickness skin grafting: A case report. Journal of Plastic, Reconstructive & Aesthetic Surgery. 2012;**65**(11):1576-1579. DOI: 10.1016/j.bjps.2012.04.002

[68] Lloyd EC, Michener M, Williams MS. Outpatient burns: Prevention and care. American Family Physician. 2013;**85**(9):25-32

[69] Philandrianos C, Andrac-Meyer L, Mordon S, Feuerstein JM, Sabatier F, Veran J, Magalon G, Casanova D. Comparison of five dermal substitutes in full-thickness skin wound healing in a porcine model. Burns. 2012;**38**(9):820-829

[70] Whitaker IS, Prowse S, Potokar TS. A critical evaluation of the use of Biobrane as a biologic skin substitute: A versatile tool for the plastic and reconstructive surgeon. Annals of Plastic Surgery. 2008;**60**(3):333-337

[71] Greenwood JE, Clausen J, Kavanagh S. Experience with biobrane: uses and caveats for success. Eplasty. 2009 Jun 26;**9**:e25

[72] Lal S, Barrow RE, Wolf SE, Chinkes DL, Hart DW, Heggers JP, Herndon DN. Biobrane improves wound healing in burned children without increased risk of infection. Shock. 2000;**14**(3):314-318

[73] Hubik DJ, Wasiak J, Paul E, Cleland H. Biobrane: A retrospective analysis of outcomes at a specialist adult burns centre. Burns. 2011;**37**(4):594-600

[74] Nihsen ES, Johnson CE, Hiles MC. Bioactivity of small intestinal submucosa and oxidized regeneratem cellulose/collagen. Advances in Skin & Wound Care. 2008;**21**(10):479-486

[75] Hodde JP, Badylak SF, Brightman AO, Voytik-Harbin SL. Glycosaminoglycan content of small intestinal submucosa: A bioscaffold for tissue replacement. Tissue Engineering. 1996;**2**(3):209-217

[76] Hodde JP, Record RD, Liang HA, Badylak SF. Vascular endothelial growth factor in porcine-derived extracellular matrix. Endothelium. 2001;**8**(1):11-24

[77] Shi L, Ronfard V. Biochemical and biomechanical characterization of porcine small intestinal submucosa (SIS): A mini review. International Journal of Burns and Trauma. 2013;**3**(4):173-179

[78] Shi L, Ramsay S, Ermis R, Carson D. In vitro and in vivo studies on matrix metalloproteinases interacting with small intestine submucosa wound matrix. International Wound Journal. 2012;**9**(1):44-53

[79] Moore M, Samsell B, Wallis G, Triplett S, Chen S, Linthurst Jones A, et al. Decellularization of human dermis rusing non-denaturing anionic detergent and endonuclease: A review. Cell and Tissue Banking. 2015;**16**:249-259

[80] Dumville JC, Keogh SJ, Liu Z, Stubbs N, Walker RM, Fortnam M. Alginate dressings for treating pressure ulcers. Cochrane Database of Systematic Reviews. 2015;**3**:CD011277

[81] O'Meara S, Martyn-St James M, Adderley UJ. Alginate dressings for venous leg ulcers. Cochrane Database of Systematic Reviews. 2015;**19**:CD010182

[82] Kawecki K, Pawlik-Kanpik D, Glik J, Misuga M. Oparzenia. Blizny jako problem w chirurgii oparzeń. In: Dziki A, editor. Przegląd Piśmiennictwa Chirurgicznego 2015. Warszawa: Fundacja Polski Przegląd Chirurgiczny ed.; 2016

[83] Wójcicka P, Gadomska-Krasny J, Zawodny JP. Zastosowanie Laserów w Medycynie Estetyczne J. Fotoodmładzanie w terapii przebarwień oraz rozszerzonych naczyń krwionośnych – cz. 1. OPM. 2010;**12**:46-49

[84] Kurkus B, Kuliński W. Laseroterapia w medycynie fizykalnej. Borgis – Balneologia Polska. 2005;**3**(4):76-83

[85] Borzęcki A, Cielica W. Zastosowanie lasera CO2 w praktyce dermatologicznej. Borgis-Nowa Medycyna. 2000;**11**:1-14

[86] Miturska R, Borzęcki A. Papilloma condylomatoides okolic narządów płciowych i odbytu leczona laserem CO2. Dermatologia Estetyczna. 2009;**11/6**(65):481-485

[87] Stocka A, Huryń A, Królicki A, Orzechowska B, Maleszka R. Laseroterapia ablacyjna w leczeniu skórnej manifestacji stwardnienia guzowatego – opis przypadku. Dermatologia Estetyczna. 2010;**12/6**(71):367-372

[88] Macedo JL, Santos JB. Predictive factors of mortality in burn patients. Revista do Instituto de Medicina Tropical de São Paulo. 2007;**49**(6):365-370

Chapter 9

Treatment of Skin Laxity Using Multisource, Phase-Controlled Radiofrequency

Yohei Tanaka

Additional information is available at the end of the chapter

http://dx.doi.org/10.5772/intechopen.71749

Abstract

Regardless of age, sex and skin type, skin tightening is a common procedure requested by patients seeking cosmetic treatments to improve facial contours and skin laxity. Radiofrequency has been proven to penetrate deeper than optical light sources independent of skin color and to be beneficial for skin tightening. I previously reported on the efficacy of multisource phase-controlled radiofrequency treatment and noninsulated microneedle radiofrequency applicator with fractionated pulse mode. The evaluation process was both subjective and objective; I evaluated objectively using three-dimensional color schematic representation with quantitative volume measurements. These three-dimensional results showed significant improvement after the treatments. The post-treatment volume was drastically reduced as compared to the pretreatment volume. Most of the patients reported satisfaction with the improvement of skin laxity. The advantages of these multisource phase-controlled radiofrequency treatments are their long-lasting high efficacy of tightening effects, and the reduction of discomfort and side effects. These characteristics facilitate repeated treatments as well as provide safe and effective treatment of skin tightening.

Keywords: skin tightening, skin laxity, multisource phase-controlled radiofrequency, noninsulated needles, noninvasive fractional radiofrequency, quantitative volume measurement, three-dimensional imaging, wrinkles

1. Introduction

Demand for a noninvasive, effective, and long-lasting treatment to improve laxity has grown dramatically over the past decades as new esthetic technologies have been introduced. Although invasive procedures such as facelifts can achieve skin tightening quickly, they do not rejuvenate the skin and subcutaneous tissues and are accompanied with prolonged downtime and potential adverse effects. Ablative procedures such as traditional skin resurfacing with CO_2 laser devices are also effective for skin tightening, however they are associated with extended recovery time, bleeding, oozing, and risk of post-treatment hyper- or hypopigmentation [1, 2]. In addition, laser treatments can be very problematic for treating darker skin types or sensitive Asian skin.

A major cause of wrinkles and laxity is the reduction in the quantity and quality of collagen fibers in the dermis and hypodermis [3]. Therefore, various devices have been introduced to stimulate collagen production. I previously reported that near-infrared can penetrate deep into human tissue, achieve skin tightening and muscle thinning, and nonthermally induce various responses in the skin and subcutaneous tissues [4–11]. In addition, I previously reported that near-infrared or radiofrequency (RF) treatments stimulate collagen and elastin production while safely and effectively promoting long-lasting skin tightening results that decrease wrinkles and laxity [12, 13].

RF treatments for skin tightening are common, as they heat the dermis and subcutaneous tissues, thereby stimulating dermal collagen remodeling. It is well documented that dermal heating induces an immediate change in collagen structure followed by a long-term stimulation of neocollagenesis [14]. These thermal effects can improve wrinkle appearance, skin laxity and contour of both face and body.

RF has been shown to overcome several disadvantages inherited in optical light-based treatments by offering enhanced tissue penetration that is independent of skin color, and beneficial skin tightening effects. The working principle of RF devices is to heat the dermis and subcutaneous tissues [15], and to induce both collagen remodeling and skin tightening. RF techniques have been proven to be safe and effective for both nonablative skin tightening and fractional RF skin resurfacing [16–18].

The thermal effects of different RF technologies such as monopolar and bipolar RF have been proven to be beneficial in skin tightening. Nevertheless, these effects were frequently partial or unpredictable because of the uncontrolled nature of monopolar or unipolar RF and the superficial nature of energy flow for bipolar, tripolar or multipolar configurations. These first-generation RF systems lack adaptation of delivered power to address the differences in individual skin impedances. Therefore, I have been using a multisource phase–controlled system, which allows continuous real-time measurement of skin impedance and delivers constant adjusted energy to the patient skin, independent of changes in its impedance.

In fractional laser or skin resurfacing treatments, thermally ablated or coagulated microscopic zones from the epidermis to the dermis are spaced in a grid over the skin surface with the nonablated zones in the undamaged surrounding tissue serving as a reservoir of cells that accelerate and promote rapid healing [19]. Same principle is implemented with microneedling, as a healthy tissue reservoir assists to reduce downtime.

The first generation of microneedle RF delivery technology used insulated needles to provide skin rejuvenation and treat acne scars. With insulated RF microneedles, the energy flows only through the tip of the needle, resulting in a small, coagulated sphere-like shape in the dermis. However, insulated RF microneedles can have several disadvantages, including: (i) micro-bleeding during treatment; (ii) the need for several passes at different lengths to affect the entire depth of the dermis [15, 18, 20]; (iii) ineffective for skin laxity.

http://dx.doi.org/10.5772/intechopen.71749

Therefore, in my studies I have been using a tapered, noninsulated microneedle radiofrequency (NIMNRF) applicator with novel fractionated pulse mode. This device achieves cylindrical micro zones of coagulation in the papillary and reticular dermis with minimal damage to the epidermis. The needles are inserted into the skin by a specially designed smooth motion motor that is electronically controlled to minimize patient discomfort. Furthermore, RF emission delivered throughout the whole dermal portion of the needle allows for effective coagulation, resulting in minimal or no bleeding, together with bulk volumetric heating.

RF technology is now considered to be one of the standard options for esthetic treatments, and as such I would like to provide clinical evidence of skin tightening using multisource phase-controlled RF treatment in this chapter. Many previous studies have reported the efficacy of various types of esthetic devices, but these studies have not included sufficient objective evaluations. Conventional evaluations using before and after treatment photographs have been widely used, but they do not provide accurate objective assessment [12, 13, 21]. For quantitative volume measurements, I have used a 3-dimensional photographic system to objectively evaluate the amount of post-treatment volume change in my clinical research.

2. Radiofrequency (RF)

RF is a part of the electromagnetic spectrum. RF can induce thermal effects in the deep tissue, whereas nonablative intense pulse light only reaches the superficial dermis, which is not clinically sufficient to treat laxity (**Figure 1**).

RF has been traditionally used for tissue heating in the field of surgery, especially as a method of coagulation for hemostasis. Tissue heating for skin tightening is achieved through tissue resistance to RF conductivity current (Joule's law). A major cause of wrinkles, laxity and cellulite is the reduction in the quantity and quality of collagen in the dermis and hypodermis. A loss of normal elastic fiber function is a common age-associated feature of both photoaging and intrinsic aging processes. The accelerated aging and sagging of the skin seen in several

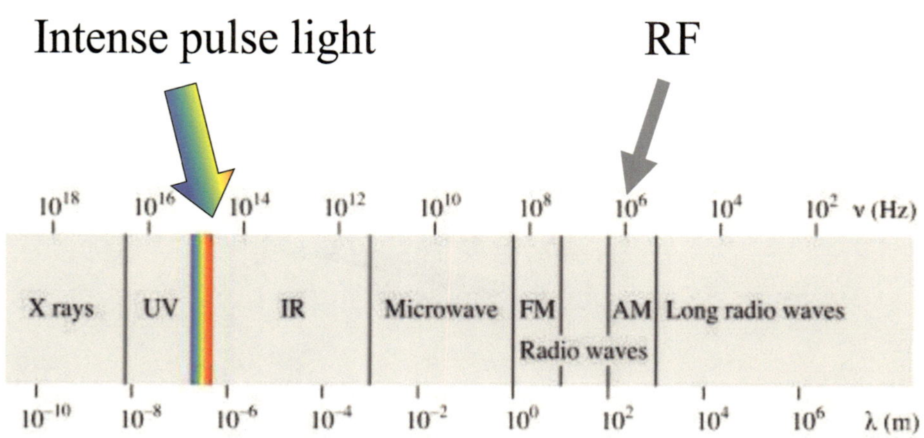

Figure 1. The electromagnetic spectrum covers a wide range of energy radiation types.

hereditary disorders involves collagen or elastin deficiency. RF is considered to be safe and very effective procedure to stimulate production of water-binding proteins, such as collagen and elastin. The effects induced by RF treatment are independent of skin color.

2.1. Monopolar RF

Monopolar RF was the first nonablative RF technology shown to be effective for skin tightening. Although deep penetration could be more effective, the treatment by use of monopolar RF is painful. Due to the uncontrolled RF flow, the treatment is less safe and requires high energy of RF and intense cooling to protect the epidermis (**Figure 2**). Finally, because the device has a disposable tip, cost effectiveness is another important concern.

2.2. Bipolar and multipolar RF

Bipolar and multipolar devices have one RF generator, which connects to two or more electrodes. Because the RF energy delivery is superficial, following the shortest path between the electrodes, the treatment is relatively safe. However, with these devices, RF energy does not penetrate to the required depth and therefore is less efficient for skin tightening (**Figure 3**). Bipolar RF devices require active cooling of electrodes to prevent epidermal burns, whereas multipolar RF devices does not need cooling because the energy is split between two or more

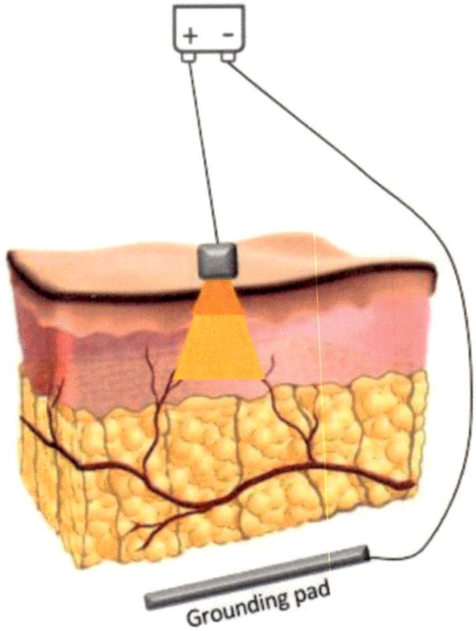

Figure 2. Monopolar RF technologies. One RF generator controls one electrode. Penetration is deeper than bipolar, since there is a flow of energy through the body to the grounding pad. Monopolar RF energy delivery results in high temperature near the electrode, requiring intense epidermal cooling, and uncontrolled energy spreading toward the grounding pad. Monopolar RF may be painful since higher power is required to "push" the RF from the single electrode into the skin.

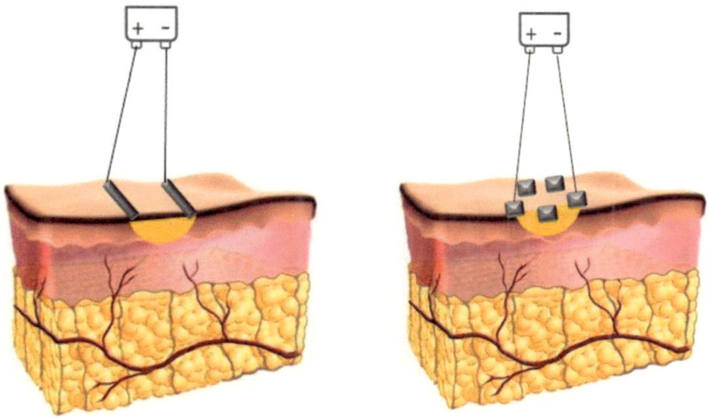

Figure 3. Bipolar RF technologies (left). One RF generator controls two electrodes. There is only superficial penetration since the energy flows along the shortest path, between the two electrodes. It requires active cooling of electrodes to prevent epidermal burns. "Multi-polar" RF Technologies (right). One RF generator controls 3–5 electrodes. There is only superficial penetration since the energy flows along the shortest path, between the 3–5 electrodes (similar to bipolar RF). No cooling is needed because the energy is split between two or more receiving electrodes.

receiving electrodes. Moreover, at any given moment during treatment only a single path is made between two electrodes.

2.3. Multisource phase-controlled RF

The effects induced by monopolar, bipolar, and multipolar RF devices have been frequently partial or unpredictable because of the uncontrolled nature of monopolar or unipolar RF and the superficial nature of energy flow for bipolar, tripolar or multipolar configurations. These first-generation RF systems lack adaptation of delivered power to differences in individual skin impedance.

Due to this lack of efficacy in these traditional RF technologies, I have been using a multisource phase–controlled RF system, which allows continuous real-time measurement of skin impedance and delivers constant energy to the patient skin independent of changes in its impedance. The RF device I have been using is an EndyMed PRO™ 3DEEP treatment platform (EndyMed Medical, Caesarea, Israel), a phase-controlled, multisource RF system that emits at 1 MHz at 1–65 W. This RF device has a unique way to deliver energy to the deep dermis and hypodermis while minimizing epidermal heating. It has six phase-controlled RF generators, allowing a complex 3D interaction between the electromagnetic fields produced in the tissue. The inner electrodes current acts as a potential barrier, which forces the next set of electrode current to penetrate deep below, and so on, creating a 3DEEP energy complex. In addition, due to the repulsion of electrical fields with the same polarity, no current is created between these electrodes on the skin surface, allowing minimal epidermal flow (**Figures 4** and **5**).

I typically perform treatments using approximately 33 W output, which is low enough that the sensation of excessive heat would not be felt. If the patient reports a strong sensation of heat, treatment movement can be performed slightly faster and/or the handpiece head can be

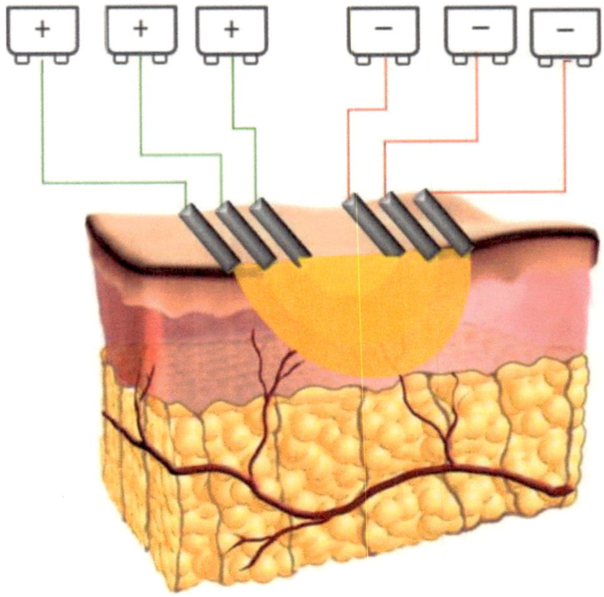

Figure 4. Multisource phase-controlled, RF system. This system can deliver RF energy to deep layers of the skin. Focused & contained deep energy flow. Minimal surface energy flow eliminates the need for intense cooling. Totally safe & painless. Personalized parameters based on multiple unique automatic skin sensing feedback mechanisms.

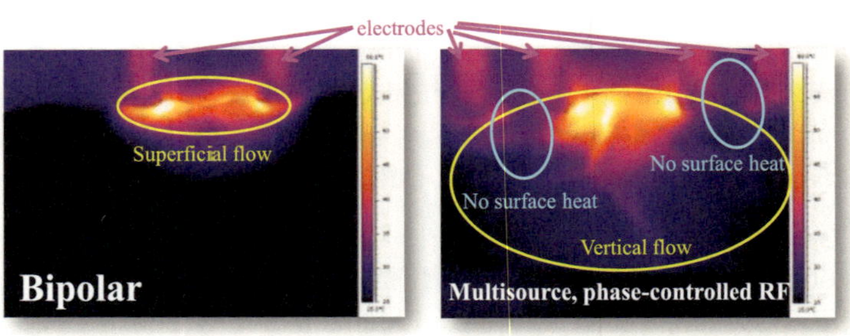

Figure 5. Comparison of bipolar vs. multisource phase-controlled RF system. With bipolar device (300 W, 1 s), superficial flow of energy, penetrates only to 1.5 mm depth. Multisource phase-controlled RF system (4 electrode, 2 × 150 W, 1 s) shows vertical flow of energy, penetrates to 6 mm depth. Absolutely no surface heat between the external electrodes. The surface flow is only between the two middle electrodes.

moved slightly away from the point of heat sensation. No topical anesthetics or oral analgesics are needed before, during, or after the treatment, and skin cooling is not required.

2.4. Noninsulated microneedle RF

I have been using the tapered noninsulated microneedle radiofrequency (NIMNRF) applicator operating with a novel fractionated pulse mode (Intensif Handpiece, EndyMed Medical,

http://dx.doi.org/10.5772/intechopen.71749

Caesarea, Israel) for tightening and acne scar treatments (**Figures 6** and **7**) [22–25]. The system platform (1MHZ) incorporates six independent phase controlled RF generators that allow the RF microneedles to induce skin remodeling through controlled dermal coagulation. The needle penetration depth is up to 3.5 mm in digitally controlled increments of 0.1 mm. The power is adjustable from 0 to 25 W with increments of 1 W. The pulse duration can be changed in 30 ms increments (maximal pulse duration is 200 ms) [15].

Thermography during a laboratory model simulation taken by a thermal camera (FLIR SC640, FLIR, Boston, MA, USA) using a laboratory skin model with an impedance that is similar to that of the human dermis. The penetration depth is 2.5 mm. The temperatures shown in this figure are relatively low because this is a laboratory model simulation wherein low power RF was used to obtain qualitative imaging. In vivo temperatures would be higher than those of a laboratory model simulation, as demonstrated by histology and coagulative effects on capillaries. Patients undergoing Intensif treatment received from 500 to 1000 pulses with the following parameters: pulse duration 80–110 ms, power 10–14 W and 1.5–2.5 mm penetration depth.

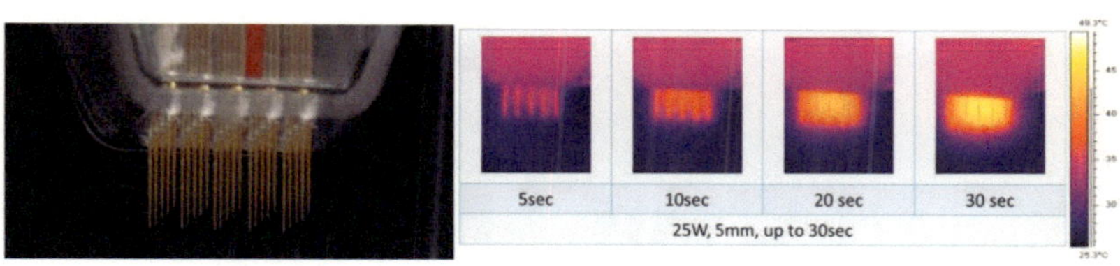

Figure 6. FDA-cleared, very sharply tapered noninsulated gold plated microneedle RF applicator operating with a novel fractionated pulse mode (above). Sterilized treatment tip with 25 microneedles (300 micron diameter at the base that gradually tapers to an especially sharp edge. Microneedles are inserted into the skin by a specially designed smooth motion motor that is electronically controlled to minimize patient discomfort (below).

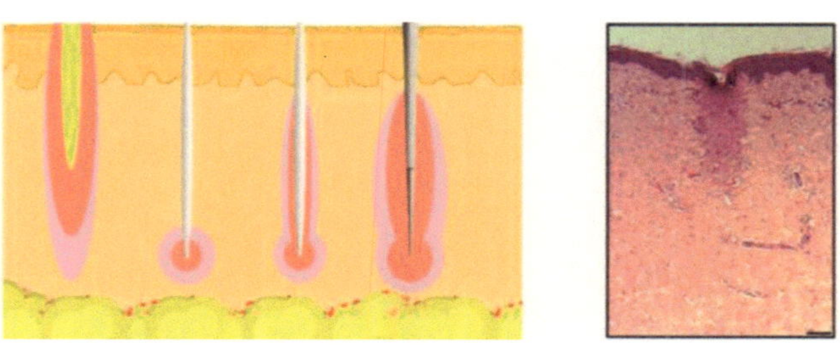

Figure 7. A heat schematic of fractional lasers and microneedles. Images from left to right show fractional lasers, insulated needles, noninsulated needles, and very sharply tapered noninsulated gold plated microneedles. (left). RF emission delivered over the whole dermal portion of the needle allows effective coagulation resulting in minimal or no bleeding, together with bulk volumetric heating. Histology of in vivo pig skin (right). This biopsy was taken immediately after treatment. The protocol was approved by the institutional ethics committee. H & E staining show dermal coagulation that matches the needle penetration depth. The parameters are 15 W, 140 ms, 2.5 mm. Scale bar = 500 μm. Cited from **Figure 7** (Ref. [22]).

3. Clinical results after RF treatments

3.1. Clinical study results after multisource phase-controlled RF treatments: "Objective Assessment of Skin Tightening Using Multisource, Phase-Controlled Radiofrequency in Asians"

Twenty Japanese patients (18 females and 2 males) aged 26–69 years (mean age, 42.4 ± 9.92 years) with Fitzpatrick skin type III to V were enrolled.

None of the subjects had a history of any type of skin disease or any cosmetic procedures affecting the treatment areas within the last 3 years. No topical pretreatment was used, and the post-treatment skin care regimen consisted of a gentle cleanser and sunblock. All patients gave written informed consent for participation in the study after reading the experimental protocol and being advised about the risks of treatments.

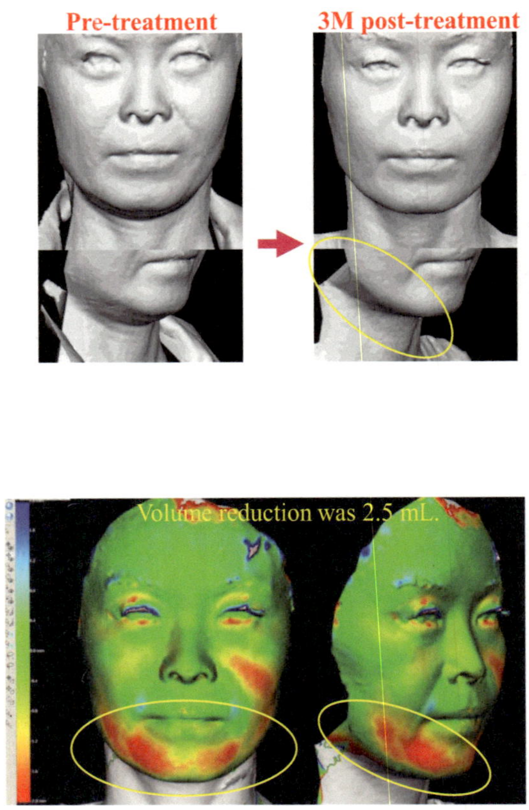

Figure 8. Representative photographs of tightening effects treated with multisource phase-controlled RF treatments. Pretreatment (above, left), a 44-year-old Japanese woman exhibited skin laxity in cheek, mental portion, and neck, and wrinkles such as nasolabial fold. Cheek and neck were treated. Three treatments at 33 W. Three months post-treatment (above, right), significant improvements were noted in both skin laxity and wrinkles. Three-dimensional color schematic representation shows the varying degrees of tightening achieved in colors yellow to red (below). Green areas remain unchanged. These images indicate significant improvement of appearance, skin laxity, and wrinkles after multisource phase-controlled RF treatments.

http://dx.doi.org/10.5772/intechopen.71749

3.1.1. *Evaluation by gray scale images and 3-dimensional imaging with quantitative volume measurements*

Objective assessments, evaluated by gray scale images and 3-dimensional color schematic representation with quantitative volume measurements, showed significant improvement after the multisource phase-controlled RF treatment (**Figures 8-10**).

3.1.2. *Histological assessments*

Human skin specimens from the face (3–5 from each patient) were obtained for microscopic investigation. Biopsies were taken pretreatment as a control and at 2 month after the final treatment. The specimens were fixed in 20% neutral buffered formalin, processed for paraffin embedding and serially sectioned along the sagittal plane (3–4 μm thickness). Tissue sections were stained by Victoria Blue staining (**Figure 11**). Elastin densities stained by Victoria Blue

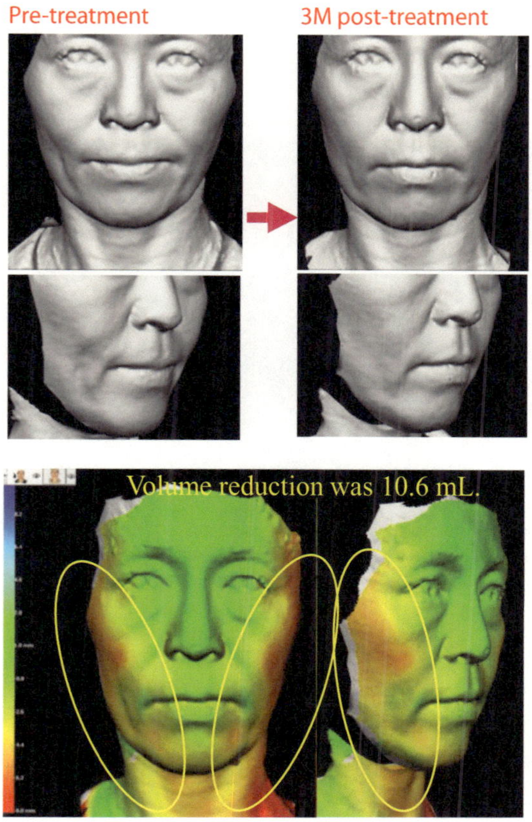

Figure 9. Representative photographs of tightening effects treated with multisource phase-controlled RF treatment. Pretreatment (above, left), a 50-year-old Japanese woman exhibited skin laxity in cheek, mental portion, and neck, and wrinkles such as nasolabial fold. Cheek and neck were treated. Three treatments at 33 W. Three months post-treatment (above, right), significant improvements were noted in both skin laxity and wrinkles. Three-dimensional color schematic representation shows the varying degrees of tightening achieved in colors yellow to red (below). Green areas remain unchanged. These images indicate significant improvement of appearance, skin laxity, and wrinkles after multisource phase-controlled RF treatments.

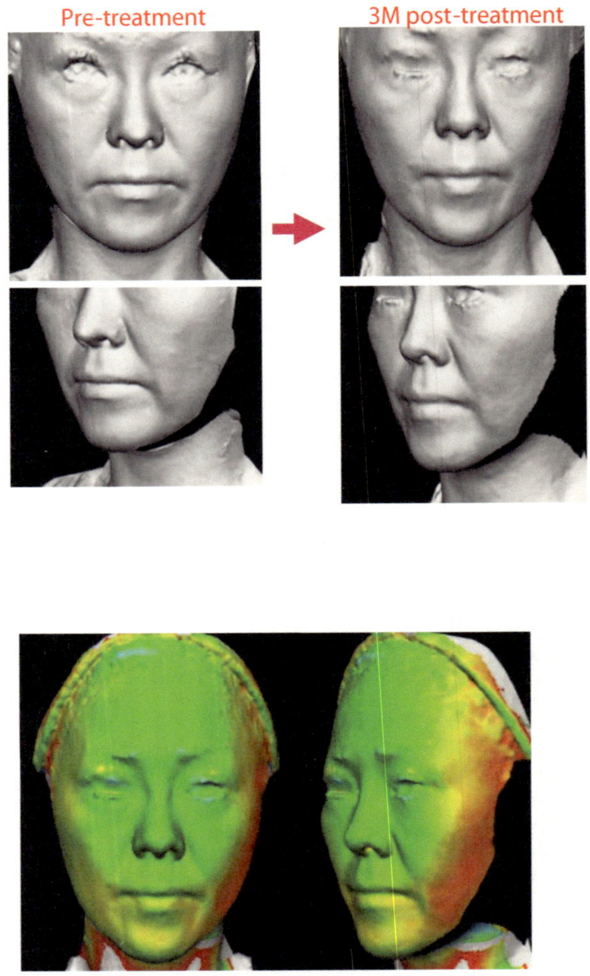

Figure 10. Representative photographs of tightening effects treated with multisource phase-controlled RF treatment. Pretreatment (left), a 43-year-old Japanese woman exhibited skin laxity in cheek, mental portion, and neck, and wrinkles such as nasolabial fold. Cheek and neck were treated. Three treatments at 33 W only to patient's left cheek. Three months post-treatment (right), significant improvements were noted in both skin laxity and wrinkles. Three-dimensional color schematic representation shows the varying degrees of tightening achieved in colors yellow to red (below). These images indicate significant improvement of appearance, skin laxity, and wrinkles after multisource phase-controlled RF treatments.

staining in the dermis were calculated after an optimized color threshold was applied to each image to distinguish between the stained areas and background. Images were scanned and quantified in five representative fields per section, and subsequently averaged to obtain a final score (**Figure 12**). The sections were photographed under an Olympus BX50 microscope (Olympus, Tokyo, Japan). The digital photographs were processed using Adobe Photoshop (Adobe, San Jose, CA, USA).

Cited from **Figure 4**. (Ref. [13]).

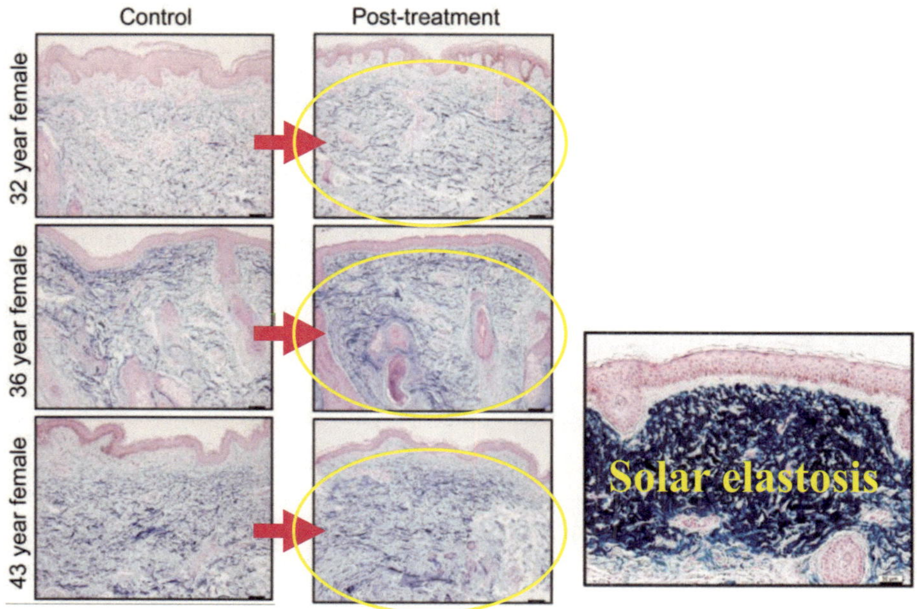

Figure 11. A representative histology of Japanese patients' cheek skin evaluated by Victoria blue staining. The amount of elastin stained in blue significantly increased post-treatment compared with control. Scale bars = 100 μm. Histological studies showed that the amount of elastin was significantly increased after the multisource phase-controlled RF treatment compared with controls in all five Japanese patients. Induced elastin appeared to be relatively fine and delicate, compared with irregular elastic fibers, such as solar elastosis.

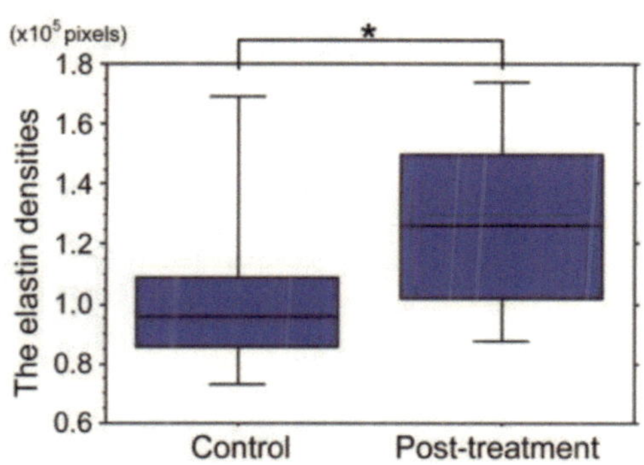

Figure 12. Mean densities of elastin in the dermis. Skin biopsies were taken from five Japanese female patients who had visited the Clinica Tanaka Anti-Aging Center to remove some pigmented nevi (more than one pigmented nevus on both control and treated side of the cheek) and achieve skin rejuvenation on their faces. The densities of elastin were significantly increased compared with controls (p = 0.0013). Data represents the means ± SD. Significant differences compared with control are indicated (*$p < .05$).

3.2. Clinical study results after RF microneedle treatments: "Long-term Nasal and Perioral Tightening by a Single Fractional Noninsulated Microneedle Radiofrequency Treatment"

Fifteen Asian patients (14 females and 1 male) aged 31–66 years (mean age, 43.4 ± 9.0 years) with Fitzpatrick skin type III-V were enrolled. All of the patients had visited the Clinica Tanaka Anti-Aging Center to achieve full facial skin tightening. None of the patients had a history of any type of skin disease or cosmetic procedure that affected the treatment areas. Topical anesthetic cream was applied to the patient's skin for 60 min before the treatment. The post-treatment skin care regimen consisted of a gentle cleanser and sunblock. Patients did not use any specific skin care products and had no specific diet. Patients who exhibited weight loss during the study period were excluded from volumetric measurement analyses because changes in diet and/or exercise may affect volumetric changes. After reading the experimental protocol and being advised of the treatment risks, all patients gave written informed consent for participation.

3.2.1. Evaluation by gray scale images and 3-dimensional imaging with quantitative volume measurements

Objective assessments evaluated with a superimposed 3-D color schematic representation showed long-lasting and significant volumetric reduction after the treatment. Representative 2-D color, and superimposed 3-D color images and volumetric reductions are shown in **Figures 13-16**.

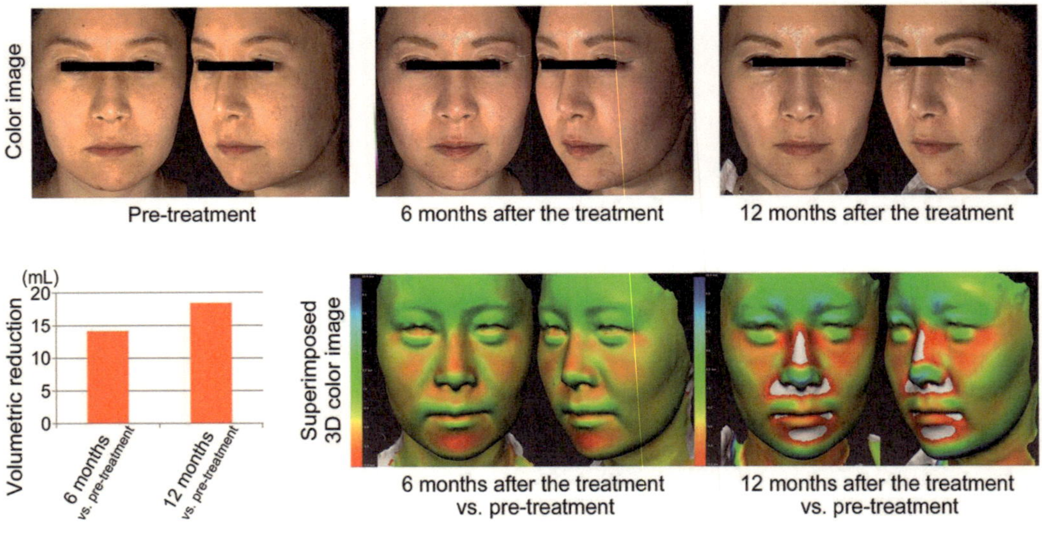

Figure 13. A 31-year-old female. Cheek mode: Pulse width; 110 ms, 14 W, 2.5 mm, 200 shots + Periorbital mode: 80 m, 10 W, 1.5 mm, 100 shots. Images from left to right show the appearance pretreatment to 12 months after the treatment. Improvement of skin texture and dilated skin pores was observed after treatment with time (above). Volumetric reduction (ml) at 6 and 12 months follow up point relative to the pretreatment volume (below, left). Superimposed 3-D color images that show the volumetric change distribution 6 and 12 months after the treatment compared to pretreatment (below, right). The varying degrees of tightening are artificially colored and range from yellow to red (red, −5 mm change). Green areas indicated no changes to the face, and gray areas indicate changes over −5 mm. Significant volumetric reduction in the nasal and perioral areas was observed. Cited from **Figure 1** (Ref. [25]).

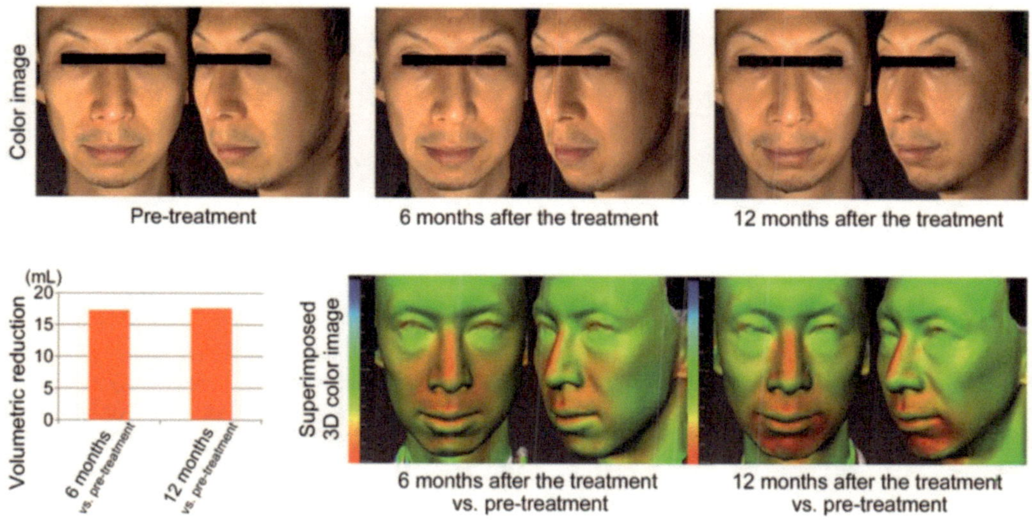

Figure 14. A 40-year-old male. Cheek mode: Pulse width; 110 ms, 14 W, 2.5 mm, 300 shots + Periorbital mode: 80 ms, 10 W, 1.5 mm, 200 shots. Images from left to right show the appearance pretreatment to 12 months after the treatment. Improvement of skin texture and dilated skin pores was observed after treatment with time (above). Volumetric reduction (ml) at 6 and 12 months follow up point relative to the pretreatment volume (below, left). Superimposed 3-D color images that show the volumetric change distribution 6 and 12 months after the treatment compared to pretreatment (below, right). The varying degrees of tightening are artificially colored and range from yellow to red (red, −5 mm change). Green areas indicated no changes to the face, and gray areas indicate changes over −5 mm. Significant volumetric reduction in the nasal and perioral areas was observed. Cited from **Figure 2** (Ref. [25]).

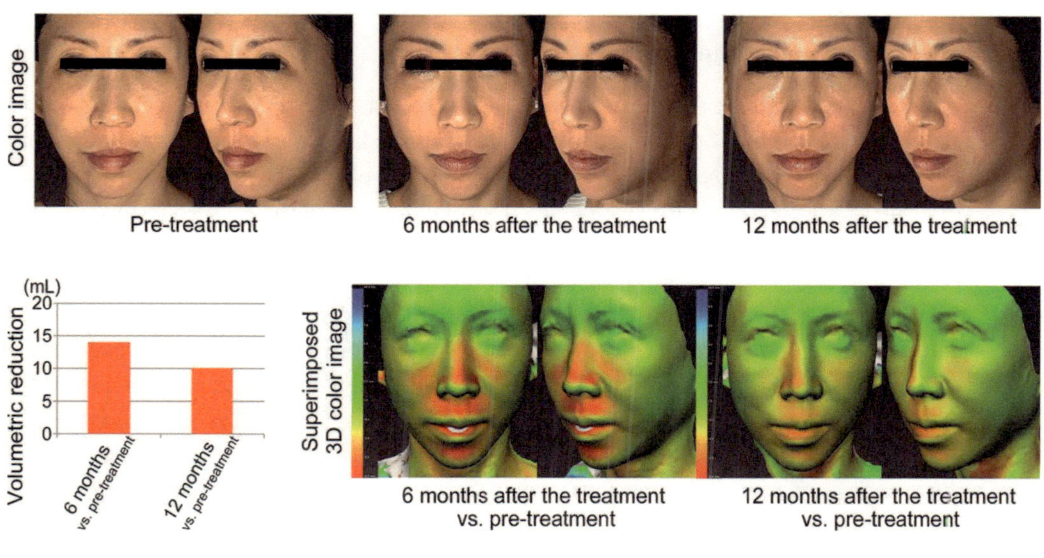

Figure 15. A 47-year-old male. Cheek mode: Pulse width; 110 ms, 14 W, 2.5 mm, 300 shots + Periorbital mode: 80 ms, 10 W, 1.5 mm, 200 shots. Images from left to right show the appearance pretreatment to 12 months after the treatment. Improvement of skin texture and dilated skin pores was observed after treatment with time (above). Volumetric reduction (ml) at 6 and 12 months follow up point relative to the pretreatment volume (below, left). Superimposed 3-D color images that show the volumetric change distribution 6 and 12 months after the treatment compared to pretreatment (below, right). The varying degrees of tightening are artificially colored and range from yellow to red (red, −5 mm change). Green areas indicated no changes to the face, and gray areas indicate changes over −5 mm. Significant volumetric reduction in the nasal and perioral areas was observed. Cited from **Figure 3** (Ref. [25]).

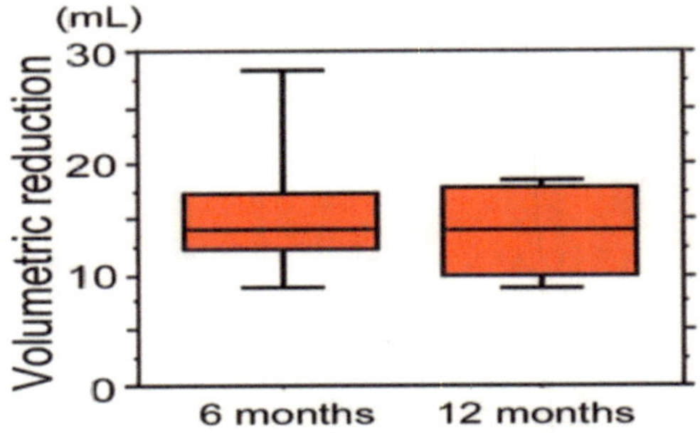

Figure 16. Median volumetric reductions at 6 and 12 months post-treatment were 14.1 and 13.8 ml, respectively. Significant volumetric reductions were observed at 6 and 12 months post-treatment compared with pretreatment ($p = 0.0033$). In contrast, statistical significance was not observed between 6 and 12 months post-treatment ($p = 0.3281$). Post-treatment volumes were significantly reduced compared with pretreatment volumes in all patients. The tightening effects appeared to be stable from 6 to 12 months post-treatment. Cited from **Figure 5** (Ref. [25]).

4. Discussion

4.1. Multisource phase-controlled RF treatments

Objective assessments of skin laxity showed significant improvements, and most patients were satisfied with the results after multisource phase-controlled radiofrequency RF treatments. The advantages of the multisource RF treatments are the reduction in discomfort and side effects. The results indicate that multisource phase-controlled radiofrequency RF treatments provide safe and effective long-term stimulation of elastin, which is beneficial for skin rejuvenation by improving skin laxity and wrinkles.

A multisource phase-controlled radiofrequency RF treatments system was used in this study, which allows continuous real-time measurement of skin impedance and the delivery of constant energy to the patient skin, independent of changes in its impedance. By using this multisource phase-controlled radiofrequency RF system, less thermal damage of the dermis and subcutaneous tissues occurred compared to monopolar or unipolar RF treatments. Multisource phase-controlled radiofrequency RF technology is based on the fact that due to the use of six RF generators, the energy flow on the skin surface is minimal, since all the energy is directed to the depth of the tissue. This is achieved by repulsion between electrical field of the same polarity on each side of the handpiece electrodes [14]. Since multisource phase-controlled radiofrequency RF handpiece delivers energy in constant circulatory motion, the effect will be an average lower temperature on the epidermis (<42°C) and higher temperature in the lower skin layers, without the need for cooling. This technology allows the system to keep epidermal temperature bellow 42°C while reaching up to 57°C in the depth of the tissue 14.

Furthermore, most of the patients did not report feeling pain during the treatment, even though it was performed without anesthesia and contact cooling. A 33 W output was used, which was low enough so that the sensation of heat was not felt. According to peer-reviewed papers, even higher energies used with EndyMed systems were well tolerated by patients without any adverse events.

Side effects, such as epidermal burns, adipose tissue atrophy, and contraction, were not observed, and the patients felt comfortable during multisource phase-controlled radiofrequency RF treatment.

4.2. RF microneedle treatments

The results obtained by RF microneedle treatments appear to be significant even though patients were only treated once. This significant efficacy can be explained by three specific features of the tested RF microneedle device. First, this procedure produced deeper skin penetration of the microneedles (up to 3.5 mm) relative to fractional lasers that usually have a penetration of no more than 1.6 mm. Electronically controlled penetration allows exact monitoring of the penetration depth, which can be customized for different treatment areas. Second, the gold plated noninsulated needles have a smooth insertion that provides a significant advantage over first generation insulated and stainless steel needles. The clinical efficacy of insulated needles is limited due to the small volume of heat produced by RF emission only at the noninsulated area near the tip and significant micro-bleeding induced by the treatment. In contrast, the noninsulated gold plated needles used here emit RF throughout the whole length, thus allowing heating of three times the volume [26]. After the needle is inserted to its maximal depth, due to the lower impedance in the dermis relative to the epidermis, the RF will flow through the dermis with no epidermal coagulation and thus there is no need for needle insulation.

Third, smooth insertion of the needle by an electronically controlled motor that was used in the system tested here resulted in minimal patient pain and downtime while also minimizing trauma to the epidermis and bleeding. Other technologies that use fixed needles, which are inserted by hand or by a spring mechanism, are frequently more damaging to the epidermis and may increase the incidence of post-treatment hyperpigmentation [26].

Most of the patients in this study reported no severe pain during the treatment, even though it was performed without oral or intravenous anesthesia and contact cooling. This reduction in reported pain seen for the fractional RF microneedle treatment may be related to the sharpness of the needles and the unique motorized needle insertion.

Post-treatment complications include burning sensation and mild erythema, but these were minor and lasted less than 5 hours. Furthermore, PIH, epidermal burns and scar formation were not observed.

Nonthermal epidermis penetration performed with a tapered microneedle inserted by smooth motion is less traumatic to the epidermis and epidermal-dermal junction, and in turn decreases the likelihood of extended post-treatment erythema and PIH as compared to ablative and nonablative lasers or other manual or fixed microneedle RF systems. In addition, RF emission through the length of the needle provides for shorter treatment times and a coagulation effect that eliminate micro-bleeding and improve the patient experience [22–26]. Digital control of the needle penetration depth with automatic motorized insertion improves the patient experience by reducing discomfort and side effects [22–26].

5. Conclusions

Significant improvements in skin laxity were observed through objective and histological assessments after receiving EndyMed 3DEEP RF treatments. The results indicate that these RF treatments provide safe and effective stimulation of elastin, which is beneficial for skin rejuvenation by improving skin laxity and rhytids. The advantages of EndyMed RF treatments are long-lasting high efficacy with minimal downtime or side effects. Furthermore, EndyMed RF treatments are convenient for patients and require almost no downtime. Because of these advantages, it will be easily accepted by even socially active individuals regardless of age or sex.

Author details

Yohei Tanaka

Address all correspondence to: info@clinicatanaka.jp

Clinica Tanaka Plastic and Reconstructive Surgery and Anti-aging Center, Nagano, Japan

References

[1] Bernstein LJ, Kauvar AN, Grossman MC, Geronemus RG. The short- and long-term side effects of carbon dioxide laser resurfacing. Dermatologic Surgery. 1997;**23**:519-525

[2] Nanni CA, Alster TS. Complications of carbon dioxide laser resurfacing. An evaluation of 500 patients. Dermatologic Surgery. 1998;**24**:315-320

[3] Elman M, Harth Y. Novel multi-source phase-controlled radiofrequency technology for nonablative and micro-ablative treatment of wrinkles, lax skin, and acne scars. Laser Therapy. 2011;**20**:139-144

[4] Tanaka Y, Matsuo K. Non-thermal effects of near-infrared irradiation on melanoma. In: Tanaka Y, editor. Breakthroughs in Melanoma Research. Croatia: InTech; 2011. p. 597-628. ISBN: 978-953-307-291-3. Available from: http://www.intechopen.com/books/breakthroughs-in-melanoma-research

[5] Tanaka Y, Tatewaki N, Nishida H, Eitsuka T, Ikekawa N, Nakayama J. Non-thermal DNA damage of cancer cells using near-infrared irradiation. Cancer Science. 2012;**103**:1467-1473

[6] Tanaka Y. The impact of near-infrared radiation in dermatology. Review. World Journal of Dermatology. 2012;**1**:30-37

[7] Tanaka Y, Tsunemi Y, Kawashima M, Nishida H, Tatewaki N. Objective assessment of skin tightening using water-filtered near-infrared (1000–1800 nm) device with a contact cooling and freezer stored gel in Asians. Clinical, Cosmetic and Investigational Dermatology. 2013;**6**:167-176

[8] Tanaka Y, Gale L. Beneficial applications and deleterious effects of near-infrared from biological and medical perspectives. Optics and Photonics Journal. 2013;**3**:31-39

[9] Tanaka Y, Nakayama J. Up-regulated epidermal growth factor receptor expression following near-infrared irradiation simulating solar radiation in a 3-dimensional reconstructed human corneal epithelial tissue culture model. Clinical Interventions in Aging. 2016;**11**:1027-1033

[10] Tanaka Y, Nakayama J. Up-regulated expression of La ribonucleoprotein domain family member 6 and collagen type I gene following water-filtered broad-spectrum near-infrared irradiation in a 3-dimensional human epidermal tissue culture model as revealed by microarray analysis. Australasian Journal of Dermatology. 2016 In Press

[11] Calderhead G, Tanaka Y. Photobiological basics and clinical indications of phototherapy for skin rejuvenation. In: Photomedicine: Advances in Clinical Practice. Croatia: InTech; 2017. p. 215-252. Available from: https://www.intechopen.com/books/photomedicine-advances-in-clinical-practice

[12] Tanaka Y. Objective assessment of skin tightening using multisource, phase-controlled radiofrequency in Asians. Journal of Cosmetics, Dermatological Sciences and Applications. 2013;**3**:110-116

[13] Tanaka Y, Tsunemi Y, Kawashima M, Tatewaki N, Nishida H. Treatment of skin laxity using multisource, phasecontrolled radiofrequency in Asians: Visualized three-dimensional skin tightening results and increase in elastin density shown through histological investigation. Dermatologic Surgery. 2014;**40**:756-762

[14] Sadick NS, Sato M, Palmisano D, Frank I, Cohen H, Harth Y. In vivo animal histology and clinical evaluation of multisource fractional radiofrequency skin resurfacing (FSR) applicator. Journal of Cosmetic and Laser Therapy. 2011;**13**:204-209

[15] Harth Y, Frank I. In vivo histological evaluation of non-insulated microneedle radiofrequency applicator with novel fractionated pulse mode. Journal of Drugs in Dermatology. 2013;**12**:1430-1433

[16] Ong MW, Bashir SJ. Fractional laser resurfacing for acne scars: A review. The British Journal of Dermatology. 2012;**166**:1160-1169

[17] De la Torre JR, Moreno-Moraga J, Muñoz E, Navarro PC. Multisource, phase-controlled radiofrequency for treatment of skin laxity: Correlation between clinical and in-vivo confocal microscopy results and real-time thermal changes. The Journal of Clinical and Aesthetic Dermatology. 2011;**4**:28-35

[18] Elman M, Vider I, Harth Y, Gottfried V, Shemer A. Non invasive therapy of wrinkles, lax skin using a novel multisource phase controlled radiofrequency system. Journal of Cosmetic and Laser Therapy. 2010;**12**:81-86

[19] Clementoni MT, Gilardino P, Muti GF, Beretta D, Schianchi R. Non-sequential fractional ultrapulsed CO_2 resurfacing of photo aged facial skin: Preliminary clinical report. Journal of Cosmetic and Laser Therapy. 2007;**9**:218-225

[20] Cho SI, Chung BY, Choi MG, Baek JH, Cho HJ, Park CW, Lee CH, Kim HO. Evaluation of the clinical efficacy of fractional radiofrequency microneedle treatment in acne scars and large facial pores. Dermatologic Surgery. 2012;**38**:1017-1024

[21] Tanaka Y. Three-dimensional volumetric assessment of body sculpting using a uniform heating radio frequency device in Asians. Journal of Cosmetic and Laser Therapy. 2015; **17**(4):194-199

[22] Tanaka Y. Long-term three-dimensional volumetric assessment of skin tightening using a sharply tapered non-insulated microneedle radiofrequency applicator with novel fractionated pulse mode in Asians. Lasers in Surgery and Medicine. 2015;**47**(8):626-633

[23] Tanaka Y. Long-term skin tightening effects of a sharply tapered non-insulated microneedle radiofrequency applicator with novel fractionated pulse mode shown through three-dimensional volumetric assessment. Australasian Journal of Dermatology. 2016;**57**(1):78

[24] Gold M, Taylor M, Rothaus K, Tanaka Y. Non-insulated smooth motion, micro-needles RF fractional treatment for wrinkle reduction and lifting of the lower face: International study. Lasers in Surgery and Medicine. 2016;**48**(8):727-733

[25] Tanaka Y. Long-term nasal and peri-oral tightening by a single fractional non-insulated microneedle radiofrequency treatment. The Journal of Clinical and Aesthetic Dermatology. 2017;**10**(2):45-51

[26] Harth Y, Elman M, Ackerman E, Frank I. Depressed acne scars- effective, minimal downtime treatment with a novel smooth motion non-insulated microneedle radiofrequency technology. Journal of Cosmetics,Dermatological Sciences and Applications. 2014;**4**:212-218

Chapter 10

The Wonder Tool Platelet Rich Plasma in Cosmetic Dermatology, Trichology and Hair Transplant

Garg Suruchi, Manchanda Shweta and Garg Chandi

Additional information is available at the end of the chapter

http://dx.doi.org/10.5772/intechopen.70287

Abstract

Platelet-rich plasma or PRP therapy is a form of regenerative medicine where body's own cells, tissues or organs can be utilized by replacing, regenerating or engineering to restore or establish normal function. Various published articles demonstrating the role of PRP therapy in cosmetic procedures like scar revision, facial rejuvenation, stretch mark removal, androgenetic alopecia, alopecia areata and hair transplant were analyzed in depth to understand its efficacy based on facts and figures along with inputs from personal experience. PRP therapy is one of the most upcoming forms of regenerative medicine with the potential to improve the homeostasis of the treated cells and tissues, provided that harvesting standards are maintained.

Keywords: platelet-rich plasma, wound healing, platelet growth factors, vampire facelift, scar revision, hair transplant, hair fall

1. Introduction

Platelet-rich plasma or PRP therapy is a form of regenerative medicine where body's own cells, tissues or organs can be utilized by replacing, regenerating or engineering to restore or establish normal function. While the role of PRP therapy is already established in sports injuries, dental and oral surgery and pain relief, it also comes as a promising option in various procedures in cosmetic dermatology, trichology and more recently hair transplant.

2. Main body of the paper

Synonyms: Autologous platelet gel, plasma-rich growth factors, platelet-concentrated plasma, platelet-rich concentrate, platelet releasate [1, 2].

Definition: Platelet-rich plasma is volume of the plasma fraction of autologous blood with an above baseline platelet concentration (usually more than 1,000,000 platelets/μl), leading to 300–700% enrichment [3, 4].

3. What is PRP?

Whole blood consists of 93% red blood cells, 6% platelets and 1% white blood cells. In PRP, the proportion of these cells in blood is inverted, that is, the red cell layer is reduced to 5% and platelets and leucocytes are increased to about 94% to stimulate tissue regeneration [5].

The cellular response to injury occurs in four stages: hemostasis, inflammation, proliferation and remodeling. In each phase, there is an enhanced cellular or molecular activity involving the platelets. Platelets and plasma are responsible for hemostasis, leucocytes and activated platelets mediate the inflammation, and growth factors derived from platelet alpha granules influence regeneration of tissues. Leucocyte content of PRP influences the inflammatory process, and angiogenic and mitogenic growth factors aid tissue regeneration [6].

Various growth factors are secreted from the α-granules of concentrated platelets activated by aggregation inducers [3]. These factors are known to regulate processes of cell migration, attachment, proliferation and differentiation and promote extracellular matrix (ECM) accumulation by binding to specific cell surface receptors [7].

Regenerative potential of PRP depends on the levels of released growth factors (GFs). PRP contains more than 20 GFs and other proteins, such as adhesion molecules, chemokines, etc., which interact, leading to inflammation, cell proliferation, differentiation and regeneration [3].

Activation of the platelets causes degranulation, leading to transformation of secretory proteins (e.g., Platelet derived growth factor (PDGF), Transforming growth factor-β (TGF-β) etc.) to a bioactive state by the addition of histones and carbohydrate side chains. Then, active proteins are secreted, which bind to transmembrane receptors of target cells, including mesenchymal stem cells, osteoblasts, fibroblasts, endothelial cells and epidermal cells. The agonist bound transmembrane receptors then activate an intracellular signal protein, leading to expression of a gene sequence which directs cellular proliferation, formation of matrix, collagen synthesis, etc., thereby provoking tissue repair and tissue regeneration (**Table 1**) [8].

The mean blood platelet level is approximately 200,000 ± 75,000/μl. Platelet concentration of more than 1 million/μl (about four to seven times the mean levels) is regarded as concentration of PRP that is therapeutically effective. A bell-shaped response curve which indicates a dose-dependent nature is associated with PRP. Lower or higher concentrations than 1.5 million platelets/μl inhibit the angiogenic potential in human endothelial cells. In vitro studies on dermal papilla cells also support that PRP should be used at the concentrations of 5–10 times the mean levels [2].

http://dx.doi.org/10.5772/intechopen.70287

Platelet growth factor	Biological actions
PDGF αα,αβ,ββ	Mitogenic factor for mesenchymal cells, proliferation of fibroblasts/smooth muscle cells, secretion of collagenase and synthesis of collagen, macrophage proliferation and chemotaxis of neutrophils
TGF (alpha-beta)	Stimulates mesenchymal cells proliferation; regulates mitogenesis of endothelial cells and fibroblasts; secretion of collagenase and synthesis of collagen, regulates mitogenic effects of other growth factors, stimulates angiogenesis, inhibition of proliferation of macrophage and lymphocyte
VEGF	Stimulates angiogenesis, increases vessel permeability and stimulates mitogenesis of endothelial cells
EGF	Stimulates angiogenesis, regulates secretion of collagenase and stimulates epithelial and mesenchymal mitogenesis
FGF	Promotion of growth and differentiation of fibroblasts and mesenchymal cells
CTGF	Promotes neoangiogenesis, regeneration of cartilage, fibrosis and platelet adhesion
IGF-1	Chemotactic for fibroblasts stimulates protein synthesis, in combination with PDGF, and enhances rate and quality of wound healing
HGF	Mediates regeneration
FGF-9	Aids generation of new follicles

Table 1. Growth factors present in alpha granules of platelets and their biological actions [2, 36, 37].

The platelets actively secrete growth factors within 10 min after activation, and more than 95% of the presynthesized growth factors are secreted within 1 h [8].

Therefore, PRP should be used within 10 min of activation. The viability of the concentrated platelets remains for up to 8 h, and it stays sterile if placed on a sterile surgical table [2].

The platelets remain viable for 7–10 days and continue releasing the growth factors in tissue during this period [6].

4. Method

Centrifugation separates the blood components, depending on their specific gravities, that is, RBCs are the heaviest, followed by WBCs, whereas platelets are the lightest. The first centrifugation is slow, so that the spinning down of platelets is avoided and isolation of plasma occurs easily. Platelets are mostly concentrated right on the top of buffy coat layer. Subsequent centrifugation is faster, so that platelets are spun down, leading to separation as a pellet at the bottom of the tube from the platelet-poor plasma (PPP) above. The final concentration of platelets depends on volume reduction of the PPP. About three-fourth of the supernatant is discarded, and the platelet-rich pellet is resuspended in rest of the plasma. The suspension formed is used as PRP. Double-spin method is preferred over the single-spin method, as the therapeutic concentration of platelets is not achieved by using the latter [2].

4.1. Manual method

4.1.1. PRP method

1. Whole blood is collected by venipuncture in acid citrate dextrose (ACD) tubes [8].
2. Blood is not chilled at any time before or during platelet separation.
3. Blood is centrifuged using a 'soft' spin.
4. Supernatant plasma containing platelets is transferred into another sterile tube (without anticoagulant).
5. Centrifuge the second tube at a higher speed (hard spin) to get a platelet concentrate.
6. The lower one-third is PRP, and upper two-thirds are called platelet-poor plasma. Platelet pellets are formed at the bottom of the tube.
7. PPP is removed, and the platelet pellet is suspended in a minimum quantity of plasma (2–4 ml) by gently shaking the tube.

4.1.2. Buffy coat method

1. Whole blood is stored at 20–24°C before centrifugation.
2. After storage, blood is centrifuged at a 'high' speed.
3. Three layers are formed because of the density: The bottom layer consists of RBCs, the middle layer consists of platelets and WBCs and the top is PPP layer.
4. Supernatant plasma is removed from the top of the container.
5. The buffy-coat layer is transferred to another sterile tube.

4.1.3. Automated method

There are various automated devices and kits available in the market.

4.1.4. Our experience

We use YCell Bio kit and REMI centrifuge for preparation of PRP.2 Vials, each containing 13.5 ml of whole blood mixed with 1.5 ml of ACD-A solution and centrifuged for 4 min at 3000 RPM. A total of 5–6 ml of buffy coat along with PRP is harvested from these two vials and injected as required. It gives five to seven times concentration of the baseline platelet count.

5. Classification

Ehrenfest et al. proposed a classification in 2009 according to which platelet concentrates can be classified into four main families depending on their cell content and fibrin architecture [9].

1. Pure platelet-rich plasma (P-PRP) or leucocyte-poor platelet-rich plasma-preparations which are leucocyte poor and have a low-density fibrin network on activation. They can be used as liquid solutions or as an activated gel. Therefore, it can be injected (as used in sports medicine) or can be placed during gelling on a wound or suture (similar to fibrin glue). Following the first slow spin centrifugation, only the superficial buffy coat layer is aspirated out and taken for second centrifugation [2]. Example: PRGF (plasma rich in growth factors or preparations rich in growth factors).

2. Leucocyte- and platelet-rich plasma (L-PRP) products-preparations with leucocytes and with formation of low-density fibrin network on activation. Largest number of commercial or experimental systems belongs to this group. During preparation of L-PRP, PPP, entire buffy coat layer and upper 1–2 mm of red blood cell layer are pipetted out after the first centrifugation [2]. Like P-PRP, they can be in liquid or gel form.

3. Pure platelet-rich fibrin (P-PRF) or leucocyte-poor platelet-rich fibrin-preparations which are leucocyte poor and with a fibrin network which is of high density. They exist only in a strongly activated gel form. To make P-PRF, P-PRP is mixed with an activator and a specific separator gel is used. After incubating for some time, a stable platelet-rich fibrin matrix (PRFM) clot is formed [2]. It cannot be injected or used like traditional fibrin glue but as it has a strong fibrin matrix, it can be handled like a real solid material and used for various other applications.

4. Leucocyte- and platelet-rich fibrin (L-PRF) or second-generation PRP product-preparations with leucocytes and a high-density fibrin network. Blood is centrifuged immediately after collection without any anticoagulant, thrombin or $CaCl_2$. Natural coagulation process leads to formation of three layers—lowest RBC layer, middle L-PRF layer and topmost plasma layer which is acellular. The PRF clot is pressed between two gauzes to form a strong membrane [2]. Like P-PRF, it exists in strongly activated gel form only.

6. Factors which influence yield of PRP

6.1. Blood withdrawal technique

In most of the protocols, large bore needles (>22) are used for withdrawal of the blood to avoid unintentional activation of platelets [10].

Waters and Roberts, in their study, found that there was decrease in platelet counts with longer draw time [11].

6.2. Centrifugal force

Separation of blood's cellular constituents is achieved by the process of differential centrifugation. In differential centrifugation, acceleration force is adjusted, leading to sedimentation of certain cellular constituents, whereas other constituents are left in suspension. Relative centrifugal field or RCF is the force which is required for separation of two phases. RCF is expressed as multiples of the earth's gravitational field (g). On accelerating g, speedy sedimentation is achieved. 'g' is the actual force being exerted on the spinning rotor's contents, which leads to separation of the aqueous solutions [8].

Revolutions per minute (rpm) is calculated using the equation [12].

$$g = (1.118 \times 10^{-5}) R\, S^2 \quad (1)$$

where 'g' is the RCF, R is radius of the rotor from center of rotor to the sample (cm) and S is speed of the centrifuge (revolutions per minute).

The RCF calculation is dependent on radius of the centrifuge rotor used [8].

6.3. Temperature

AABB manual recommends temperature of 21–24°C for blood centrifugation for the purpose of obtaining PRP [13]. Macey et al. reported that cooling may retard the platelet activation, and therefore, it may be essential to obtain PRP with viable platelets [14].

6.4. Anticoagulants

An ideal anticoagulant should preserve best functionality, integrity and morphology of platelets [8].

Anticoagulants with citrate and dextrose of sodium citrate are recommended for the PRP preparation [15].

Ethylene diamine tetra acetic acid (EDTA) is not preferred because it can damage the platelet membrane [8].

ACD binds calcium and prevents the clotting cascade initiation by the coagulation proteins. Citrate also makes blood more acidic than is physiological. As some growth factors are influenced by the tissue pH, some protocols recommend that PRP should be buffered back to a physiologic range before injection [16].

6.5. Activation of PRP

PRP is exogenously activated by thrombin, calcium chloride or mechanical trauma. Collagen is a natural activator; thus, when PRP is used in soft tissue, there is no need to be exogenously activated [10].

On activation of PRP, a fibrin network begins to form and solidification of the plasma occurs, leading to fibrin clot or membrane formation. If PRP is activated too strongly, the fibrin network formed will be a bivalent, unstable network. If it is activated in a more physiologic manner, there is formation of a tetramolecular stable network that enhances cells and growth factor enmeshment. It is undesirable to have overly viscous PRP when injecting into the soft tissue [16].

6.6. Utility of inhibitor of platelet aggregation

Anticoagulants do not interrupt platelet aggregation. This has been overlooked in preparing conventional PRP. Aggregated platelets stick to the syringe wall and do not get easily detached from them. The primary aggregation of platelets is reversible, so the platelets come off from the wall and float in the plasma again after several hours. Waiting for such a long time is not feasible in the daily practice. So platelet aggregation inhibitor (PGE1) can be used to prevent this aggregation [17].

6.7. Contraindications

Absolute contraindications:

1. Platelet dysfunction syndrome.
2. Critical thrombocytopenia.
3. Hemodynamic instability.
4. Septicemia.
5. Local infection at the site.
6. Patient unwilling to accept risks.

Relative contraindications:

1. Consistent use of NSAIDs within 48 h of procedure.
2. Corticosteroid injection at treatment site within 1 month.
3. Systemic use of corticosteroids within 2 weeks.
4. Use of tobacco.
5. Recent fever/illness.
6. Cancer—especially hematopoietic or bone.
7. Hemoglobin < 10 g/dl.
8. Platelet count < 10^5/μl.

6.8. Complications

1. Pain in the injected area, headache, heaviness of head.
2. Swelling and redness.
3. Infection-PRP is antimicrobial and is effective against most bacteria except *Klebsiella*.

4. *Enterococcus* and *Pseudomonas*.
5. Allergic reaction—urticarial rash.
6. Skin discoloration, bruising.
7. Bleeding.
8. Cross labeling of samples—leading to serious side effects, for example, severe hypersensitivity reaction [18].

7. Indications of PRP in cosmetic dermatology, trichology and hair transplant

7.1. Trichology

7.1.1. Androgenetic alopecia (AGA)

Growth factors from platelets act on stem cells present in the bulge area of the follicles, stimulating the new follicular development and promotion of neovascularization. They activate the proliferation and transdifferentiation of hair and stem cells and produce new follicular units. Basic fibroblast growth factor promotes the proliferation of papilla cells in vitro and, therefore, plays a key role in hair shaft elongation. Activated PRP promotes the proliferation and prevents apoptosis of dermal papillary cells [19].

Singhal et al. found out that by the end of 3 months, all 10 androgenetic alopecia (AGA) patients treated with PRP had a good hair growth with reduction in number of hair pulled out by average 65%. New hair growth was observed in six patients as early as 7 days and in four patients in 15 days. Three patients developed mild headache after the procedure. There was no inflammation or infection [20].

In an another study on PRP in 11 AGA patients, the hair pull test after four sessions (once in 2 weeks) of PRP became negative in nine patients. Moderate improvement in hair volume and coverage was reported [19].

Greco and Brandt in their study, involving five patients who were given PRP therapy and five patients in non-PRP group (10 AGA patients in total), concluded that PRP used as mesotherapy in AGA patients leads to a significant increase in hair diameter and hair density [21].

Various modes of PRP therapy for AGA are as follows [2]:

1. Interfollicular PRP injection—an amount of 0.05–0.1 ml/cm^2, in a retrograde fashion from deep to superficial, at distance of a centimeter, throughout the treated site.
2. PRP mesotherapy—microneedling with a roller of 1–1.5 mm long needles followed by interfollicular PRP injections (or using mesogun) over the treated area, and later, PRP is sprayed on top of the scalp and left overnight. It is usually repeated at an interval of 1–3 months.
3. PRP as an adjunct to hair transplantation:

http://dx.doi.org/10.5772/intechopen.70287

a. The follicular grafts are dipped into PRP for about 15 min, before implantation to increase their rate of survival following implantation [22].

b. PRP is injected into the recipient area of scalp before or just after graft implantation [23].

c. PRP is injected at and around the donor strip excision line, in follicular unit transplantation (FUT), to decrease bleeding, stimulation of wound healing and reduction of scarring.

7.1.2. Our experience

At our institute, we studied the effects of PRP therapy in 30 male patients with grade I to IV androgenetic alopecia. Three sessions of PRP at an interval of 1 month were given. Along with PRP, multivitamin supplements, peptide-based topical serum and high protein diet were also advised. Growth of new hair was observed to start at about 4–6 weeks after first session in 60% of the patients. By 8 weeks, increase in hair diameter was noted in 80% of the patients. There was significant improvement with perceptible difference in diameter and density of hair at 3 months after the completion of PRP sessions (**Figure 1**).

There were nine cases of female pattern hair loss in whom, we observed that more number of sessions were required for perceptible improvement to occur, that is, mean of six PRP sessions was required. New hair growth was seen as early as 6–8 weeks. On video-microscopy, moderate increase in density and diameter of hair was noted at about 6–10 months. Marked improvement in skin texture was observed. We also noted gradual diminution of the perifollicular halo with successive PRP therapy. Reduction in active hair fall was noticed as early as 4–6 weeks (**Figure 2**).

7.1.3. Our experience in FUE with PRP therapy

We conducted a randomized control study of 40 patients with androgenetic alopecia undergoing hair transplant, and 20 patients each were allocated to PRP and the control group. In the PRP group, after harvesting and slitting, 0.2–0.3 ml PRP was injected at 1 cm gap to the depth of dermis and subcutis in freshly done slits, whereas the non-PRP group received normal saline instead of PRP. There was more than 75% growth in all patients in PRP group after

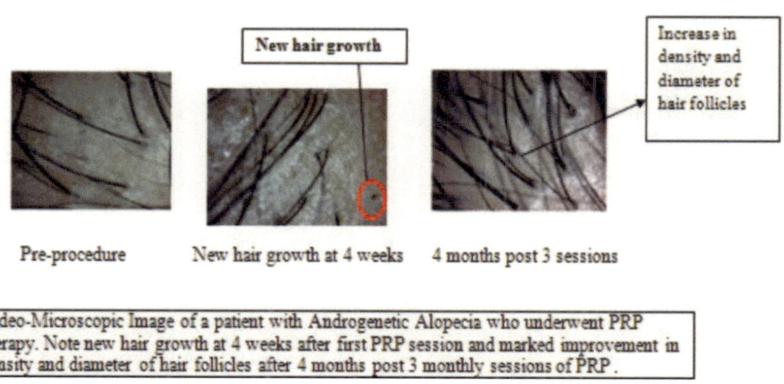

Figure 1. Video-microscopic image of a patient with androgenetic alopecia who underwent PRP therapy. Note new hair growth at 4 weeks after first PRP session and marked improvement in density and diameter of hair follicles after 4 months post 3 monthly sessions of PRP.

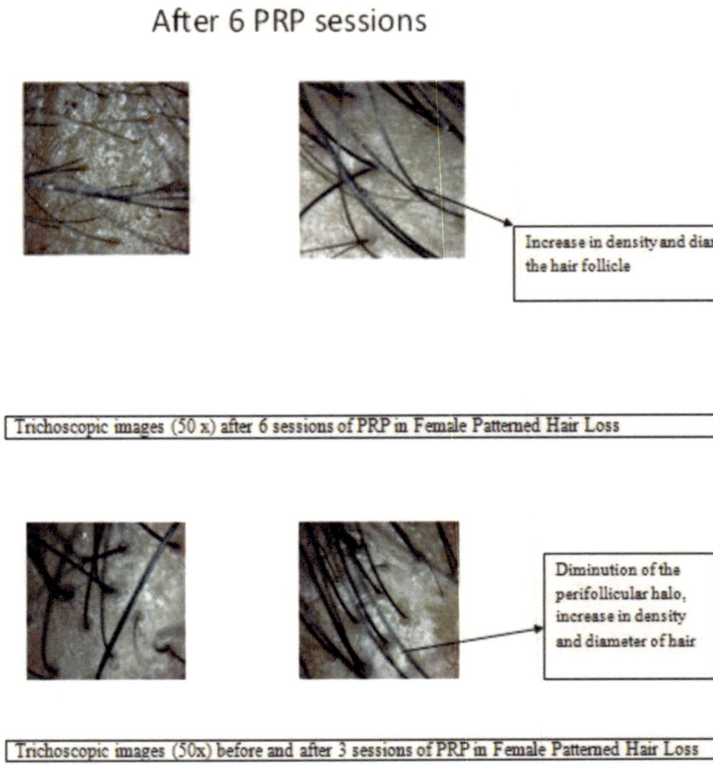

Figure 2. Trichoscopic images (50×) after six sessions of PRP in female patterned hair loss. Trichoscopic images (50×) before and after three sessions of PRP in female patterned hair loss.

6 months, whereas only 20% of non-PRP group had similar growth. PRP group had much denser and lengthier follicle growth. Also, in PRP group, number of multiple grafts was more, shafts were longer, better texture of hair was seen, posttransplant catagen fall was less and there was absence of redness after 3 months. PRP therapy during hair transplant was found to play a significant role in regrowth of hair and remarkably improved the density and quality of hair growth 8 months after transplantation (**Figure 3**).

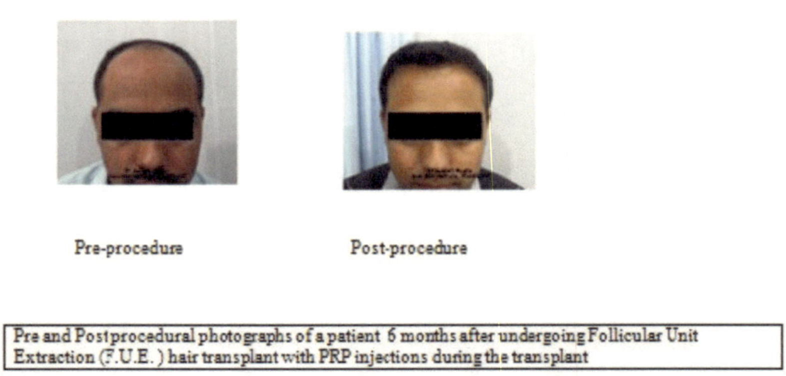

Figure 3. Pre- and post-procedural photographs of a patient 6 months after undergoing follicular unit extraction (F.U.E.) hair transplant with PRP injections during the transplant.

http://dx.doi.org/10.5772/intechopen.70287

8. Alopecia areata

A double-blinded, placebo and active-controlled, half-head, parallel group study on 45 patients designed to evaluate the efficacy of PRP in alopecia areata concluded that PRP is a safe and alternative treatment for AA. PRP was found to significantly increase hair regrowth and to decrease hair dystrophy and burning or itching sensation without any side effects. Ki-67 levels, which are a cell proliferation marker, were significantly higher in PRP group [24].

Singh found in their study that out of 20 patients with alopecia areata treated with PRP, only one had a relapse. There were no side effects, and all patients well tolerated the procedure [25].

8.1. Scars and dermal augmentation

A study done to determine the efficacy of single injection autologous PRFM for deep nasolabial folds (NLFs) correction concluded that PRFM provides significant long-term deep NLFs diminution. No fibrosis, irregularity, hardness, restricted movement or lumpiness was seen [26].

PRP has a high concentration of platelets with neovascularization properties and, thus, has the potential to promote survival of fat graft. Fat graft volume and weight were found to be significantly higher in the PRP group than in the control group. Histologic evaluation showed greater vascularity, fewer cysts and vacuoles, and lesser fibrosis in the PRP group [27].

8.1.1. Post-acne atrophic scars

PRP injections combined with fractional carbon dioxide resurfacing provide good results in treatment of acne scars as revealed by a simultaneous split face trial [28].

8.1.2. Our experience

We find combination of PRP therapy with Er:YAG laser resurfacing to be effective therapeutic modality for the treatment of post acne atrophic scars. This combination also helps in decreasing the downtime and incidence of adverse effects like post-inflammatory hyperpigmentation which are conventionally associated with usage of Er:YAG lasers alone. So, higher fluences can be used for treatment with less chances of post-inflammatory hyperpigmentation (**Figure 4**).

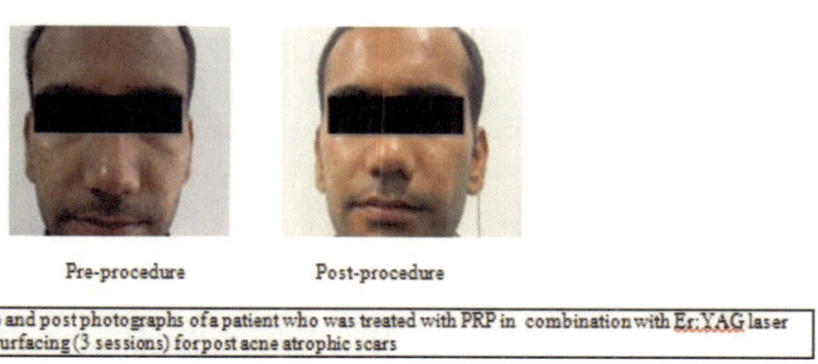

Figure 4. Pre- and post-photographs of a patient who was treated with PRP in combination with Er:YAG laser resurfacing (three sessions) for post-acne atrophic scars.

8.1.3. Skin rejuvenation (vampire facelift)

A study on skin rejuvenation with autologous platelet-rich plasma demonstrated good results with increase in the skin homogeneity and the patient satisfaction without serious side effects [29].

PRP enhances gene expression of matrix molecules, such as collagen and stimulates fibroblast proliferation ex vivo in the experimental models, thereby increasing total protein synthesis. PRP enhances elastin production by fibroblasts and stimulation of myofibroblast [29].

PRP and activated platelet poor plasma (aPPP) treatment increased the proliferation of human dermal fibroblasts, increased procollagen type I carboxy-terminal peptide production by human dermal fibroblasts, increased expression of type 1 collagen, alpha1 and type 1 collagen, alpha2, increased Matrix Metalloproteinase-1 (MMP-1) and MMP-3 proteins expression. MMPs digest various structural components of the ECM and are centrally involved in dermal remodeling. PRP can be topically applied or directly injected into the skin [7].

Skin remodeling can be enhanced by increasing the penetration and inducing mild inflammatory reactions through use of microneedles and lasers along with PRP [7].

PRP helps in remodeling of the skin.

As an adjuvant to lasers or microneedling, it is usually done once in every 4–6 months for 1 year and then yearly as maintenance therapy [30].

Fractional nonablative (Erbium glass) laser therapy combined with topical application of PRP resulted in objective improvement in elasticity of skin, a lower erythema index and an increased density of collagen. Histologically, an increase in length of dermo-epidermal junction, in amount of collagen and fibroblasts, was seen in the treated skin [31].

PRP can be combined with fractional ablative lasers (carbon dioxide) for treatment of deep wrinkles and severe photodamaged skin. The combination helps in reducing transient adverse effects like erythema and decreases the downtime, leading to rapid healing [32].

PRP injections once a month for 3 months, have shown good results for infraorbital rejuvenation, without any obvious adverse effects in a split face blinded trial [33].

8.1.4. Our experience

We found combination of PRP therapy with Er:YAG laser to be efficacious for facial and periorbital rejuvenation without much adverse effects. It is performed once every month for a total duration of 3 months. It promotes neocollagenogenesis and provides an environment for vascularization, leading to reduction in fine lines and improvement in texture and complexion as seen in **Figure 5**.

8.2. Striae distensae

For treatment of striae distensae, a combination of intradermal radiofrequency (RF) device with autologous PRP was synergistically effective, had fewer adverse effects and was well tolerated.

http://dx.doi.org/10.5772/intechopen.70287

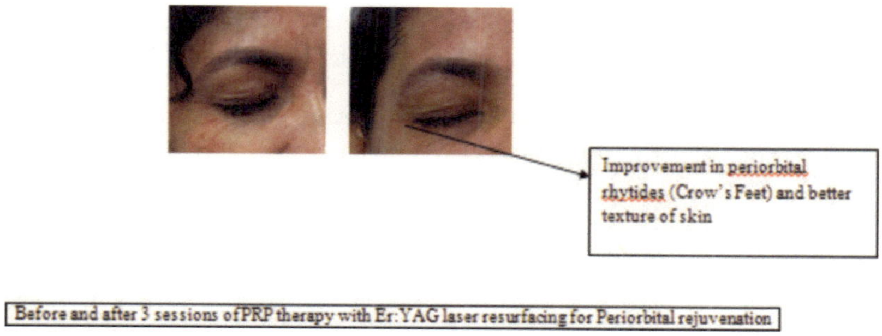

Figure 5. Before and after three sessions of PRP therapy with Er:YAG laser resurfacing for periorbital rejuvenation.

No significant side effects other than transient bruising were noted. Bipolar RF generated thermal energy, thereby denaturing the elastic fibers and collagen bundles, while PRP stimulated wound healing, leading to synergism and good cosmesis [34].

Combined enhanced penetration platelet-rich plasma and ultrasound following plasma fractional radiofrequency were also found to be useful in treatment of striae distensae in a study [35].

9. Conclusion

PRP therapy is one of the most upcoming forms of regenerative medicine with the potential to improve the homeostasis of the treated cells and tissues, provided that harvesting standards are maintained. Since it belongs to one's own body, safety is always ensured unlike various plant- and animal-derived stem cells or medications which may prove deleterious to human body. There is negligible risk of reacting to one's own cells and the procedure is minimally invasive with down time of or two days. It can give very promising results for facial rejuvenation, and nonsurgical face lifts minimizing and delaying the requirement of botulinum toxin and fillers. Results are, similarly, quite promising in burn and scar removal as monotherapy or in combination with lasers and micro-needling. PRP therapy also helps in hair strengthening and regrowth as monotherapy or in combination with hair transplant.

Author details

Suruchi Garg*, Shweta Manchanda and Chandi Garg

*Address all correspondence to: gargsuruchi01@gmail.com

Aura Skin Institute, Chandigarh, India

References

[1] Banihashemi M, Nakhaeizadeh S. An introduction to application of platelet rich plasma (PRP) in skin rejuvenation. Reviews in Clinical Medicine. 2014;**1**(2):38-43

[2] Arshdeep, Kumaran MS. Platelet-rich plasma in dermatology: Boon or a bane? Indian Journal of Dermatology, Venereology, and Leprology. 2014;**80**:5-14

[3] Maria-Angeliki G, Alexandros-Efstratios K, Dimitris R, Konstantinos K. Platelet-rich plasma as a potential treatment for noncicatricial alopecias. International Journal of Trichology. 2015;**7**:54-63

[4] Marwah M, Godse K, Patil S, Nadkarni N. Is there sufficient research data to use platelet-rich plasma in dermatology? International Journal of Trichology. 2014;**6**:35-36

[5] Lana JFSD, Vicente EF, Weglein A, Belangero WD, Assis FD, Mansano AM. Platelet-rich plasma in pain medicine. In: Maffulli N, editor. Platelet Rich Plasma in Musculoskeletal Practice. 1st ed. London: Springer-Verlag; 2016. p. 32. DOI: 10.1007/978-1-4471-7271-0

[6] Da Silva RT, Heidrich F. Therapy with use of platelet-rich plasma in orthopedics and sports traumatology: Literature review, evidence and personal experience. In: Lana JFSD, Andrade Santana MH, Dias Belangero W, Malheiros Luzo AC, editors. Platelet-Rich Plasma. Regenerative Medicine: Sports Medicine, Orthopedic, and Recovery of Musculoskeletal Injuries. 1st ed. Berlin: Springer; 2014. p. 154

[7] Kim DH, Je YJ, Kim CD, et al. Can platelet-rich plasma be used for skin rejuvenation? Evaluation of effects of platelet-rich plasma on human dermal fibroblast. Annals of Dermatology. 2011;**23**(4):424-431. DOI: 10.5021/ad.2011.23.4.424

[8] Dhurat R, Sukesh M. Principles and methods of preparation of platelet-rich plasma: A review and author's perspective. Journal of Cutaneous and Aesthetic Surgery. 2014;**7**(4):189-197. DOI: 10.4103/0974-2077.150734

[9] Dohan Ehrenfest DM, Andia I, Zumstein MA, Zhang C-Q, Pinto NR, Bielecki T. Classification of platelet concentrates (Platelet-Rich Plasma-PRP, Platelet-Rich Fibrin-PRF) for topical and infiltrative use in orthopedic and sports medicine: Current consensus, clinical implications and perspectives. Muscles, Ligaments and Tendons Journal. 2014;**4**(1):3-9

[10] Marlovits S, Mousavi M, Gäbler C, Erdös J, Vécsei V, et al. A new simplified technique for producing platelet-rich plasma: a short technical note. European Spine Journal. 2004;**13**(Suppl 1):S102-S106. DOI: 10.1007/s00586-004-0715-3

[11] Waters JH, Roberts KC. Database review of possible factors influencing point-of-care platelet gel manufacture. Journal of Extra-Corporeal Technology. 2004;**36**:250-254

[12] Jain SK, Soni V. Bentley's Textbook of Pharmaceutics—An Update. Chapter 17, 1st ed. India: Elsevier India; 2014. pp. 556-565

[13] Sweeny J, Grossman BJ. Blood collection, storage and component preparation methods. In: Brecher M, editor. Technical Manual. 14th ed. Bethesda, MD: American Association of Blood Banks (AABB); 2002. pp. 955-958

[14] Macey M, Azam U, McCarthy D, Webb L, Chapman ES, Okrongly D, et al. Evaluation of the anticoagulants EDTA and citrate, theophylline, adenosine, and dipyridamole

(CTAD) for assessing platelet activation on the ADVIA 120 hematology system. Clinical Chemistry. 2002;**48**:891-899

[15] Anitua E, Prado R, Sánchez M, Orive G. Platelet-rich-plasma: Preparation and formulation. Operative Techniques in Orthopaedics. 2012;**22**:25-32

[16] Harmon K, et al. Guidelines for the Use of Platelet Rich Plasma [Internet]. The International Cellular Medical Society. Version 1.0. 2011. Available from: http://www.cellmedicinesociety.org/attachments/370_Section%2010%20-%20Platelet%20Rich%20Plasma%20(PRP)%20Guidelines.pdf [Accessed: March 23, 2016]

[17] Fukaya M, Ito A. A new economic method for preparing platelet-rich plasma. Plastic and Reconstructive Surgery Global Open. 2014;**2**(6):e162

[18] Godse K, Mahajan A. Platelet-rich plasma. In: Pai GS, editor. Complications in Cosmetic Dermatology Crafting Cures. 1st ed. New Delhi: Jaypee Publications; 2016. pp. 174-177

[19] Khatu SS, More YE, Gokhale NR, Chavhan DC, Bendsure N. Platelet-rich plasma in androgenic alopecia: Myth or an effective tool. Journal of Cutaneous and Aesthetic Surgery. 2014;**7**(2):107-110. DOI: 10.4103/0974-2077.138352

[20] Singhal P, Agarwal S, Dhot PS, Sayal SK. Efficacy of platelet-rich plasma in treatment of androgenic alopecia. Asian Journal of Transfusion Science. 2015;**9**:159-162

[21] Greco J, Brandt R. The effects of autologous platelet rich plasma and various growth factors on non-transplanted miniaturized hair. Hair Transplant Forum International. 2009;**19**:49-50

[22] Uebel CO, da Silva JB, Cantarelli D, Martins P. The role of platelet plasma growth factors in male pattern baldness surgery. Plastic and Reconstructive Surgery. 2006;**118**:1458-1466

[23] Garg S. Outcome of intra-operative injected platelet-rich plasma therapy during follicular unit extraction hair transplant: A prospective randomised study in forty patients. Journal of Cutaneous and Aesthetic Surgery. 2016;**9**:157-164

[24] Trink A, Sorbellini E, Bezzola P, Rodella L, Rezzani R, Ramot Y, et al. A randomized, double-blind, placebo- and active-controlled, half-head study to evaluate the effects of platelet-rich plasma on alopecia areata. British Journal of Dermatology. 2013;**169**:690-694

[25] Singh S. Role of platelet-rich plasma in chronic alopecia areata: Our centre experience. Indian Journal of Plastic Surgery : Official Publication of the Association of Plastic Surgeons of India. 2015;**48**(1):57-59. DOI: 10.4103/0970-0358.155271

[26] Sclafani AP. Platelet-rich fibrin matrix for improvement of deep nasolabial folds. Journal of Cosmetic Dermatology. 2010;**9**:66-71

[27] Oh DS, Cheon YW, Jeon YR, Lew DH. Activated platelet-rich plasma improves fat graft survival in nude mice: A pilot study. Dermatologic Surgery. 2011;**37**:619-625

[28] Lee JW, Kim BJ, Kim MN, Mun SK. The efficacy of autologous platelet rich plasma combined with ablative carbon dioxide fractional resurfacing for acne scars: A simultaneous split-face trial. Dermatologic Surgery. 2011;**37**:931-938

[29] Mikhael NW, El-Esawy FM. Skin rejuvenation with autologous concentrated platelet-rich plasma. Egyptian Journal of Dermatology and Venereology. 2014;**34**:5-9

[30] Konda D, Thappa DM. Mesotherapy: What is new? Indian Journal of Dermatology, Venereology, and Leprology. 2013;**79**:127-134

[31] Shin MK, Lee JH, Lee SJ, Kim NI. Platelet-rich plasma combined with fractional laser therapy for skin rejuvenation. Dermatologic Surgery. 2012;**38**:623-630

[32] Na JI, Choi JW, Choi HR, Jeong JB, Park KC, Youn SW, et al. Rapid healing and reduced erythema after ablative fractional carbon dioxide laser resurfacing combined with the application of autologous platelet-rich plasma. Dermatologic Surgery. 2011;**37**:463-468

[33] Kang BK, Lee JH, Shin MK, Kim NI. Infraorbital rejuvenation using PRP (platelet-rich plasma): A prospective, randomized, split-face trial. Journal of the American Academy of Dermatology. 2013;**68**:SAB24

[34] Kim IS, Park KY, Kim BJ, Kim MN, Kim CW, Kim SE. Efficacy of intradermal radiofrequency combined with autologous platelet-rich plasma in striae distensae: A pilot study. International Journal of Dermatology. 2012;**51**:1253-1258

[35] Suh DH, Lee SJ, Lee JH, Kim HJ, Shin MK, Song KY. Treatment of striae distensae combined enhanced penetration platelet-rich plasma and ultrasound after plasma fractional radiofrequency. Journal of Cosmetic and Laser Therapy. 2012;**14**:272-276

[36] Sunitha Raja V, Munirathnam Naidu E. Platelet-rich fibrin: Evolution of a second-generation platelet concentrate. Indian Journal of Dental Research. 2008;**19**:42-46

[37] Middleton KK, Barro V, Muller B, Terada S, Fu FH. Evaluation of the effects of platelet-rich plasma (PRP) therapy involved in the healing of sports-related soft tissue injuries. The Iowa Orthopaedic Journal. 2012;**32**:150-163

Section 4

Perspectives

Chapter 11

Oral Naturally Derived Agents as an Adjuvant Photoprotection after Dermatologic Surgery

Premjit Juntongjin and Chavanatda Chanyasak

Additional information is available at the end of the chapter

http://dx.doi.org/10.5772/intechopen.71750

Abstract

To be effective in protecting against the harmful effects of ultraviolet radiation (UVR), many photoprotective strategies have been used. Inadequate physical protection, amount of topical application, and allergic reactions to topical agents are limitations associated with current photoprotective strategies. Systemic agents are an emerging alternative, providing promising protection against UVR. This chapter will thoroughly review photoprotective outcomes of oral naturally derived agents from randomized controlled trials using evidence-based method. From total 24 clinical trials with 850 participants, two categories of naturally derived agents were identified. Plant-derived agents include beta-carotene, green tea, golden serpent fern, tomato, cocoa bean, and vitamin E, whereas animal-derived products consist of nicotinamide and omega-3 polyunsaturated fatty acids. In conclusion, systemic plant and animal-derived photoprotective agents may be a promising alternative in addition to conventional photoprotection.

Keywords: oral photoprotection, sunscreen, natural products

1. Introduction

Ultraviolet radiation (UVR) can cause various adverse effects to the skin including pigmentary changes, epidermal hyperplasia, free radical formation, photoaging, immunosuppression, and photocarcinogenesis [1]. Physical and topical protective agents are the standard photoprotective strategies especially after dermatologic surgery. Sunscreen is the most widely used protective agent, providing protection only to the areas in which the agents are applied upon. However, the protection is only limited to the few hours subsequent to their applications. In addition, topical protective agents may cause allergic reactions on some individuals [2].

Systemic or oral protective agents in the form of supplementation, preventing free radicals formation and its harmful effects would be an alternative option for photoprotection. Several researches have studied the effects of oral agents to show the protective abilities against UV exposure. This chapter will demonstrate those extensive studies systematically.

All studies included only adult healthy participants aged 18 years and older. In vitro or animal studies were not included into the review. Minimal erythema dose (MED) or changes in UV-induced erythema (UIE) intensity was assessed in most of the studies providing measurement for clinical outcomes. Photoprotective effects of systemic products can be clinically observed through increased MED and decreased UIE intensity. In some studies, physical changes in skin, histopathology, and immunohistochemistry were identified as biomarker outcomes. Two main groups were categorized regarding to their natural sources (**Tables 1** and **2**).

	Dose/duration	Subjects	Comparison	Clinical outcomes	Histology/biomarker outcomes
Beta-carotene					
Heinrich et al. [3]	β-carotene 24 mg (from an algal source) daily vs. mixed carotenoids (β-carotene 8 mg, lutein 8 mg, and lycopene 8 mg) daily for 12 weeks	36	Placebo	Decreased UIE in both groups ($p < 0.001$)	N/A
Stahl et al. [4]	Total carotenoids 25 mg daily vs. carotenoids 25 mg with α-Toc 500 IU daily for 12 weeks	17	carotenoids	Decreased UIE in combination of carotenoids and α-Toc ($p < 0.01$) and in carotenoids alone ($p < 0.05$)	N/A
Mathews-Roth et al. [5]	β-Carotene 180 mg daily for 10 weeks	30	Placebo	Increased MED ($p < 0.05$), less pigmentary changes after sun exposure ($p < 0.05$)	N/A
Camellia sinensis					
Farrar et al. [6]	GTCs 540 mg with 50 mg vitamin C, twice daily for 12 weeks	50	Placebo	No significant changes in MED	No significant difference in leukocyte infiltration
Heinrich et al. [7]	Total catechins 1402 mg daily for 12 weeks	60	Placebo	Decreased UIE ($p < 0.05$)	Decreased skin elasticity ($p < 0.05$), TEWL ($p < 0.001$), roughness, scaling, wrinkles ($p < 0.05$). Increased hydration, cutaneous blood flow, and O2 saturation ($p < 0.05$).

	Dose/duration	Subjects	Comparison	Clinical outcomes	Histology/biomarker outcomes
Chow et al. [8]	EGCG 800 mg daily vs. EGCG 400 mg twice daily vs. EGCG as Polyphenon E 800 mg daily vs. EGCG as Polyphenon E 400 mg twice daily for 4 weeks	40	Placebo	No significant changes in MED	N/A
Polypodium leucotomos					
Nestor et al. [9]	PL extract 480 mg daily for 60 days	40	Placebo	Increased MED ($p = 0.01$), decreased UIE ($p < 0.01$)	Decreased sunburn cells ($p = 0.04$)
Villa et al. [10]	PL extract 480 mg before 2–3 MED exposure	10	Placebo	N/A	Decreased common deletion of mtDNA ($p = 0.06$). No significant difference in histology
Gonzalez et al. [11]	PL extract 1080 mg before UV exposure	23	Placebo	Increased MED ($p < 0.001$), IPD ($p < 0.01$)	Preservation of CD1a-expressing epidermal LCs
Solanum lycopersicum					
Sokoloski et al. [12]	Tomato paste (16 mg lycopene) vs. lycopene capsule (16 mg lycopene) daily for 10 weeks	20	Lycopene capsule	Decreased UIE in both groups ($p = 0.054$). No significant changes in MED in both groups.	N/A
Rizwan et al. [13]	Tomato paste 55 g (16 mg lycopene) in olive oil vs. olive oil alone daily for 12 weeks	20	Placebo	Increased MED ($p = 0.03$)	Reduced UV-induced MMP-1 ($p = 0.04$), increased in pCI deposition ($p = 0.05$), decreased mtDNA 3895-bp deletion ($p = 0.01$)
Aust et al. [14]	Tomato extract (9.8 mg lycopene) vs. drink containing solubilized tomato extract (8.2 mg lycopene) vs. synthetic lycopene (10.2 mg lycopene) daily for 12 weeks	36	Synthetic lycopene	Decreased UIE of both tomato extract ($p < 0.001$) and drink containing tomato extract ($p < 0.001$) but not in synthetic lycopene group	N/A
Stahl et al. [15]	Tomato paste 40 g (16 mg lycopene) in olive oil vs. olive oil alone daily for 10 weeks	19	Placebo	Decreased UIE ($p = 0.02$)	N/A

	Dose/duration	Subjects	Comparison	Clinical outcomes	Histology/biomarker outcomes
Theobroma cacao					
Mogollon et al. [16]	HFC 600 mg vs. LFC <30 mg daily for 12 weeks	74	LFC	Increased MED in both groups; however, no significant difference between HFC and LFC group	Increased skin elasticity and hydration in both groups
Williams et al. [17]	HFC 600 mg vs. LFC <30 mg daily for 12 weeks	30	LFC	Increased MED in HFC group ($p = 0.005$) but not in LFC. Significant difference between HFC and LFC group ($p \leq 0.05$).	N/A
Heinrich et al. [18]	HFC 329 mg vs. LFC 27 mg daily for 12 weeks	24	LFC	Decreased UIE ($p < 0.05$) in HFC group but not in LFC group. Significant difference between HFC and LFC group ($p < 0.05$)	Increased skin density, thickness and hydration, and decreased skin roughness, scaling and TEWL in HFC ($p < 0.05$). No different changes in LFC
Tocopherol					
McArdle et al. [19]	α-Toc 400 IU daily vs. β-carotene 15 mg daily for 8 weeks	16	β-Carotene	No significant changes in MED in both groups	Decreased skin malondialdehyde concentration in α-Toc ($p < 0.05$)
Mireles-Rocha et al. [20]	α-Toc 1200 IU daily vs. Asc 2 g daily vs. α-Toc 1200 IU with Asc 2 g daily for 1 week	45	Asc	Increased MED in α-Toc alone ($p = 0.002$) and in Asc with α-Toc ($p = 0.0001$). No significant changes in Asc alone group	N/A
Fuchs et al. [21]	α-Toc 2 g daily vs. Asc 3 g daily vs. α-Toc 2 g with Asc 3 g daily vs. placebo for 50 days	40	Placebo	Increased MED only in α-Toc with Asc group ($p < 0.005$)	N/A
Werninghaus et al. [22]	α-Toc 400 IU daily for 6 months	67	Placebo	No significant change in MED	No significant difference in sunburn cells

Abbreviation: Asc = ascorbic acid, EGCG = epigallocatechin gallate, GTCs = green tea catechins, HFC = high-flavanol chocolate, IPD = immediate pigment darkening, LCs = Langerhans cells, LFC = low-flavanol chocolate, MED = minimal erythema doses, MMP-1 = matrix matelloprotenase-1, mtDNA = mitochondrial DNA, PL = *Polypodium leucotomos*, SPT = skin phototype, TEWL = transepidermal water loss, UIE = UV-induced erythema, and α-Toc = D-α-tocopherol.

Table 1. Plant-derived photoprotective agents.

	Dose/duration	Subjects	Comparison	Clinical outcomes	Histology/biomarker outcomes
Nicotinamide					
Thanos et al. [23]	Nicotinamide 500 mg twice daily for 1 week	30	Crossover study	Reduced MIE ($p < 0.0001$)	Reduced Mantoux diameter ($p < 0.0001$)
Yiasemides et al. [24]	Nicotinamide 500 mg three times daily (high dose) vs. once daily (low dose) vs. placebo for 1 week	61	Crossover study	No significant changes in MED	Reduced Mantoux diameter ($p < 0.001$) in both groups
ω-3 polyunsaturated fatty acids					
Rhodes et al. [25]	95% EPA 4 g vs. 95% oleic acid 4 g daily for 12 weeks	42	Oleic acid	Increased MED ($p < 0.01$) in EPA but not in OA.	Reduced UV-induced p53 expression ($p < 0.01$) in EPA but not in OA. No statistical difference in CPDs changes. Decreased in tail moment by comet assay ($p < 0.05$) in EPA but not in OA.
Orengo et al. [26]	Fish oil (2.8 g EPA + 1.2 g DCHA) daily for 4 weeks	20	Placebo	Increased MED ($p < 0.02$)	No significant changes in PGE2

CPDs = cyclobutane pyrimidine dimers, DCHA = docosahexaenoic acid, EPA = eicosapentaenoic acid, MED = minimal erythema doses, MIE = Mantoux induced erythema, OA = oleic acid, PGE2 = prostaglandin E2, and SPT = skin phototype.

Table 2. Animal-derived photoprotective agents.

2. Plant-derived photoprotective agents

2.1. Beta-carotene

Previous study reported an increase in the ability to tolerate sunlight among photosensitive subjects, especially in erythropoietic porphyria after high-dose administration of beta-carotene [27]. However, only three RCTs of beta-carotene reported significant decrease in UIE intensity and increased MED after 10–12 weeks of supplementation in healthy subjects [3–5]. The major source of beta-carotene in two studies was from *Dunaliella salina*, a unicellular biflagellate green alga [3, 4]. Heinrich et al. [3] compared the administration of 24 mg of beta-carotene daily versus mixed carotenoids (beta-carotene 8 mg, lutein 8 mg, and lycopene 8 mg) for 12 weeks. The results showed the statistically significant decrease in UIE intensity in both groups. In another study conducted by Stahl et al. [4], a 25-mg-carotenoid supplement was given daily comparing to the supplementation of the combination of 25-mg-carotenoid and 500-IU-α-tocopherol during 12-week period. Both groups demonstrated significant decrease in UIE intensity at the end of the study. However, it seemed that in combination with vitamin E revealed more significant changes than with the carotenoid supplementation alone. Also, the study by Mathews-Roth et al. [5] suggested that high dose supplementation of a 180-mg-beta-carotene daily for 10 weeks could significantly reduce in MED and showed less pigmentary changes after sun exposure.

Beta-carotene alone, mixed of carotenoids, and in combination with α-tocopherol were effective. Nevertheless, there was no study evaluating histological changes. In animal study, *Dunaliella salina* exhibited potent protection from UV-induced oxidative damage due to the increase of antioxidative activities and the inhibition of lipid peroxidation [28].

2.2. *Camellia sinensis*

Camellia sinensis leaves that have not undergone the withering and oxidation process are commonly known as green tea. Four major polyphenols in green tea include epicatechin, epicatechin-3-gallate, epigallocatechin, and epigallocatechin-3-gallate (EGCG), the most potent antioxidant. In animal models, green tea polyphenols and EGCG demonstrated the protection against the UV-induced sunburn and photoaging of the skin [29].

A 540 mg of green tea catechins (GTCs) in combination with a 50 mg of vitamin C supplement was administered twice daily comparing to placebo group for 12 weeks [6]. There were no significant differences both in clinical outcomes of MED changes and in histological outcomes of leukocytic infiltration or the cutaneous production of proinflammatory metabolites. Similarly, supplementation of epigallocatechin gallate (EGCG) or Polyphenon E (decaffeinated green tea polyphenol mixture) at a dose of 800 mg was administered daily in comparison with placebo for 4 weeks [8]. There were no significant changes in MED after the supplementation. Therefore, these may conclude that there was no statistical effect on both clinical and histological changes of the skin basal inflammatory status or the response to acute proinflammatory UVR challenge based on histologic sunburn cells and proinflammatory mediators. However, one double-blinded RCT exhibited a significant reduction of UIE intensity following daily administration of total catechins 1402 mg for 3 months [7]. Skin elasticity, roughness, wrinkles, hydration, and cutaneous blood flow were also improved.

Green tea, a notable antioxidant product, has an extensive in vitro studies of its properties, including systemic antioxidant, anti-inflammatory activities, prevention of DNA damage [30], immunoregulation, and antiphotoaging properties. However, only one randomized, double-blind, placebo-controlled trial indicates an increase in photosensitivity threshold and improves skin physiology following a daily intake. Therefore, further clinical studies should be conducted to evaluate the exact efficacy of green tea for its photoprotective property.

2.3. *Polypodium leucotomos*

Polypodium leucotomos (PL), commonly known as golden serpent fern, is a tropical fern plant found in Central America. Its active ingredients are polyphenols including phenolic acids p-coumaric, ferulic, fumaric, vanillic, quinic, caffeic, chlorogenic, 3,4-dihydroxybenzoic, and 4-hydroxybenzoic, along with five phenolic chlorogenic acid isomers. The photoprotective properties of PL may link to its antioxidant activities, scavenging reactive oxygen species (ROS), and possessing anti-inflammatory properties.

There were three studies with a daily intake ranging from 480 to 1080 mg of PL for 1–60 days [9–11]. Two studies [9, 11] showed a statistically significant increase in MED and lower erythema intensity after UV exposure. The result was confirmed by the reduction of sunburn cells [9] and preservation of CD1a-expressing epidermal Langerhans cells [11]. For the ingestion just prior to UV exposure, a standard dose of 480 mg PL supplements did not demonstrate significant photoprotection in both clinical and histological outcomes [10].

Polyphenols are a large group of plant products occurring naturally. It prevents damages affecting cellular lipids, protein, DNA, and premature aging of the skin from photooxidative damage. Based on chemical structures, polyphenols can be classified into flavonoids, stilbenes, lignans, and phenolic acids [31]. Golden serpent fern, green tea, and cocoa bean have polyphenol structures, and they exhibited the same mechanisms of action in ROS suppression and anti-inflammation [31]. Though PL extract is one of the most well-known systemic photoprotective agents, there were only three RCTs comparing PL and placebo in healthy subjects. Daily supplements of PL at 480 mg exhibited photoprotection [9]. However, only high dose of PL at 1080 mg could prevent acute sunburn [11]. Immunomodulating effect of PL was found by the preservation of CD1a-expressing epidermal LCs in human skin [11].

2.4. *Solanum lycopersicum*

Lycopene, one of the powerful carotenoids antioxidants, is found abundantly in tomatoes, *Solanum lycopersicum*. Depending on the type of tomato and its state of ripening, lycopene contents vary significantly. Lycopene levels can reach as high as 50 mg/kg in the reddest strains of tomatoes and reach as low as 5 mg/kg in the yellow strains. Through thermal processing and dietary lipids coingestion, the bioavailability of lycopene from dietary sources increases substantially. As the bioavailability of carotenoids rises through cooking and food-processing process, an ingestion of tomato paste (processed tomatoes) yields a higher lycopene uptake than an ingestion of fresh tomatoes [32].

Four RCTs of lycopene from tomato paste or tomato extract showed similar trends of photoprotection. After 10–12 weeks of tomato paste ingestion at a dose ranging between 8.2 and 16 mg of lycopene daily, a significant decrease in UIE intensity or an increase in MED in lycopene group was noticed [12–15]. Significant decrease in MMP1 and the 3895-bp deletion in mitochondrial DNA following UV exposure were also found in histology [13]. It suggested that tomato paste may play a role in photoprotection through decreasing DNA mutagenesis.

Carotenoids, naturally fat-soluble pigments, are synthesized by plants and algae. Most of the carotenoids are from food with yellow to orange hues such as carrots, plums, and apricots. Carotenoids are usually classified into two broad classes: carotenes (lycopene, α-carotene, and β-carotene) and xanthophylls (β-cryptoxanthin, lutein, and zeaxanthin). Major biological effects of carotenoids include provitamin A activity, cellular signaling, and antioxidation [33]. Since tomato paste administration could reduce mitochondrial DNA deletion, this might also represent its role in mutagenic suppression [13].

2.5. *Theobroma cacao*

Freshly harvested cocoa beans are abundant in polyphenols. Flavonoids are the main phenolic phytochemical structure. However, during the production process of conventional chocolate, much of the antioxidant capacity of fresh cocoa beans is greatly diminished [34].

In three randomized controlled studies, daily intake of high flavanol cocoa (HFC, more than 329 mg) and low flavanol cocoa (LFC, less than 30 mg) for 3 months were compared. All studies revealed an increase in MED or a decrease in UIE intensity following HFC ingestion [16–18]. Only one research reported increasing MED in LFC administration [16]. Moreover, skin elasticity and hydration were improved after HFC administration [16, 18].

All three RCTs in cocoa bean demonstrated similar trends. Daily ingestion of chocolate with high flavanol cocoa for 3 months exhibited higher photosensitivity threshold [16–18]. Correspondingly, several in vitro studies showed antioxidative activities and anti-inflammatory properties of cocoa beans [35, 36]. These effects may be associated with the mechanisms of photoprotection of cocoa.

2.6. Tocopherol

Vitamin E is a group of compounds including tocopherols and tocotrienols. γ-tocopherol is considered to be the common form of vitamin E widely found in soybean oil, corn oil, margarine, and dressings. α-tocopherol, another form of vitamin E, can be found most abundantly in wheat germ oil, sunflower, and safflower oils. It affects oxidative stress by interrupting the free radical formation.

Four RCTs with daily supplement of α-tocopherol, at dosage between 400 and 1200 IU, alone or in combination with ascorbic acid were revealed [19–22]. The results were controversial. Two studies with daily intake of 400 IU of α-tocopherol showed no significant change in MED following the supplementation for 2 or 6 months [19, 22]. In contrast, a daily ingestion of 1200 IU or 2 g of α-tocopherol together with ascorbic acid administration could increase MED significantly [20, 21]. As a result for daily supplement of vitamin E, only high dosage could exhibit an increase of photoprotection. The mechanism of photoprotective activities may involve lipid peroxidation through the reduction of cutaneous malondialdehyde concentration after UV exposure [19].

3. Animal-derived photoprotective agents

3.1. Nicotinamide

Nicotinamide, an amide form of vitamin B3, is the precursor of nicotinamide adenine dinucleotide (NAD), an essential coenzyme for ATP production. Therefore, nicotinamide supplementation can accelerate cellular energy and elevate DNA repair, an energy-dependent cellular processes. Vitamin B3, an essential water-soluble vitamin, is generally not stored in the body. It is usually excreated in the urine on a daily basis. Maintenance is only possible through dietary consumption of vitamin B3 and tryptophan, an essential amino acid which is frequently reported in most variations of protein and makes up approximately 1% of total dietary protein. Nicotinamide are found mainly in meats, nuts, grain products, yeast extracts, eggs, and legumes. In animal studies, nicotinamide has photoprotective, anticarcinogenic, and immunosuppressive effects [37].

Using a Mantoux delayed-type hypersensitivity model, oral nicotinamide at dosage ranging from 500 to 1500 mg daily was administered in healthy subjects [23, 24]. The studies revealed the reduction of Mantoux diameter following the supplementation for a week. This might demonstrate the ability of UV-induced immunosuppression of the skin. Nevertheless, there were no significant changes in MED [24].

It has been demonstrated that nicotinamide prevents UV-induced ATP depletion, enhances UV-induced DNA repair, regulates inflammatory cytokines and mediators in human keratinocytes [38], and prevents photocarcinogenesis in animal studies [39]. In human studies, topical and oral nicotinamide administration could reduce the number of actinic keratoses [40, 41]. However, only two controlled studies could demonstrate the reduction of Mantoux-induced erythema and diameter at irradiated sites, indicating its immunosuppressive effect [23, 24].

3.2. Omega-3 polyunsaturated fatty acids

Dietary omega-3 polyunsaturated fatty acids (ω-3 PUFAs) are extracted mostly from oily fish such as mackerels, sardines, and salmons. Eicosapentaenoic acid (EPA) and docosahexaenoic acid (DCHA) are major components.

Rhodes et al. [25] reported daily intake of 4 g of purified ω-3 PUFAs comparing to a supplement of 4 g oleic acid. This trial demonstrated the significant increase in MED and UIE threshold following the supplementation of ω-3 PUFAs for 3 months. In immunohistochemical study, UV-induced p53 expression was also suppressed. Moreover, Orengo et al. [26] exhibited that daily supplements of fish oil composing of 2.8 g EPA for 1 month could significantly increase MED. Nevertheless, there was no significant change in PGE2 from immunohistological outcomes.

ω-3 PUFAs modulate NF-kB and AP-1, which control genes associated with inflammation and lipid metabolism. Dietary ω-3 PUFAs have been previously reported to reduce UVR-induced prostaglandin E_2, a mediator of UV immunosuppression, in both animals and human skins [42]. Clinical studies also indicated an increase in UIE threshold [25, 26]. Reduction in

UV-induced p53 expression indicating its effect on skin cancer reduction or DNA repair was observed in histology [25].

4. Conclusion

Conventionally, topical sunscreens, physical protection, and sun avoidance are recommended as standard photoprotection following most of the dermatologic surgery. However, several limitations including inadequate amount, reapplication needs, and photoallergic reactions limit their use in clinical practice. Regarding to the evidences of available natural product based, oral naturally derived agents are promising as an addition for photoprotection. Although, there are numerous in vitro and animal studies of the agents, the numbers of clinical studies are limited with small sample size of the subjects. Further high-quality controlled trials with higher number of participants are needed in order to get better understanding of the efficacy, mechanism of actions, and role of a natural product for photoprotection.

Author details

Premjit Juntongjin* and Chavanatda Chanyasak

*Address all correspondence to: premjitvp@yahoo.com

Division of Dermatology, Chulabhorn International College of Medicine, Thammasat University, Pathum Thani, Thailand

References

[1] Jansen R, Wang SQ, Burnett M, Osterwalder U, Lim HW. Photoprotection: Part I. Photoprotection by naturally occurring, physical, and systemic agents. Journal of the American Academy of Dermatology. 2013;**69**:853 e851-812; quiz 865-856

[2] Greenspoon J, Ahluwalia R, Juma N, Rosen CF. Allergic and photoallergic contact dermatitis: A 10-year experience. Dermatitis. 2013;**24**:29-32

[3] Heinrich U, Gartner C, Wiebusch M, Eichler O, Sies H, Tronnier H, Stahl W. Supplementation with beta-carotene or a similar amount of mixed carotenoids protects humans from UV-induced erythema. The Journal of Nutrition. 2003;**133**:98-101

[4] Stahl W, Heinrich U, Jungmann H, Sies H, Tronnier H. Carotenoids and carotenoids plus vitamin E protect against ultraviolet light-induced erythema in humans. The American Journal of Clinical Nutrition. 2000;**71**:795-798

[5] Mathews-Roth MM, Pathak MA, Parrish J, Fitzpatrick TB, Kass EH, Toda K, Clemens W. A clinical trial of the effects of oral beta-carotene on the responses of human skin to solar radiation. The Journal of Investigative Dermatology. 1972;**59**:349-353

[6] Farrar MD, Nicolaou A, Clarke KA, Mason S, Massey KA, Dew TP, Watson RE, Williamson G, Rhodes LE. A randomized controlled trial of green tea catechins in protection against ultraviolet radiation-induced cutaneous inflammation. The American Journal of Clinical Nutrition. 2015;**102**:608-615

[7] Heinrich U, Moore CE, De Spirt S, Tronnier H, Stahl W. Green tea polyphenols provide photoprotection, increase microcirculation, and modulate skin properties of women. The Journal of Nutrition. 2011;**141**:1202-1208

[8] Chow HH, Cai Y, Hakim IA, Crowell JA, Shahi F, Brooks CA, Dorr RT, Hara Y, Alberts DS. Pharmacokinetics and safety of green tea polyphenols after multiple-dose administration of epigallocatechin gallate and polyphenon E in healthy individuals. Clinical Cancer Research. 2003;**9**:3312-3319

[9] Nestor MS, Berman B, Swenson N. Safety and efficacy of oral *Polypodium leucotomos* extract in healthy adult subjects. The Journal of Clinical and Aesthetic Dermatology. 2015;**8**:19-23

[10] Villa A, Viera MH, Amini S, Huo R, Perez O, Ruiz P, Amador A, Elgart G, Berman B. Decrease of ultraviolet a light-induced "common deletion" in healthy volunteers after oral *Polypodium leucotomos* extract supplement in a randomized clinical trial. Journal of the American Academy of Dermatology. 2010;**62**:511-513

[11] Gonzalez S, Pathak MA, Cuevas J, Villarrubia VG, Fitzpatrick TB. Topical or oral administration with an extract of *Polypodium leucotomos* prevents acute sunburn and psoralen-induced phototoxic reactions as well as depletion of Langerhans cells in human skin. Photodermatology, Photoimmunology & Photomedicine. 1997;**13**:50-60

[12] Sokoloski L, Borges M, Bagatin E. Lycopene not in pill, nor in natura has photoprotective systemic effect. Archives of Dermatological Research. 2015;**307**:545-549

[13] Rizwan M, Rodriguez-Blanco I, Harbottle A, Birch-Machin MA, Watson RE, Rhodes LE. Tomato paste rich in lycopene protects against cutaneous photodamage in humans in vivo: A randomized controlled trial. The British Journal of Dermatology. 2011;**164**: 154-162

[14] Aust O, Stahl W, Sies H, Tronnier H, Heinrich U. Supplementation with tomato-based products increases lycopene, phytofluene, and phytoene levels in human serum and protects against UV-light-induced erythema. International Journal for Vitamin and Nutrition Research. 2005;**75**:54-60

[15] Stahl W, Heinrich U, Wiseman S, Eichler O, Sies H, Tronnier H. Dietary tomato paste protects against ultraviolet light-induced erythema in humans. The Journal of Nutrition. 2001;**131**:1449-1451

[16] Mogollon JA, Boivin C, Lemieux S, Blanchet C, Claveau J, Dodin S. Chocolate flavanols and skin photoprotection: A parallel, double-blind, randomized clinical trial. Nutrition Journal. 2014;**13**:66

[17] Williams S, Tamburic S, Lally C. Eating chocolate can significantly protect the skin from UV light. Journal of Cosmetic Dermatology. 2009;**8**:169-173

[18] Heinrich U, Neukam K, Tronnier H, Sies H, Stahl W. Long-term ingestion of high flavanol cocoa provides photoprotection against UV-induced erythema and improves skin condition in women. The Journal of Nutrition. 2006;**136**:1565-1569

[19] McArdle F, Rhodes LE, Parslew RA, Close GL, Jack CI, Friedmann PS, Jackson MJ. Effects of oral vitamin E and beta-carotene supplementation on ultraviolet radiation-induced oxidative stress in human skin. The American Journal of Clinical Nutrition. 2004;**80**:1270-1275

[20] Mireles-Rocha H, Galindo I, Huerta M, Trujillo-Hernandez B, Elizalde A, Cortes-Franco R. UVB photoprotection with antioxidants: Effects of oral therapy with d-alpha-tocopherol and ascorbic acid on the minimal erythema dose. Acta Dermato-Venereologica. 2002;**82**:21-24

[21] Fuchs J, Kern H. Modulation of UV-light-induced skin inflammation by D-alpha-tocopherol and L-ascorbic acid: A clinical study using solar simulated radiation. Free Radical Biology & Medicine. 1998;**25**:1006-1012

[22] Werninghaus K, Meydani M, Bhawan J, Margolis R, Blumberg JB, Gilchrest BA. Evaluation of the photoprotective effect of oral vitamin E supplementation. Archives of Dermatology. 1994;**130**:1257-1261

[23] Thanos SM, Halliday GM, Damian DL. Nicotinamide reduces photodynamic therapy-induced immunosuppression in humans. The British Journal of Dermatology. 2012;**167**:631-636

[24] Yiasemides E, Sivapirabu G, Halliday GM, Park J, Damian DL. Oral nicotinamide protects against ultraviolet radiation-induced immunosuppression in humans. Carcinogenesis. 2009;**30**:101-105

[25] Rhodes LE, Shahbakhti H, Azurdia RM, Moison RM, Steenwinkel MJ, Homburg MI, Dean MP, McArdle F, Beijersbergen van Henegouwen GM, Epe B, Vink AA. Effect of eicosapentaenoic acid, an omega-3 polyunsaturated fatty acid, on UVR-related cancer risk in humans. An assessment of early genotoxic markers. Carcinogenesis. 2003;**24**:919-925

[26] Orengo IF, Black HS, Wolf JEJ. Influence of fish oil supplementation on the minimal erythema dose in humans. Archives of Dermatological Research. 1992;**284**:219-221

[27] Mathews-Roth MM, Pathak MA, Fitzpatrick TB, Harber LH, Kass EH. Beta carotene therapy for erythropoietic protoporphyria and other photosensitivity diseases. Archives of Dermatology. 1977;**113**:1229-1232

[28] Tsai CF, FJ L, Hsu YW. Protective effects of Dunaliella Salina—A carotenoids-rich alga—Against ultraviolet B-induced corneal oxidative damage in mice. Molecular Vision. 2012;**18**:1540-1547

[29] Yusuf N, Irby C, Katiyar SK, Elmets CA. Photoprotective effects of green tea polyphenols. Photodermatology, Photoimmunology & Photomedicine. 2007;**23**:48-56

[30] Yiannakopoulou EC. Targeting DNA methylation with green tea catechins. Pharmacology. 2015;**95**:111-116

[31] Manach C, Scalbert A, Morand C, Remesy C, Jimenez L. Polyphenols: Food sources and bioavailability. The American Journal of Clinical Nutrition. 2004;**79**:727-747

[32] Gartner C, Stahl W, Sies H. Lycopene is more bioavailable from tomato paste than from fresh tomatoes. The American Journal of Clinical Nutrition. 1997;**66**:116-122

[33] Stahl W, Sies H. Bioactivity and protective effects of natural carotenoids. Biochimica et Biophysica Acta. 2005;**1740**:101-107

[34] Andres-Lacueva C, Monagas M, Khan N, Izquierdo-Pulido M, Urpi-Sarda M, Permanyer J, Lamuela-Raventos RM. Flavanol and flavonol contents of cocoa powder products: Influence of the manufacturing process. Journal of Agricultural and Food Chemistry. 2008;**56**:3111-3117

[35] Lee KW, Kundu JK, Kim SO, Chun KS, Lee HJ, Surh YJ. Cocoa polyphenols inhibit phorbol ester-induced superoxide anion formation in cultured HL-60 cells and expression of cyclooxygenase-2 and activation of NF-kappaB and MAPKs in mouse skin in vivo. The Journal of Nutrition. 2006;**136**:1150-1155

[36] Kim JE, Son JE, Jung SK, Kang NJ, Lee CY, Lee KW, Lee HJ. Cocoa polyphenols suppress TNF-alpha-induced vascular endothelial growth factor expression by inhibiting phosphoinositide 3-kinase (PI3K) and mitogen-activated protein kinase kinase-1 (MEK1) activities in mouse epidermal cells. The British Journal of Nutrition. 2010;**104**: 957-964

[37] Gensler HL, Williams T, Huang AC, Jacobson EL. Oral niacin prevents photocarcinogenesis and photoimmunosuppression in mice. Nutrition and Cancer. 1999;**34**:36-41

[38] Surjana D, Halliday GM, Damian DL. Nicotinamide enhances repair of ultraviolet radiation-induced DNA damage in human keratinocytes and ex vivo skin. Carcinogenesis. 2013;**34**:1144-1149

[39] Surjana D, Halliday GM, Damian DL. Role of nicotinamide in DNA damage, mutagenesis, and DNA repair. Journal of Nucleic Acids. 2010;**2010**

[40] Moloney F, Vestergaard M, Radojkovic B, Damian D. Randomized, double-blinded, placebo controlled study to assess the effect of topical 1% nicotinamide on actinic keratoses. The British Journal of Dermatology. 2010;**162**:1138-1139

[41] Surjana D, Halliday GM, Martin AJ, Moloney FJ, Damian DL. Oral nicotinamide reduces actinic keratoses in phase II double-blinded randomized controlled trials. The Journal of Investigative Dermatology. 2012;**132**:1497-1500

[42] Rhodes LE, Durham BH, Fraser WD, Friedmann PS. Dietary fish oil reduces basal and ultraviolet B-generated PGE2 levels in skin and increases the threshold to provocation of polymorphic light eruption. The Journal of Investigative Dermatology. 1995;**105**:532-535